Benjamin Brandreth

The Doctrine of Purgation

Curiosities from ancient and modern literature: a collection of quotations on the

use of purgatives, from Hippocrates and other medical writers

Benjamin Brandreth

The Doctrine of Purgation
Curiosities from ancient and modern literature: a collection of quotations on the use of purgatives, from Hippocrates and other medical writers

ISBN/EAN: 9783337386177

Printed in Europe, USA, Canada, Australia, Japan

Cover: Foto ©Thomas Meinert / pixelio.de

More available books at **www.hansebooks.com**

THE

DOCTRINE OF PURGATION.

Curiosities from Ancient and Modern Literature.

A COLLECTION OF QUOTATIONS ON THE USE OF PURGATIVES,

FROM

HIPPOCRATES,

AND OTHER MEDICAL WRITERS,

COVERING A PERIOD OF OVER TWO THOUSAND YEARS,

PROVING

Purgation is the Corner-stone of all Curatives.

COMPILED BY B. BRANDRETH, M. D., SING SING, N. Y.

THIRD EDITION.

NEW YORK:
BAKER & GODWIN, PRINTERS,
PRINTING-HOUSE SQUARE.
1873.

INTRODUCTION TO AUTHORITIES

FOR

DOCTRINE OF PURGATION,

AND

OPINION AS TO CAUSE OF DISEASE AND PREMATURE DEATH.

LIFE may be considered the union of soul and body. It is one of the most impenetrable secrets of Him who lives in all things, and in whom all live, and move, and have their being; who, in His goodness, has led man, as by the hand, to the path whereby he may arrive at a knowledge of his bodily infirmities and death; and how he may reduce the one, and thereby keep the other at bay. All nature is God's work, but man is the only living creature that appears to be endowed with cumulative reason. The Bible tells us he is fallen from his primitive condition of happiness, and in consequence of this fall, he receives at his birth a germ or principle of corruptibility, which continues to be propagated throughout all time. For the child receives from his parents the principle of his life, and also that of his death—corruption. From long study and experience, we are convinced that the death principle is corruption, or therein contained. The examination of the dead proves this; the putrefaction we observe tells us plainly that if that had been removed in time, life would not have been extinguished. The principles of life and death occupy the same body, and one or the other must rule. In order, therefore, that we continue in health, the principle of life must have the balance in its favor. Our method teaches this important knowledge. Some writers fix old age at between fifty and sixty years. Every five years that a man lives after this period may be set down as a degree added to old age. If there are so few who reach an advanced period of life, it is because the innate principle of corruption becomes active, and disease breaks out with more or less malignity, and the proper means not being employed, death may follow, t e individual not having reached that age he should and ought to have attained from the principle of life which he possessed. We look upon this as premature, not natural death. Natural death is a cessation of all the faculties; the man or woman falls asleep, ceasing to exist without effort or struggle.

It is true that all men must die, but no one need die of disease. Even now, human beings have a longer average of life than was their lot in the last century. This may be the consequence of a better knowledge of the laws of life. Let it be comprehended that we carry within ourselves the cause of disease and death; let us admit this fact, and not wait until convinced by the terrible manifestations of pain and inflammation.

To apply the remedy in time is the knowledge needed. It is worthy of remark, and we see with surprise, that young persons, apparently in the full vigor of health, whose complexions seem to indicate the most robust constitution, are oftener attacked by severe disease than persons always pale and feeble. These persons have more vitality, which occasions a quicker waste or change in the material of their bodies, so that when they are sick, unless the secretions are restored immediately, the death principle gains the ascendency. Prompt measures in the right direction are all that is needed, and in such cases purgation means life, and the want of it means death.

Some persons are peculiarly blessed with health. In their constitutions no impurity shows itself, often taking one hundred years or more to wear out the "spark of life." In others, life has ceased before birth, and the child is still-born.

All the solid parts of our bodies are made from fluid; first derived from the blood of the mother, then from the mother's milk. Thus solids and fluids constitute our material being.

WASTE AND REPAIR.

The body wears. Movement causes waste. The hardest steel wears away when used. So also the body wears away, but, unlike the steel, it is renewed faster than it wears away in a child, which is the occasion of its growth. It is a great truth, we die daily; but the food consumed also supplies us with new life daily. These are marvelous facts; this decay and renewal are among the wonderful mysteries of the Almighty.

We know the hair and nails grow. Mark your finger nail near the root. Day by day it advances toward the end; at length we pare the mark away. The whole nail has been renewed, the growth was supplied, the waste was repaired. The same waste, the same renewal occurs in the nose, and all other parts, though we cannot mark the change as in the finger nail.

WHERE THE REPARATIVES ARE.

The substance which is to form the nail is in the blood; as perfectly mixed as a grain of salt is dissolved in a glass of water. As the blood circulates in the small vessels at the root of the nail, this nail substance deposits and organizes itself, and replaces what is worn away. The hair is also renewed by materials from the blood deposited in the roots of the hair; so the bones; and so the flesh; and so with all other tissues and parts of man's body. Each part receives its needed supply of new material. Thus the eye retains its fire, the tongue its power of utterance, the brain the power of thought.

Analogy tells us even the brain, the organ of thought, wears, and is renewed by the blood, which circulates and renews all the parts of the body alike, whether it be brain, spinal cord, the eye, the bones, the flesh, the hair, or the nail.

The blood carries new material to repair the waste, and it reloads itself with worn-out parts which it discharges through the appropriate vents. When the new materials are greater than the waste, the child grows; or the man spreads. When the waste is exactly equal to the new material, the body remains of the same size and weight. These facts indicate that all substance of all the organs and parts of a living body are present in the blood. It is therefore important to our well-being that this life fluid should be free from imperfections.

For if the blood does not contain all the needed ingredients, or if it should contain more, it cannot renew the different parts according to their requirements. Deformed and ill-made people owe their infirmities to the blood of their parents; pure blood cannot do otherwise than make perfectly organized beings, thus we may estimate the value of certain means to make the blood perfect.

Food, by its organ the stomach, supplies all the parts of which blood is made. We now speak of this conversion.

DEFINITION.

SUBSTANCES WHICH CONTAIN AND SUPPLY NUTRITION ARE FOOD.

Healthy food possesses substance, because the stomach cannot grind it well without it possesses this quality. Too fine food makes the stomach weak; it cannot use its muscular power, and debility of the stomach follows. If we do not walk, our legs soon become weak. To be strong, organs need exercise. When food is digested, part makes blood; the refuse passes off by the bowels, the kidneys, and the skin. Our stomach, if properly supplied, continually prepares new blood, which renews all the organs, carrying vitality to the hair and nail as well as to the head, with its master-organ the brain. Every part is each moment of our lives changing, the worn-out parts carried away, and new parts supplied, whether good or bad. Here we see the necessity of eating and drinking several times a day. We constantly wear and constantly repair. Such is the law of our being.

WORN-OUT PARTS MUST BE EXPELLED.

The worn-out parts must be expelled from the body daily, or the blood will become impure. We may comprehend this by an inquiry respecting new-born children. They have taken no food by the mouth, and yet when born their bowels and bladders are full. Whence did these secretions come? They came evidently from the blood of the mother, which made their bodies. We also know that sick persons, who eat no food for days, have evacuations by the kidneys and bowels. These parts are also the worn-out parts of the blood.

The blood is, in fact, a messenger which takes to every part of the body what it needs for renewal, and also carries back to the bowels, kidneys, and skin, worn-out substance to be expelled from the body.

We therefore must admit that every part of a human body is made from blood; and that it wastes and is repaired; that food makes blood, which is distributed with singular intelligence to all the various organs.

HOW IMPURE BLOOD IS DEVELOPED.

The bowels may be costive; in this case there is an absorption into the circulation, of gases and gummy substances, which are a great cause of poison to the blood. Should the kidneys fail to do their work, another source of poison to the blood is developed. Again, should the perspiration be checked, matters flow back upon the blood which soon load it with impurities. Suppose only the feet, by cold, cannot perspire, and their fetid exhalations flow back upon the blood. If all these outlets —the skin, the kidneys, and the bowels—do their work even imperfectly only, for a short time, it is evident that the blood will be burdened with noxious matters, which must interfere seriously with the circulation, and soon clog up the smaller vessels, so that only a small amount of blood can pass. Soon the lungs, the intestines, the stomach, and the brain will sound an alarm. You will have pleurisy, inflammation of the bowels or severe cholic, violent headache, or sick stomach. Because the worn-out parts of the body, instead of being carried out by those avenues nature designed, are shut up, poisoning the blood, thus causing it to become impure.

Other causes besides these produce impurity of blood. The food may not be healthy; digestion may be imperfect; troubles, grief, anxiety, miasmas from swamps or other exhalations; breathing close air in crowded rooms; staying in too hot rooms; all these causes tend more or less to vitiate the blood. Grief, fear, and anxiety, *hurt, by making the blood to circulate slower,* and soon produce a very serious injury to the composition of the blood, occasioning stubborn fevers, and various derangements of the body and mind.

The best part of food makes chyle, which is absorbed into the circulation, to repair the waste the blood sustains in rebuilding the body, and in forming bile and all the other fluids of the body—for all the fluids are made from the blood. The coarse portions, and those not needed, are expelled daily by the bowels, the kidneys, and the skin.

The fluids, or as some writers call them, the humors, are as natural and necessary as the blood. It is not from humors we are sick, but from the humors becoming unsound; from infection, or absorption of fungi, or other poisonous vapors or matters. These produce a putrid fermentation, or chills and fever, or fevers continued or intermittent.

It is supposed that in the humors resides the germ of corruptibility, which is aroused into activity by the above causes.

To have humors is as natural as to have blood. It is not having humors that causes us to be sick, but because they become corrupted. The humors absorb infection, in consequence of their being the seat of the innate germ of corruption. When this germ or root, from any cause, receives an increase, it may show itself by colds, catarrhs, tumors, or other effects, by which life may be shortened, or a serious attack of some specific disease produced.

Corrupted humors always cause sickness; they cause death. If they are removed in time, the sickness is cured, and death prevented. We know they can be removed, and should not corruption be quickly removed from a living body? Their infectious smell tells of their hurtful nature to a living body; cleanse, sweep out from the bowels and blood the unhealthy parts, and your disease will soon be cured.

While in health, the humors and the blood are sound; but so soon as you do not feel well, be sure the humors and blood are getting deranged in their sound qualities; and when painful sensations are felt, we should at once take steps to prevent serious trouble. These steps usually are evacuation, for we cannot recover health until the blood and the humors are freed from all acrid and unhealthy qualities, however acquired.

The humors, after becoming corrupted, soon accumulate a degree of acrimony or burning heat, that the burning sensation is often almost insupportable. They often resist great quantities of purgatives, but outward applications are really useless without evacuation of the bowels.

Two hundred medical writers, running through a period of over two thousand years, agree as to the means of reducing this death principle—agree as to a general indication—agree as to the perfect innocence of purgation. We hold that this evidence is important in our intelligent age, and hope it may lead to a more uniform and a more humane method of treating patients. Perhaps a wise regard for the improvement of the human race will make purgation the principal curative reliance; other means should be only secondary. Physicians may soon be governed by this rule, because purgation may be set down as the magnet, the guide, the star of safety.

Purgation corrects errors in the digestive organs; and Dr. Abernethy observes (in *Surgical Observations*, p. 22): "By correcting the obvious errors in the state of the digestive organs, local diseases which had baffled all attempts at cure by *local means*, have speedily been removed." When local applications are applied, they should be in harmony with purgation, and incapable of doing injury.

We can remove disease in two ways: by the upper and by the lower passages— by vomiting and by purging—purging when the patient is weak, vomiting only when he is strong. We will define purgation as "cleansing," and apply to both the upper or lower ways.

For forty years I have directed my attention to the cure of disease on this plan, and facts derived from experience have long since confirmed me in the belief that this is calm Nature's own method of cure, because it assists her in removing impurities by the means and outlets she has so wisely provided for herself.

Believing that all mineral and chemical agents which can act on foreign or impure matters in the blood, invariably injure the organization of the blood itself— destroying its corpuscles, besides injuring the coats of the stomach, and producing serious effects upon the bones—I have therefore discarded minerals and chemicals entirely, and trust to vegetable remedies alone.

That which I have principally employed to enforce this theory has been Brandreth's Pills, whose permanent and wide-spread success is the strongest evidence of their distinguished merit.

The question has been asked, If the value of this medicine is so great, is it not a duty to make known its true components, so that physicians and others could prepare it? To this it may be answered, that if Brandreth's Pills certainly would be made the same as they are now, and all their healing, cleansing and innocent qualities retained, one of the reasons for their remaining a secret medicine would be removed.

But every man knows, who knows anything of the drug and medicine business, that not one box in a hundred would be prepared of such medicines as are incorporated in the Brandreth Pills prepared by me. It is true the pills might be composed of ingredients *called by the same name*, but the name would be all the resemblance they would possess to the pure extracts and medicinal preparations which comprise the composition of BRANDRETH'S PILLS.

Therefore, for the sake of the lives and health of men—for the sake of the

GREAT SANATORY THEORY OF PURGATION—

the manner of preparing Brandreth's Pills will never be divulged, until the time arrives when all the drugs of the stores shall be true and uniform preparations.

I am not without examples for this decision :

Dr. James, the celebrated author of James' Powder, left his prescription to Messrs. Newbery & Sons, of London, more than a hundred years ago, by whom they are yet made. The great Stahl and Hoffman, of Germany, Professors of Physic at Halle, without scruple confined many medicines to their own private practice. And even in our own time, there are few medical men of extensive practice who have not remedies which they carefully retain in their own families, who are more likely to prepare them with reference to securing their curative effects, without regard to profit, than they would be in the hands of strangers.

The quotations from the writings of medical men, embodied in this pamphlet, prove the talent that has been at work upon this Theory of Purgation for over a period of two thousand years—and in vain. Then what has prevented its complete success? Simply this, in my opinion: Not a single writer has given a medicine which, out of their own hands, would successfully and safely enforce the purgative theory.

The public, in Brandreth's Pills, have a medicine which it is intended shall ever be within its reach, always certain to purge only impurities from the blood, and when the upper ways require cleansing, occasion vomiting ; and that is safe for both sexes and all ages. Composed of vegetable preparations entirely—indeed, the Pills are guaranteed to contain no mineral in any form—they may, if the requirement of the constitution need them, be taken daily for any length of time, without a possibility of producing any bad effects on the body, and must reduce the sum of disease.

WARRANTEE.

That Brandreth's Pills, in all future time, are warranted to possess and contain those purgative, those cleansing and innocent qualities, which they have always heretofore possessed in so eminent a degree.

The principle of curing disease by the use of purgatives is beginning to be extensively recognized as indispensably necessary for the recovery of health by many intelligent families and individuals. To prove to them and to the world at large, as well as to physicians of all schools, the broad and deep foundations and authority this principle of cure possesses, I have printed the following extracts which, as in a mirror, is exhibited the views, and experience, and sentiments of medical men, during a period of over TWO THOUSAND YEARS.

They possess a peculiar significance for those who desire to investigate this subject, so important to the lives and health of men, because they throw a flood of light on the application of purgatives as a means of removing disease from the system.

The great aim by many of these writers is, that in the administration of medicine, we should *do good* possibly, but never *harm.*

Bleeding, Mercury, Tartar Emetic, Antimony, Veratria, Strychnine, Morphine, and a host of similar remedial agents may, nay generally do, a great deal of harm, and often are the occasion of fatal mistakes; while the great advantage of using Brandreth's Pills in sickness is, that *they never make any mistakes,* often prolonging, never shortening life.

In pleurisy, in inflammation, in fevers, and where pain is present, their prompt and energetic administration is often life-saving, and it is in evidence they have often effected cures when physicians and friends had given up all hope. Then what risk does any man or woman incur in using a medicine like Brandreth's Pills, which are the adopted remedy of millions of families living in every part of the civilized world ?

The facts given in the following pages prove that fevers, inflammations, and severe pain are only, in reality, so many evidences of healthful constitutional power, and that if purgation is enforced according to the necessities of the case, the fever, severe pain, or inflammation will be removed, provided no sedatives or narcotics are employed.

B. BRANDRETH.

SING SING, June 1, 1871.

HIPPOCRATES.

PURGATION THE CORNER-STONE OF CURATIVES.

HIPPOCRATES.—*Aphorisms, written about* 400 B. C.   *Edited by Elias Marks, M. D., New York,* 1818.

1. Life is short, art long, occasion brief, experience fallacious, judgment difficult. It is requisite that the physician exhibit what is essential, and that the patient, attendants, and all which surrounds him, concur therein (1, sect. I).

The golden rule.

2. In *diarrhea and spontaneous vomiting*, if the matter voided be of a nature that ought to be expelled, let the patient be purged, for in this case the evacuations are beneficial and are easily supported (2. sect. I).

Diarrhea. Purgation indicated by nature.

3. The greater the evil the more vigorous the remedy (6, sect. I).

The power of the remedy.

4. In acute diseases the most violent symptoms supervene; the severest regimen is, therefore, to be observed. But if these symptoms be wanting, a more generous diet is to be permitted, only we are to have recourse to it in proportion to the subsidence of the malady (7, sect. I). In the choice of regimen, more evil results from abstraction than from a small excess. A thin, frugal, and over-exact regimen accords not even with the man in health, who grievously supports the privation. Hence, in general, the superiority of a due refection over that which is deficient (5, sect. I).

On Diet.

The nutritive plan of cure.

5. In those diseases which quickly arrive at their climax, a thin regimen should immediately be adopted. In those which attain it at a somewhat later period, we should at or before that period, subtract from their diet; but, until then, sufficient nourishment should be allowed, that the strength of the patient may be supported (10, sect. I).

Diet to be regulated according to the character of the disease.

6. That which is excrementitious should be drawn off at the point to which it most tends, by the most convenient outlets (21, sect. I).

Purgatives, Diuretics, Sudorifics.

When to give purgatives. 7. Purgatives should be administered after the food on the stomach is concocted, not while it is yet crude (22, sect. I).

NOTE BY THE EDITOR.—There is no danger in administering a purgative before or after a meal, provided there be pain or dizziness, which symptoms are relieved by purgation.

How to direct the purging. 8. Depletion is not to be estimated by its copiousness but by its being judiciously used and easily supported. When it is necessary to extend it "ad deliquium animi," let it be done, but previously consult the resources of the patient (23, sect. I).

NOTE BY EDITOR.—Where there is danger of congestion, purgation may be enforced to fainting with Brandreth's Pills (see paragraph 55).

9. If the convalescent acquire not strength from the food he takes, it shows that the body needs a more plentiful supply. But if the same effect arise from an inability to partake of food, it sufficiently evinces the necessity of purgatives (8, sect. II).

Quality of evacuation. 10. When it becomes necessary to purge, the evacuations ought to be loose and free (9, sect. II).

How to direct the nourishment. 11. Impure constitutions, when most nourished, are most injured (10, sect. II).

Relapses from insufficient purgation. 12. The (morbid) matter remaining in the body after the crisis is past often produces a relapse (12, sect. II).

Change of dejections. 13. In alvine fluxes, a change in the dejections, unless they assume a vicious appearance, is beneficial (14, sect. II).

Tubercles. Examination of stools. 14. When the fauces are affected, and tubercles arise therein, we ought to examine the excretions; when they are of a bilious nature, the entire body is affected; but if they be as in health, we may safely impart nourishment (15, sect. II).

Disease from intemperance in food or drink: Purgation the cure. 15. Excess of food produces disease, and at the same time points out the remedy (17, sect. II). The sickness which arises from repletion is cured by evacuation; and that which arises from evacuation, by repletion. Thus, opposites are counteractives of each other (22, sect. II).

Sudden action against nature. Proceedings must be gradual and continued. 16. Evacuation, repletion, frigeration, and calefaction—these, or any other correspondent modifications of body, when excessive, or too suddenly accommplished, are dangerous—*nature* being ever *opposed to extremes*. That *which is gradually done is safely done*, whether we pass from one extreme to another, or otherwise (51, sect. II). Everything which is judicious being done, without success, we are not, therefore, to recede from our plan, while we still entertain the same views as we did at first (52, ibid).

17. *Some diseases accord better with some constitutions than others;* and this also obtains with certain ages, as connected with season, climate and aliment (3, sect. III). In the various seasons, if cold and heat frequently alternate with each other, we must look forward to *autumnal diseases* (4, ibid).

Predisposition . by constitution, age, season, climate, and food : change of temperature.

18. Those suffering from phthisis should avoid vomits (8, sect. IV).

Phthisis, emetics injurious.

19. The melancholic should be copiously evacuated downwards ; and, from the same principle of reasoning, those of a contrary temperament should be differently treated (9 sect. IV).

Purgatives and emetics, where to be used.

20. *Sound Doctrine.*—In very acute affection, attended with turgescence, purgatives are immediately to be used; to procrastinate here is dangerous (10, sect. IV).

Acute diseases, purge without delay.

21. Those who are tormented with severe *gripings, pains about the umbilicus, and* in the region of *the loins,* and who are neither relieved by purgatives, or any other means, usually fall into tympanites (11, sect. IV).

Gripings and pains— purgatives useful.

22. If there be *pain* immediately *above or below the diaphragm,* the former demands vomiting, the latter purging (18, sect. IV).

Internal pains—vomiting and purging.

23. Those who, during the operation of purgatives, have no thirst, ought to be purged until thirst be induced (19, sect. IV).

Degree of purging.

24. *Pain* in the *lower region of the abdomen,* with *griping* and aching of the knees, unattended with fever, indicate the necessity of purgatives (20, sect. IV).

Pain in the abdomen —purgation necessary.

25. *Dark-colored dejections,* resembling black blood, coming on spontaneously, either with or without fever, are very unfavorable ; and the more so if the color of these dejections become, with their continuance, still more depraved; but if the evacuations assume a more healthy complexion, or, if their *dark color* be *the effect of purgatives,* less evil is to be apprehended (21, sect. IV).

Evacuations critical.

26. The expectoration of blood, how small soever in quantity, is injurious; but the *evacuation of black blood downwards* is (frequently) advantageous (25, sect. IV).

Evacuation of blood different in character.

27. With those who are *deaf,* a coming on of *bilious evacuations* generally *removes* it (28, sect. IV).

Deafness, evacuations good.

28. If, in those recovering from indisposition, there occur any local pain, it foreshows the formation of an abscess (32, sect. IV).

Pain, symptom of abscesses.

29. From whatsoever part of the body sweat breaks forth, it foreshows a determination of the disease to that part (38, sect. IV).

Sweats and heat, symp-

tomatic of
disease, indi-
cate the ne-
cessity of
Purgation.
In whatever part of the body heat or cold arises there the disease seats itself (39, ibid).

Where there occur alternate changes of cold and heat, and the complexion undergoes various changes of color, we may predict extended illness (40, ibid).

Profuse sweats, during sleep, without any manifest local affection, may arise from a too plentiful diet; but if they take place notwithstanding the observance of a frugal regimen, it shows the necessity of evacuation (41, ibid).

Abscesses in
Fever must
be purged
away.
30. In fever, where abscesses have not been dispersed during the primary stages of the disease, they foreshow extended illness (51 sect. IV).

Fever, in-
dications by
the urine.
31. When, with existing fever, a thick, gummy, scant urine is followed by a thin and copious discharge, it is beneficial; but it is the more so, when, at the commencement of disease, or a little time after, the urine deposits a sediment (69, sect. IV).

Bleeding in
pregnancy
causes abor-
tion.
32. With pregnant women, *venesection produces abortion*, especially if gestation be far advanced (31, sect. V).

Brandreth's Pills are safe at every period of gestation with the generality of females.

Irregular
menstrua-
tion requires
purgation.
33. Discolored and irregular menses indicate the necessity of purgatives (36, sect. V).

Tumors,
beneficial or
malignant.
34. *Tumors* which have a soft feel are beneficial; those which are hard and callous are unfavorable (67, sec. V).

Dropsy,
purgation
the cure.
35. In dropsy, if the water pass off into the intestines, by means of the veins, the disease ceases (14 sec. VI).

Purgation brings it to the intestines and so causes the water to be evacuated.

Diseases of
the Eyes
cured by
Purgation.
36. Diarrhea supervening in *ophthalmia* is beneficial (17, sect. VI). *Pains of the eyes* are relieved by pure urine, bathing, fomentation, venesection, and purging (31, sect. VI).

Fever the
natural cure.
37. Pains in the hypochondrium, unattended with inflammation, are relieved by fever (40, sect. VI).

Effects of
neglected
purgation.
38. *Long-continued dysentery*, supervening in affections of the spleen, induces either dropsy or lientery, and consequent death (43, sect. VI).

Purging in
Spring.
39. Those with whom purgatives agree should have recourse to them in the *spring* (47, sect. VI).

Gout cured
when inflam-
mation is
purg'd away.
40. Those attacked with the *gout* are entirely freed of it in forty days after the subsidence of the inflammation (49, sect. VI).

More effects
of neglected
purgation.
41. In atrabilious affections the translation of the humors to various parts has a tendency to produce the following diseases: *apoplexy, mania, convulsion* and *blindness* (56, sect. VI).

42. When a serous collection, attended with pain, takes place between the abdomen and diaphragm, without its having an issue in either cavity, if the fluid be drawn out of the body by means of the veins, the disorder ceases (54, sect. VII; vide Aph. 14, sect. VI). *Accumulations in the intestines require purgation.*

43. Excessive perspiration, cold or hot, continually going on, is indicative of redundant moisture within; we ought, therefore, to evacuate it from the system either by vomiting, if the patient be strong, or by purgation if he be weak (61, sect. VII). *Sweat—Indicative of fluid accumulations. Cure, Purgatives.*

44. He should attend to the urinary discharge in order to ascertain whether it be conformable to what takes place in health; in proportion as it departs from the healthy state is the severity of the disease, and "vice versa" (66, sect. VII). *The urine a criterion of health or disease—its turbid condition indicative of Purgation.*

If, on suffering the urine to remain, without disturbing it, we observe a deposit resembling sawdust, the greater or less quantity of this deposit is indicative of the severity or mildness of the disease; in either case, it is necessary to have recourse to *purgatives;* in proportion as we neglect *these,* for a nutritive regimen, will be the augmentation of the disease (67, sect. VII).

45. In continued fever, the expectoration of a livid, bloody, bilious, or fœtid matter, is alike unfavorable; but, if the expectoration be good, and in due season, it is favorable. The same may be said of the alvine and urinary discharges; *furthermore,* any excrementitious matter remaining in the system, and not coming away with the evacuations, proves injurious (69, sect. VII; vide Aph. 12, sect. II). *Continued Fever — uterine and urinary evacuations early and thoroughly required.*

HIPPOCRATES, *the genuine works of. Transl. by Francis Adams, LL.D., and printed for the Sydenham Society. 2 vols. London,* 1849.

46. Medicine is, of all arts, the most noble; but, owing to the ignorance of those who practice it, and of those who inconsiderately form a judgment of them, it is at present far behind all the other arts (The Law, p. 784, vol. I). *Medical Ignorance.*

47. When nature opposes, everything else is in vain. *Nature is the physician of diseases* (p. 102, vol. I). *Nature.*

48. The physician must have his special object in view with regard to diseases, namely: TO DO GOOD or TO DO NO HARM. The art consists in three things: the disease, the patient, and the physician. *The physician's special object.*

The physician is the servant of nature, and the patient must combat the disease along with the physician (Epidemics, Book 1, § 5, p. 360, vol. II). *The servant of nature.*

49. Gentle purging of the bowels agrees with most *ulcers,* and in wounds of the head, belly, or joints, where there is danger of gangrene, in such as require sutures, in phagediac, spreading, and in otherwise inveterate ulcers (On Ulcers, pp. 796-7, vol. II). *Ulcers. Purge gently.*

Purge in plethoric diseases.   50. Disorders arising from *repletion* are removed by evacuation (On the Nature of Man, p. 262, vol. I; Aphor, 22, sect. II).

Fevers pass away when the morbid matter is removed.   51. When the discharges become thicker, more concocted, and are freed from all acrimony, then the fevers pass away, and the other symptoms which annoyed the patient (Ancient Medicine, p. 174, vol. I).

Many painful symptoms removed by natural or artificial purgation, the only true cure.   52. When there is an overflow of the bitter principle, which we call yellow bile, what anxiety, burning heat, and loss of strength prevail! But if relieved from it, either by being purged spontaneously, or by means of *medicine seasonably administered*, the patient is decidedly relieved of the pain and heat. But while these things float on the stomach unconcocted and undigested, no contrivance could make the pains and fever cease; and where there are acidities of an acrid and eruginous character, what varieties of frenzy, gnawing pains in the bowels and chest, and inquietude prevail! And these do not cease until the acidities be purged away (p. 174, vol. I, ibid.)

The bad humors of various kinds.   53. The coction, change, attenuation, and thickening into the form of humors, take place through many and various forms (p. 174, ibid.)

What to purge.   54. We must purge and move such humors as are unconcocted (p. 703, vol. II).

Purge until evacuations are healthy, even to fainting.   55. The evacuations are not to be judged of by their quantity, but whether they be such as they should be, and how they are borne. And when proper to carry the evacuation to "liquidium animi" (faintness), this, also, should be done, provided the patient can support it (p. 704, vol. I; Aph. 23, sect. I).

NOTE BY EDITOR.—To give the patient an opportunity of doing so, have gruel or light broth ready for him to sip a little at a time. Intelligent nursing must go alongside of the purgative method, then success is moderately certain.

Purgative axiom.   56. If the matters which are purged be such as should be purged, the evacuation is beneficial (p. 704, vol. II; Aph. 2, sect. I).

Effects of insufficient purgation.   57. Bodies not properly cleansed, the more you nourish, the more you injure (p. 706, vol. II; Aph. 10, sect. II). What remains in diseases, after the crises is past, is apt to produce relapses (p. 707, vol. II; Aph. 12, sect. II).

Purgative axiom.   58. In purging we should bring away such matters from the body as it would be advantageous had they come away spontaneously (p. 723, vol. II).

Acute Diseases. Purge only.   59. *Our Doctrine.*—In very acute disease, purge on the first day, for it is a very bad thing to procrastinate in such cases (p. 724, vol. II; Aph. 10, sect. IV).

60. In convalescents from diseases, if any parts be pained, there are deposits being formed. But if any part be in a painful state previous to the illness, there the disease fixes (p. 728, vol. II ; Aph. 32, sect. IV). *Deposits from imperfect purgation.*

61. N. B.—The translator says: " Hippocrates was strictly the physician of experience and common sense." *Experience and common sense.*

62. Nature finds out ways for herself without consultation ; nature, untaught and without learning, does what is needful (Epidem., lib. VI, S. 5, Edinb. ed.) *Nature's ways to cure.*

63. *Asclepiades*, about 100 years B. C., the earliest hydropathist, contrived easy methods, and such ones as any one might use without the help (and cost) of a physician. This made them very acceptable, and Plinius (Lib. XXVI, Cap. III, p. 444) writes about him the following : " Five things of most common benefit he held to: Occasional abstinence from meat, at other times from wine, the use of the flesh-brush, the exercise of walking and of riding ; which, as every one believed he could prescribe for himself such remedies as these, and as it is natural to wish those things true that are most easy, made all people flock unto him as to one sent from heaven." He disapproved of the then popular practice of frequently using violent emetics and purgatives, for which he substituted the *clyster* as the *safest way* to obtain—what appeared to him *the first measure* to be taken in most of diseases—*evacuation of the bowels.* His method of employing *simple remedies*, for the sake of their safety and innocence, but producing the effect wished for, and his extraordinary skill in a quick diagnostic, gained him a fame that almost overthrew the old heroic method of the then practitioners of Rome, as we read of him in Plinius, XXVI, 8; Celsus, III, 4, II, 6, Carlius Aurelianus, Morb. acert., I, 15; Aquilejus, Florid., IV, 362 ; Plinius, Hist. Nat., VII, 37; and Saleh Beu Balah, Chap. 12. *Simple and safe purgative remedies. MEDICINE OF THE PEOPLE, combined with wholesome food, personal cleanliness, temperance, and exercise of the body preserve health and cure disease.*

He recommended clysters of cold water for the aged, and for persons troubled with stone or gravel, for females having falling or other affections of the womb, and in all kidney affections when the bowels require moving. *Water clysters for the aged.*

64. RHAZES OR RASIS, *on Pestilence, written about* 890 *at Corduba·* This book of Rhazes' is a curious and valuable record of the Arabian practice in *small-pox* and *measles.* The best edition in Arabic and Latin is that by I. Channing, London, 1766. The doctor's theory is that of fermentation, and his practice is of the *cooling* kind, together with *free evacuation of the bowels.* *Small-pox and measles —powerful purges.*

There is also another translation of this book in English from the Arabic text by Dr. Greenhill (8vo., London, 1847).

65. AVICENNA, *or Abu Ali Al Hosain Ebn Abdallah Ebn Sina,* who was born in the year of the hegira 370 or 987 A. D., the *first writer who formed a complete system of medicine,* was of opinion that *evacuation of the bowels, actively and perseveringly employed, was the main principle in the cure of disease.* He was, however, more in favor of clysters than *Intestinal disorders — powerful evacuation the cure.*

of internal purgative remedies, not considering that that method of purgation, often repeated in a proportionately short space of time, by its
mechanical action, must prove injurious, causing ulcerations in the in-

Colic. testinal canal. Thus, when subject to a severe attack of *colic*, he took
eight clysters in one day, which producing ulcers in the intestines, together with an epilepsy, a consequence of intemperance and sensuality,
that had weakened his vital forces, thus causing his early death. Of
his numerous books, said to be more than one hundred, his " *Canon*"
and some tracts were printed in 1593 in Rome.

PAREY, AMBROSE, M. D., *Physician to Henry III., King of France
and Poland. Paris,* 1579. *Transl. Thos. Johnson, M. D. London,* 1634.

*Experience
the mother of
the science.*   66. Although indeed we cannot deny but that experience has much
profited this art, as it has and does many others. For, as men perceived that some things were profitable, some unprofitable for this or
that disease, they set it down, and so by diligent observation and mark-
ing of singularities, they established universal and certain precepts, and
so brought it into an art (Pref.)

*Disease
from impur-
ity of the
blood.*   67. There is no disease which arises not from some one, or the mixture of more, *humors*. Which thing Hippocrates understanding,
wrote every creature to be either *sick or well according to the condition
of the humors*. And certainly all *putrid fevers* proceed *from the
putrefaction of humors*. Nor do any acknowledge any other original
and distinctive of the differences of *abscesses* or *tumors;* neither do
*Purgatives
correct and
remove mor-
bid matter
from the
blood.*   ulcerated, broken, or otherwise wounded members hope for the restoration of continuity, from other than from the sweet falling down of
humors to the wounded part, which is the cause that often in the cure
of these affects. The physicians are necessarily busied in tempering the
blood; that is, bringing to a mediocrity the humors composing the mass
of the blood, if they at any time offend in quantity or quality. For if
anything abound or digress from the wonted temper, none of the accustomed functions will be well performed. . . . *Purging corrects and
draws away the vicious quality of the blood* (pp. 11, 12; cf. Hippoc. 29,
30).

*To preserve
health, keep
the blood in
its normal
state.*   68. But with the blood at one and the same time, all the humors
are made, whether alimentary or excrementitious. Therefore the blood,
that it may perform *its office*, that is, the faculty *of nutrition*, must
necessarily be purged and cleansed from the excrementitious humors.
. . . The parts of which the blood is composed ought to be tempered
and mixed among themselves in a *certain proportion, which remaining,*
health remains, *but violated, disease follows* (p. 12).

*Diarrhea
and vomit-
ing. The nat-
ural ejection
of morbid
matter must*   69. *Evacuation* is no other thing than the expulsion or effusion of
humors which are troublesome, either in quantity or quality. Of evacuations some are universal, which expel superfluous humors from the
whole body; such are purging, vomiting, perspiration, sweats; some

particular, which are performed only to evacuate one part, as the be assisted by art. stomach by vomiting and stools, the guts by stools, the liver and spleen by urine and ordure. These evacuations are sometimes *performed by nature, freeing itself of that which is troublesome* to it; otherwhiles by the *art* of the physician *in imitation of nature* (p. 37).

70. *The causes of congestion* are two principally, as the weakness of Tumors from morbid accumulations. Cure by Purgation. the *concoctive faculty*, which resides in the part, by which the assimilation into the substance of the part of the nourishment flowing to it is frustrated, and the weakness of the *expulsive faculty;* for while the part cannot expel superfluities, their quantity continually increases (p. 250). Those humors which are rebellious rather offend in quality than in quantity, and undergo the divers forms of things dissenting from nature, which are joined by no similitude or affinity with things natural (p. 252). A convenient *diet and purging* must be used; ill humors are amended by *diet and purging* (p. 253).

71. *Cancer.*—The antecedent cause depends upon the default of Cancer from impurity of the blood. irregular diet, *generating and heaping up gross and feculent blood;* by the morbific affection of the liver disposed to the generation of that blood; by the infirmity or weakness of the spleen in attracting and purging the blood; by the suppression of the courses or hemorrhoides, or any such accustomed evacuation. The conjunct cause is that gross and melancholic humor sticking and shut up in the affected part, as in a strait (pp. 279–80).

72. The glands at the root of the tongue are very subject to inflam- Sore-throat. Cure by purgation and external applications. mations and swelling from crude, viscous humors. Swallowing is painful to the patient, and commonly he has a fever. Often the neighboring muscles of the throat and neck are so swollen together with these glandules that the passage of air and breath is stopped and the patient strangled. We resist this imminent danger by purging, by applying cupping-glasses to the neck and shoulders, by frictions and ligatures of the extreme parts, and by washing and gargling the mouth and throat with astringent gargarisms (pp. 293, 94).

73. The dropsy is a tumor against nature by the abundance of Dropsy— Its causes. waterish humors, of flatulences, or of phlegm, gathered one while in all the habit of the body, otherwhiles in some part, and that especially in the capacity of the belly, between the peritoneum and the entrails. From this distinction of places and matters there arise *divers kinds* of dropsies. . . . Yet they *all arise from the same cause ; that is, the weakness or defect of the altering or concocting faculties,* especially of the liver, which has been caused by a scyrrhus, or any great distemper (pp. 299, 300).

74. The beginning of the cure must be with gentle and mild medi- Cure by purgatives and diuretics. cines; neither must we come to a paracentesis, unless we have formerly used and tried these; therefore, it shall be the part of the physician to prescribe a drying diet, and such medicines as carry away water, *both by stool and urine* (p. 301).

Tetanus, from excrementitious matters.

75. *Tetanus* — Causes.—Abundance of humors causes repletion; dulling the body by immoderate eating and drinking, and omission of exercise or any accustomed evacuation, as suppression of the hemorrhoides and courses, for hence are such like *excrementitious humors* drawn into the nerves with which they, being replete and filled, are dilated more than is fit, whence, necessarily becoming more short, they *Cure by purgatives and local medicines, &c.* suffer convulsion. . . . It is cured by discussing and evacuating remedies, as purging, digestive local medicines, exercise, frictions, and other things which may consume the superfluous excrementitious humors that possess the substance of the nerves and habit of the body (pp. 329, 30).

NOTE.—Allcock's Porous Plasters applied along the spine from neck to os sacrum, and Brandreth's Pills two every two hours, is good treatment for lockjaw.

Palsy from obstruction by morbid matter.

76. *Palsy.*—The cause are humors obstructing one of the ventricles of the brain, or one side of the spinal marrow, so that the animal faculty—the worker of sense and motion—cannot, by the nerves, come to the part to perform its action (p. 332).

Purgation cures.

In the cure of the palsy we must not attempt anything, unless we have first used general remedies, *diet and purging*, all which care lies upon the learned and prudent physician (p. 333).

Erysipelas. Purge, but do not bleed.

77. *Erysipelas.*—The cure of such an effect must be performed by two means; that is, *evacuation and cooling* with humectation. If bile alone cause this tumor, we must easily be induced to let blood, *but we must purge* him with medicine *evacuating bile* (p. 353).

NOTE.—Bleeding must never be resorted to in Erysipelas; it is dangerous, never does any good, and is certain to retard the cure.

Gangrene. The superfluous humors must be evacuated.

78. The cure of *gangrene*, caused by the too plentiful and violent defluxion of humors suffocating the native heat, by reason of great phlegmons, is performed by *evacuating and drying* up the humors, which putrify by delay and collection in the part (p. 456). . . . If the body be plethoric, or full of ill humors, you *must purge* (p. 455).

Ulcers require always purgation, then external applications.

79. An *ulcer* has one, and that a simple indication, that is, exsiccation. . . . Before you do anything about the ulcer, you must first use general means; for in *Galen's* opinion, if the whole body require preparation, that must be done first, for in some ulcers *purgation alone* will be sufficient (p. 470). . . . Dry ulcers you shall correct by humeating medicines, as fomenting it with warm water, &c., but *always you must first purge*. . . . Then you must have recourse to refrigerent things (p. 471).

NOTE.—The Gum Elimi Universal Cerate should be procured. We can recommend it. It contains no grease or oil, but is a vegetable production, and very useful in all affections of the skin ; as an application to a felon or otherwise it is superior to bread or linseed meal as a poultice.

Inflammation of the eyes. Purge before all.

80. *Ophthalmia* can proceed from different causes, external and internal, producing the settling of humors to the eye. The evacuations

of the matter flowing into the eye, shall be performed by *purging medi-cines*, cupping the neck and shoulders with scarification or *without*; and lastly by frictions, as the physician shall think it fit (p. 645).

Allcock's Porous Plasters are superior, applied to back and shoulders, to cupping, scar-ifications or frictions.

81. The *Diabetes* is a disease wherein presently, after one has drunk, the urine is made in great plenty, by the dissolution of the retentive fac-ulty of the veins, and the deprivation or immoderation of the attractive faculty. The causes are the inflammation of the liver, lungs, spleen, but especially of the kidneys and bladder. . . . For the cure of so great a disease, the *matter must be purged* which *causes or feeds the inflammation* (p. 688).

Diabetes. Evacuate the morbid mat-ter which causes in-flammation.

82. Whenever the guts, being obstructed or otherwise affected, the excrements are hindered from passing forth, if the fault be in the small guts, the effect is termed "Voloutus, Iteos, or miserere mei;" but if it be in the greater guts, it is called the "colic," from the part affected, which is the colon. Therefore *Avicen* rightly defines the colic as "a pain in the guts, wherein the excrements are difficultly evacuated by the fundament." *Taulus Eleginata* reduces all the causes of colic to four heads, to wit: to the grossness or toughness of the humors impact in the coats of the guts; flatulencies hindered from passage forth; inflammation of the guts; and, lastly, the collection of acrid and bit-ing humors. . . . Over-eating and taking in of nourishments that do not agree with each other, or with the constitution of the body, produce crudity and obstruction, and at length the collection of flatulencies, whereon a tensive pain ensues. . . By the use of crude fruits and too cold drinks the stomach and guts are refrigerated, and the humors and excrements therein contained are congealed, and, as it were, burned up (p. 689). . . .

Colic. The causes and physiol-ogy.

83. There is also another cause of the colic which is not so common, to wit, the twining of the guts, that is, when they are so twined, folded and doubled, that the excrements, as it were, bound in their knots, can-not be expelled.* . . . The colic is cured, the *humors being first atten-uated and diffused, and at length evacuated by medicines taken by the mouth and otherwise* (pp. 690, 91).

Ente-ocele. Cure by pur-gation.

* *Some sweet oil, followed by a dose of Brandreth's Pills,* is the simple remedy by which to relieve such painful state of the bowels. Also, clysters of water, about summer heat, should be given.

84 *Arthritis*, or *Gout*, is a disease occupying and harming the sub-stance of the joints by the falling down and collection of a virulent matter and humors. When there is a great abundance of humors in a body, and the patient leads a sedentary life, not some one, but all the joints of the body are at once troubled with the gout (p. 697).

Gout. Its physiolo-gy. It is a general dis-ease, mani-festing itself in different locations.

The causes. Intemperance, untimely sleep, want of exercise, produce accumulation of morbid matter.

85. The causes of gout are unprofitable humors which are generated and heaped up in the body, and in the process of time acquire a virulent malignity. Such humors arise from an inordinate diet; they offend in feeding who eat much meat, drink strong wine, sleep presently after exercise, and use little exercise. For hence a fullness and obstruction of the vessels, crudities, and the increase of excrements, especially serous, and, if they flow down into the joints, without doubt they cause this disease. Besides, also, the suppression of excretions accustomed to be voided at certain times.

Imperfect purgation in diseases also produces gout.

. . . Those who recover of great and long diseases, unless they be fully and perfectly purged, these humors falling into the joints, which are the relics of the disease, make them become gouty. The humor impact and shut up in the capacities and cavities of the joints, it cannot be easily digested and resolved. The humor then causes pain by reason of distention or solution of continuity, distemper, and besides the virulency and malignity which it acquires. The concourse of flatulencies and hinderance of transpiration increase the morbific painful distention in the membranes, tendons, ligaments and other bodies of which the joints consist (p. 700).

Cure: Purgation, regular to be had in spring and autumn.

86. To cure the gout there are two indications: the first is *the evacuation and alteration of the peccant humors*, the other the strengthening of the weak joints, accompanied by a fit diet. . . . A fit time for purging is the spring and autumn, because gouts reign chiefly in these seasons (p. 704 ; cf. Hipp. Aph. 55, S. VI).

GOLDEN WORDS.

Purgation must be strong, gradually increasing. It cures also the incident fever, and is the treatment required through out the course of the disease.

87. Now, it is convenient that the purge be stronger than ordinary, for if it should be too weak it will stir up the humors, but not carry them away, and they thus agitated will fall into the pained and weak joints, and cause the gout to increase. . . . The *fever* accompanying the gout easily becomes continual, unless the belly being first gently purged, nature be freed by stronger p⬤es of the troublesome burden of the humors. . . . Seeing that *physic is the addition of that which nature wants, and the taking away of those things that are superfluous, and the gout is a disease* that has its essence *from the abounding humor*, certainly, *without the evacuation of them, we cannot hope to cure either it or the pain which accompanies it. Metrius*, in his treatise of the gout, writes, that it must be cured by *purging, used not only in the declination but also in the height of the disease*, WHICH WE HAVE FOUND TRUE BY EXPERIENCE (p. 710; cf. Hipp. Aph. 23, sect. I, and Aph. 8, sect. II.)

Sciatica. Strong purges and vomits.

88. *Sciatica.—Strong purgatives* are here also useful, such as used in phlegmatic causes. Often vomitings do not only evacuate the humors, but also make a revulsion (p. 720).

89. The *heat* or *scalding of the water* arises from repletion, inanition or contagion. That from repletion proceeds from too great abundance

of blood, causing tension and heat in the urinary parts, whence proceeds the inflammation of them and the genital parts. . . . *Purgings are convenient*, and a diet abstaining from heating articles, together with cooling external applications (pp. 738, 740).

Strangury. Cure by purgation.

90. *Buboes, or Swellings in the Groins.*—The matter of these for the most part is abundance of *cold, tough and viscous humors*, as you may gather from the hardness and whiteness of the tumor, the poverty of the pain and contumacy of cure; which also is a reason why the virulency of this disease may be thought to fasten itself in a phlegmatic humor. The cure shall be performed by detergent medicines, and *the humor evacuated by a purging medicine* (p. 746).

Buboes. Evacuate the cause by purgation.

91. *Tetters, Ring-worms or Chops.*—For general remedies, the distemper of the liver and habit of the body must be corrected. This may be done by diet conveniently appointed, by purging and alterative medicines, as they acquire their matter from salt phlegm or adust bile (p. 754).

Tetters, Ring-worm, &c. Purge.

92. Now, the *Small-Pox is pustules*, and *the Measles spots*, which arise in the top *of the skin*, by reason of the impurity of the corrupt blood sent there by the force of nature (p. 757). You must neither purge nor draw blood, the disease increasing or being at its height, unless peradventure there be a great plentitude, or else the disease complicate with others, as with a pleurisy, inflammation of the eyes, or a squinancy* which require it, lest the motion of nature should be disturbed, but you shall think it sufficient to loose the belly with a gentle clyster; but when the height of the disease is over, you may with cassia, or some stronger medicine, evacuate part of the humors and the relics of the disease (p. 759).

Small-Pox and Measles from impurity of the blood.

The use of purgatives.

* Quinsy.

Parey was plainly unacquainted with the good effect of purgation in the early stage of Small-Pox,.when the purgative employed was efficient yet innocent.

In many thousand cases the BRANDRETH PILLS have been administered, more or less during the course of Small-Pox, and with evident advantage in every case.

These Pills are very useful where patients cannot obtain a doctor, and there are thousands of towns in the United States where there is not a medical man within one hundred miles.

The following letter from Daniel Bissell, of Newcomb, Essex County, New York, who was supervisor of the town for twenty years, may be important. I consider it my duty to publish it here :

MR. BISSELL'S LETTER.

Four persons cured of Small-Pox by purging with Brandreth's Pills.

NEWCOMB, ESSEX Co., N. Y., Sept. 13th, 1861.

DOCTOR BENJAMIN BRANDRETH, New York.

Dear Sir : In our family we have used your excellent Pills for several years, and have found them to be a never-failing remedy in mild and severe cases of sickness, but their full value we did not fully appreciate until last winter, when the Small-Pox visited so many families in this and the surrounding towns. I was first attacked, and supposed I had a cold ; took four Pills and some warm drinks; next day no better, took four more; still no better, and my wife said I should take eight—did so, and then the Small-Pox began to show itself. On the fifth day took to my bed, and in less than four days was covered from head to foot with pustules. I continued to use the Pills daily, and took no other medicine whatever except your Vegetable Universal Pills. The Pox was less than four days in coming to a head, and in about the same time they dried up. I began to attend some to my stock in about two weeks, but in three weeks I was attending to my regular farming business, having quite recovered my usual health. I took eighty Pills during my sickness, in doses of four to eight Pills, according to effect, being careful to procure two or three evacuations a day; and though covered from head to foot with the disease, yet it has not left a mark upon me, which is one of the benefits said certainly to be secured by the use of Brandreth's Pills. I and my family found this to be so in our experience of their effects in this fell disease.

My wife, well known as Aunt Polly for one hundred miles around us, was attacked with the disease about the time I was getting well of it. From the first she understood it was the Small-Pox, and prepared herself to combat its virulence by a free use of the Pills. In six days, and while confined to her bed, and scarcely able to move from excessive weakness, she used twenty-six Pills, or a little over an average of four Pills per day. And what was the consequence of this continued purging with Brandreth's Pills? On Tuesday she was obliged to take to her bed; by Friday the pustules were all filled; and by the following Tuesday she had dressed herself! and in one week after was attending to her regular household duties, to the astonishment of all her neighbors. One fact deserves notice: although she was covered with the disease, yet it has left no mark whatever on her skin, which bears no evidence of the awful ordeal it has passed under.

Mrs. Wetherbee, my daughter, her husband, and their only child, were all stricken down by the Small-Pox. Mrs. W. had it light, and only some seven pustules came out. She used thirty Pills in fourteen days. Alonzo, her husband, had a severe attack, and took the Pills all through it, the number not noted. They both recovered in fourteen days from its commencement. Their little boy, Daniel, about fifteen months old, had the disease badly; we had little hope to save him. He was covered from head to feet; he was like a huge scab; and for days he lay insensible. We all supposed he would die—that nothing could save him. His bowels had been confined for several days, and my wife said this must be remedied—that perhaps if the boy could be purged he might revive. She read over yours and Dr. Lull's experience, and gave him one Pill, crushed, in some warm water. The Pill produced no effect, but she was impressed with your remarks upon the necessity and importance of having the bowels purged in Small-Pox, and in all serious sickness whatever; so she gave him another Pill. Still no effect. She then pounded three Pills, and added warm water, and gave them to the boy at once. Still no effect. There the little sufferer lay without motion, except the rapid breathing and peculiar signs of speedy dissolution evident to all. If he died, it would be said he might have got well had his bowels only been opened, and we then commenced to give him three Pills in two hours, or at the rate of one and one-half per hour. When this child of fifteen months had taken thirteen Pills, they operated, and most fully. *The stools were black as pitch, and most offensive.* Every one was satisfied that it was DEATH and MORTIFIED matter which the Pills had brought away, and that the Pills had saved another life, through the Providence of God.

In an hour after the Pills commenced to operate he began to revive, and took some refreshment. He continued to improve until he got well. He is not marked with the disease. It seems proper to state that, though it took thirteen Pills to open his bowels, yet two days after he had a full natural evacuation without medicine, and his bowels have been regular up to this day, which is nearly nine months from the time of his sickness, nor has he used a Pill since. He is as lively, intelligent, and healthy a boy as can be seen. His parents will ever be grateful to you, and they and myself and wife desire you to publish this letter, which, if need be, can be certified to by all the residents of this and the adjoining towns.

I am, respectfully, yours,
DANIEL BISSELL,
For many years Supervisor of the Town.

We certify to the truth of the above. (Signed)—POLLY BISSELL; ALONZO WETHERBEE; MARY WETHERBEE; RUSSELL ROOT, Postmaster, Schroon River; ERASTUS P. ROOT; Thomas R. CAREY, Justice of the Peace, Town of Long Lake; CYRUS H. KELLOGG, Supervisor of Town of Long Lake, 1860; WILLIAM WOOD, Commissioner of Roads, Town of Long Lake; JOSIAH WOOD, Raquette Lake; WM. HELMS, Forked Lake; W. H. PLUMBLEY, Forked Lake; AMOS HOUGH, Forked Lake; EZEKIEL PALMER, Long Lake Hotel.

ANOTHER CURE OF SMALL-POX.

HOW TWO MEN WERE TREATED.

I may also in this connection introduce the following statement of Joseph Daily, of No. 4 Union Square, New York:

Joseph Malone and Henry Downs, acquaintances, on the same day were taken sick. Malone took ten Pills of Brandreth's; next day, feeling no better, he took six more: still feeling no better, he took four more the third day; fourth day better, got up and dressed himself, when, to his great astonishment, he observed large pimples on his face; it was in fact covered with Pox. Upon a further examination he found that they were coming out all over him; even the soles of his feet were full. Malone used the Pills more or less every day until he was perfectly recovered, which was within three weeks from the first day of sickness, when he was again at his business. Though covered from head to foot with the Pox they did not leave a mark behind.

Henry Downs when taken sick called in a doctor, who discovered on the third day the true nature of the disease, and sent his patient to the Small-Pox Hospital on Blackwell's Island. There he remained two months, and then was discharged cured. He lost an eye while in the Hospital, and was so marked that his nearest friends hardly knew him. These facts will bear the strictest investigation.

WORMS.

93. A *gross, viscid and crude humor* is the *material cause of worms*, which having got the beginning of corruption in the stomach, is quickly carried into the guts, and there it putrefies, having not acquired the form of laudable chyle in the first concoction. This, for that it is viscid, tenaciously adheres to the guts, neither is it easily evacuated with the other excrements; therefore, by delay it further putrefies, and by the efficacy of heat, it turns into the matter and nourishment of *worms* (p. 765). In this disease there is but one indication, that is the casting out of the worms forth of the body, as being such that in their whole kind are against nature. . . . Now as such things breed of a putrid matter, *the patient shall be purged*, and the putrefaction repressed. . . . OIL OF OLIVES KILLS WORMS, AND SO DO ALL BITTER THINGS (p. 767). *(margin: Worms from viscid humors accumulated in the intestines; ejected by purgatives.)*

Brandreth's Pills are infallible as a cure for worms, with or without olive oil.

94. *Leprosy proceeds from impurity of blood.*—You must understand that the cause of the *leprosy* by the *retention of the superfluities*, happens because the corrupt blood is not evacuated, but regurgitates over the whole body, and corrupts the blood that should nourish all the members, wherefore the assimilative faculty cannot well assimilate by reason of the corruption and default of the juice, and thus, in conclusion, the leprosy is caused. The antecedent causes are the humors disposed to adustion and corruption into melancholy by torrid heat. . . . *Galen* (ad Glauconem, lib. 1, cap. II.) defines it: " An effusion of troubled or gross blood into the veins and habit of the whole body " (pp. 769, 70). A cooling diet and *purging* shall be prescribed *to evacuate the impurity of the blood* and mitigate the heat of the liver (ibid.; cf. 68; cf. 71, 82, 93; Hippoc. 42, 60). *(margin: Elephantiasis or Leprosy—from impurity of the blood. Evacuate the impurity and prevent its regeneration.)*

95. *Hydrophobia.*—Such as have not their animal faculty as yet overcome by the malignity of the raging venom must have *strong purgatives* given them. For it is a part of extreme and dangerous madness to hope to overcome the cruel malignity of this poison already admitted into the bowels by gentle purging. . . Neither shall they let blood, lest so the poison should be drawn further into the veins. But it is good that the patient's body be soluble from the very first (p. 789). *(margin: Hydrophobia. Strong purgatives from beginning. Bleeding dangerous.)*

NOTE.—BRANDRETH'S PILLS, four every two hours, until twenty pills be taken, is the best means, and will hardly fail if resorted to in season.

Plague from corrupted air and predisposition of the body.

96. The general and natural causes of the *plague* are absolutely two, that is the *infection of corrupt air*, and a *preparation* and fitness *of corrupt humors* to take that infection (p. 819).

Humors putrify either from fullness which breeds obstruction, or by distemperate excess, or by admixture of corrupt matter (p. 820).

Abscesses the cure of nature.

97. I say that the pestilence does depend on the default of the air; this default, being drawn through the passages of the body, does at length pierce into the entrails, as we may understand by the abscesses that break out, by reason that nature using the strength of the expulsive faculty, drives forth whatever is noisome and hurtful (p. 845).

Bleeding kills.

Strong and immediate purging saves.

98. The physician must not let blood, for when nature is debilitated by this evacuation and the *spirits, together with the blood, exhausted,* the venomous air will soon pierce and be received into the empty body, where it exercises its tyranny to its utter destruction. . . . If there be great fullness in the body, especially in the beginning, . . then it is lawful to *purge strongly.* . . . If you call to mind the proper indications, purging shall seem necessary, and that must be prescribed as the case requires, rightly *considering that the disease is sudden,* and requires medicines that may *with all speed drive out* of the body the hurtful humor wherein the noisome quality does lurk and is hidden (pp. 846, 47).

Concussion of the brain. Purgation indicated.

99. *Concussion of the Brain.*—By a heavy blow or the like occasion, the veins and arteries of the head may be broken. From hence proceeds the afflux of blood running between the skull and membranes, or else between the membranes and brain. The blood congealing there, causes vehement pain, and the eyes become blind, vomiting is caused, the mouth of the stomach suffering together with the brain, by reason of the nerves of the sixth conjugation, which run from the brain thither, and from thence are spread all over the ventricle; whence, becoming a partaker of the offense, it contracts itself, and is presently, as if it were, overturned; whence first these things that are therein contained are expelled, and then such as may flow thither from the neighboring parts, as the liver and gall, from all which bile is first expelled (p. 351).

Brandreth's Pills in these cases purge in from thirty to sixty minutes.

In fractures of bones and all surgical operations purge to purify the blood

100. To cure a *broken and dislocated bone* is to restore it to its former figure and site; that is, first to restore the bone to its place; second, to bring it to stay, being so restored; third, to hinder the increase of malign symptoms and accidents, or else if they happen to temper and correct their malignity. . . . For this purpose we *drive away the defluxion* ready to fall down upon the part by medicines, repelling the humor and strengthening the part, or by appointing a good diet, hinder the begetting of excrements in the body, and *divert them by purging* (pp. 565, 66).

NOTE.—The importance of purging and the reasons therefor are strongly presented by Ambrose Parcy, and will have weight with sensible men, in or outside of the profession

Sanctorius, M. D., *Prof. of Physic at Venice ; Ars. de Statica medi-cina, Venice*, 1614. *Aphorisms, translated by John Quincy, M. D. London*, 1720

101. *If there daily be an addition of what is wanting, and a subtraction of what abounds, in due quantity and quality, lost health may be restored, and the present preserved.* (Aph. 1, sect. 1.) *The great principle of health : a systematic disorganization and reorganization.*

He only who knows how much and when the body does more or less insensibly perspire, will be able to discern when and what is to be added or taken away, either *for the recovery* or preservation of health (Aph. 3).

Note.—Nature herself does all these things, provided we relieve the body by purgation ; for innocent purgatives take out no humors but those *which are depraved.*

102. *Insensible perspiration* is either made *by the pores* of the body, which is all over perspirable, and covered with a skin like a net, or it is performed *by respiration through the mouth*, which usually in the space of one day amounts to about half a pound (Aph. 5). *Insensible perspiration, how it is performed.*

Note.—Should either of these processes of the skin or the lungs be partially suspended, we have only to increase by purgation the activity of the bowels, this organ measurably taking upon itself their work, they partially resting the while ; then both lungs and skin will soon regain their healthy functions.

103. If the body increases beyond its usual weight without eating or drinking more than customary, there must either be a retention of the sensible excrements, or an abstraction of the perspirable matter (Aph. 9). *Static medicine : its fundamental principles.*
The body continues in the same state of health as long as it returns to its wonted weight, without any increase of the sensible evacuations ; but if it comes to its standard by larger discharges, either by stool or urine, than ordinary, it then begins to decline from its former health. (Aph. 10; cf. Parey, 71, 82, 93, 94 ; cf. Hippoc., 44, 45.)

104. From too great fullness arise bad qualities, but none vice versa (Aph. 18). Too great a weight and fullness may be lessened by sensible or insensible evacuations, either of digested or undigested matter, and it is good so to do (Aph. 19). *Plethora requires evacuation.*

105. That perspiration which is beneficial, and most clears the body of superfluous matter, is not what goes off with *sweat*, but that insensible steam or vapor (Aph. 21). . . . which becomes sensible when there is too great a supply, *or upon faintings*, or upon violent motions (Aph. 22). Insensible perspiration accompanied with sweat is bad, because sweat diminishes the strength of the fibers. (Aph. 23 ; cf., Hipp. 29, 43.) *Sweat (or visible perspiration) unhealthy.*

When persons faint from severe purging, I have always observed that when they came to, the countenance appeared relieved from great anxiety ; perhaps a congestion was broken up, or some troublesome humor removed.

106. The body is not presently thrown into a disease by an external injury, unless some of the viscera be first disposed to receive its impres- *Predispo-*

sition for, and symptoms of advancing disease. Remore crudities and prevent disease by purgation. sions, which predisposition may be known by a greater or less weight than is customary, and that not without some considerable uneasiness (Aph. 39). The first impressions of a disease are much more easily discernible from the changes of an unusual perspiration, than from the disorders of any of the other functions (Aph. 42). If, upon weighing, the perspirable matter appears to have been obstructed, and there is neither increase of sweat nor urine for some days after, there is a great deal of danger of a putrefaction of the detained crudities (Aph. 43). If the obstructed matter can neither be removed by nature nor a feverish heat, there is immediate danger of a malignant fever. (Aph. 46; cf. Hipp. 17; cf. Hipp., 37.)

107. The excrements of the guts which are well digested, are large
Evacuations, when healthy. in bulk, but light in weight; they swim because of the included air, and what is ejected at once seldom exceeds the third of a pound (Aph. 72).

108. *Importance of Ventilation to Imperceptible Pores.*—Nothing more tends to prevent a corruption of the humors than plentiful ventila-
Double action of the lungs and pores (active and negative). tion; not only by that which is drawn in by the lungs, but what is drawn in through the imperceptible pores. (Aph. 120; cf. Hipp., 10, 55 and 13, 26.)

109. The plague is communicated not by any immediate contact, but
Pestilential infection, how propagated, prevented and cured by purgation. either by drawing in infectious air or the steams of tainted furniture; and it is thus: the vital spirits are infected by the air, and from the infected spirits *the blood is coagulated,* which produces *black* spots, *carbuncles* and *buboes,* and if *not sufficiently discharged,* occasion death; but if it be all thrown out, they escape. (Aph. 127; cf. Parey, 94).

The above shows the absolute necessity of Brandreth's Pills in Plague, because they purge safely.

Air—Its influence upon the body. 110. The external air which passes through the arteries into the body may render the body heavier or lighter; lighter if it be subtle and warm, and heavier when thick and moist (Aph. 3, sect. II). In a foggy air perspiration is lessened, the pores are obstructed, and the fibers weakened and not rendered more firm; and the weight of the retained matter is both perceivable and injurious. (Aph. 8; cf. 103, 106, 109.)

Summer-complaint: how it ensues. Its cure by gentle purging to remove obstructed matter. 111. Temperate persons weigh in *summer time* about three pounds less than in the winter (Aph. 23). That lassitude or weariness which is perceivable in summer time is not because the body is then heavier, but because it is then rendered weaker (Aph. 24). In summer time the body is not uneasy from the heat of the air immediately, for every part of the body is even then hotter than the external air, but because at such times there is not a sufficient coldness to *concentrate the natural heat.* By which means it becomes so scattered that it cannot drive out *the perspirable matter,* in its own nature hot, by insensible steams; which matter, by being retained, acquires a sharpness, and is really the cause of that uneasiness we are under from a sense of the summer heat (Aph. 27, sect. 1)

112. *When to Purge.*—The *autumn* is unhealthful, both because perspiration lessens upon the supervening cold, and because that which is obstructed acquires an *acrimony* and a *corrosive quality* (Aph. 42). They who are accustomed to a distemper in winter, that arises *from a fullness of humors*, ought to purge in autumn (Aph. 48). *Autumnal disease—Its causes; cure by evacuating the acrimonious accumulations.*

NOTE.—Our experience is, purge only when the body calls for it—when we have pain or oppression, or the bowels are costive.

113. But for such diseases as arise from *noxious qualities*, purging ought rather to be used in the spring than autumn, because in the hot weather such qualities grow worse more than in the winter (Aph. 49; cf. Parey, 86). *Spring the season for purging for constitutional diseases.*

114. If the obstructed perspirable matter acquires an *acrimony*, it *produces fevers and inflammations;* but when it offends only in *quantity*, it causes *apostumations, distillations*, and *cachexies* (Aph. 51). *Acrimony is corrected and superabundance carried off by purgation.*

115. When a full meal is not perfectly digested, it is to be known by an increase of weight, for the body will not then perspire well; but an empty stomach is filled with vapors (Aph. 12, sect. 3 ; cf. Apo. 5, sect. 1.) Robust persons discharge their food for the most part by perspiration; those not so strong by urine; and the weak chiefly by an indigested chyle (Aph. 14). A full or an empty stomach lessens perspiration ; for a full one diverts it by corruption of the aliment, and an empty one draws it back, that it may be filled (Aph. 11), and the obstructed matter will acquire a sharpness, whence the body will be subject to distempered heat (Aph. 15). *Insensible and visible excretion—their equilibrium depending on constitutional strength.*

116. When a person seems to himself lighter than he really is, it is a very good sign, because it arises from a perfect digestion of all the juices (Aph. 19). *Sensation of health.*

117. That sort of food best perspires, and affords the most suitable nourishment, whose weight is not perceived in the belly (Aph. 28). *What is suitable food.*

118. Nothing more frequently interrupts sleep than a putrefaction of the food, such is the sympathy between the stomach and the brain (Aph. 40, sect. 4). From eating comes sleep; from sleep digestion, and from digestion a good perspiration (Aph. 59 ; cf. Parey, 99). *Watchfulness from morbid matter—purge. Sympathy of brain and stomach.*

119. By exercise bodies are rendered lighter ; for all the parts, especially ligaments and muscles, are cleared of their excrements by motion; the perspirable matter is fitted for exhalation, and the spirits rendered firmer (Aph. 9, sect. 5). Exercise promotes both the sensible and insensible evacuations ; but rest only the insensible (Aph. 10). *Digestion requires exercise of the body.*

120. The heavy part of the perspirable matter being more than usually retained in the body, it will dispose a person to fear and sorrow ; but the lighter part being obstructed, to anger or joy (Aph. 5, sect. 7). *"Nervousness" from obstructed exertion— therefore purge.*

HARVEY, WILLIAM, DR.—*The works of, written 1628–51; transl. by Robt. Willis, M. D., and published by the Sydenham Society. London, 1846–47.*

HARVEY, WILLIAM, DR.—*The works of, written 1628–51; transl. by Robt. Willis, M. D., and published by the Sydenham Society. London, 1846–47.*

Harvey on the blood. 121. The blood acts with forces superior to the forces of the elements. As the instrument of the Great Workman, no one can ever sufficiently extol its admirable, its divine faculties. . . . It penetrates everywhere, and is ubiquitous; abstracted, *the soul or the life, too, is gone,* so that the blood does not seem to differ in any respect from the soul, or the life (anima) itself. At all events it is to be regarded as the substance whose act is the soul or the life. . . .*In one way the blood is part of the body, but in another way is the beginning and cause of all that is contained in the animal body.* . . That which is abundantly nourished by it, increases; what is not sufficiently supplied, shrinks; what is perfectly nourished, preserves health; what is not perfectly nourished, falls into diseases (pp. 510, 11).

Vitiated blood. 122. Vitiated states and plethora of the blood are causes of a whole host of diseases (p. 391; cf. Hippocr. Works, p. 262, Vol. I., Aphor. 22, sect. 2; cf. Parey, 68–99).

Nature the teacher of medicine. 123. The physiological consideration of the things which are according to nature is to be first undertaken by medical men, since that which is in conformity with nature is right, and serves as a rule both to itself and to that which is amiss (p. 90; Hippocr. Works, p. 102, Vol. I., p. 360, Vol. I).

The timid concert to the new doctrine. 124. Not yielding implicitly to the truth, he fears to speak out plainly, "lest he offend the ancient physic" (p. 91).

The old fogies of Harvey's time. 125. Who will not see that the precepts he has received from his teachers are false; or who thinks it unseemly to give up accredited opinions; or who regards it as in some sort criminal to call in question doctrines that have descended through a long succession of ages, and carry the authority of the ancients; to all these I reply: that *the facts cognizable by the senses wait upon no opinions,* and that *the works of* *Nature the oldest authority.* *nature bow to no antiquity; for, indeed, there is nothing either more ancient or of higher authority than nature* (p. 123; cf. Hippocr. 47).

The blood again. 126. *The blood is the generative part, the fountain of life, the first to live, the last to die, and the primary seat of the soul* (p. 377).

The blood is both *the author and preserver of the body;* it is the principal element, moreover, and that in which the vital principle (anima) has its dwelling place. . . The blood, moreover, is that alone which lives and is possessed of heat while life continues (p. 379; cf. pp. 510, 11).

COLLINS, SAMUEL, M. D., *System of Anatomy. London*, 1685.

127. *Cathartics do not only affect the blood at a distance*, but also the villous coat and nervous filaments, which do immediately disturb them with troublesome stroaks proceding from the pungent particles of purgatives, vellicating the inward coat of the stomach as a tender compage beset with nervous fibrils, which, irritated by sharp medicines, spew out serous liquor out of the excretore ducts, derived from the glands of the intestines. *How purgative medicines act on the stomach and intestines, by irritation of the intestinal nerves, stimulating the peristaltic motion and cleansing off the mucous matter.*

The purgation extract of medicines first produced by the ferments of the stomach, and afterwards imparted to the intestines, does highly excite the nervous and carnous fibers, and gives a most troublesome sensation to the inward coat of the guts finely dressed with fibrils; and afterwards affects the excretory vessels of the pancreas and hepatic ducts with a kind of convulsive motion, making them disgorge their pancreatic and bilious recrements, into the larger receptacle of the intestines.

And not only the *feces of the blood*, secreted from it in the glands of the liver and pancreas, are thrown into the guts by the excitement of the nervous and carnous fibers, but also *the extremities of the arteries and excretory vessels* belonging to the glands, *are opened* by the sharp and aperient qualities of the purgatives, *unlocking the* secret *pores of the inward coat of the intestines* lined with a *mucous matter*, which *is scraped off by the cleansing qualities of purgatives*, leaving the intestines exposed to the active power of raking medicines, which force open the extremities of the arteries (p. 369, vol. I).   .

128. The *concoctive faculty* of the intestines is disaffected; first, as it is *wholly abolished, when no chyle*, or very little, *is extracted* in the stomach or intestines. This evil proceeds from the want of natural heat deficient primarily in the blood, and from a defect of good succus pancreaticus, and bilious liquor, and a laudable serous and nervous juice, not being imparted by the extremities of the arteries and nerves to the crude aliment lodged in the guts. This disorder is commonly called *lienteria*, an unnatural excretion of the aliment, little or no ways altered, wherein its compage is not well opened by due ferments, and a secretion made of the alimentary liquor from the grosser feces (p. 370). This *obstruction of the hepatic and pancreatic ducts* is cured by *aperient medicines* (p. 371). *Pathology of the intestines. Lienteria from obstruction of the hepatic and pancreatic ducts. Cure by purgatives.*

129. Another disorder of the intestines near akin to the former, as differing from it in degree, is the *lessened concoction*, commonly styled *caeliac affection*, wherein the food is in some sort digested, and remains confused, as not secreted from the gross parts, because the chyle is not well attenuated by the pancreatic and bilious liquor, and serous and nervous juice, which are destitute of volatile salt, oily and spirituous particles, so as to render the chyle fluid in the intestines; whereupon the clammy chyle embodying with the crude aliment, is excreted by the expulsion faculty (p. 370). This distemper is cured by the same means as a lienteria (p. 371). *Caeliac affection is imperfect digestion from defective composition of the circulating fluid. Cure by purgative medicine.*

130. The third indisposition of the concoctive faculty of the intestines *Imperfect digestion*

30 THE DOCTRINE OF PURGATION.

from acrid humors. Purge. is its *depraved action*, produced by ill ferments of *sharp bilious, and acrid pancreatic liquor*, vitiating the extracted aliment in the guts, and afterwards *spoiling the mass of blood*, when it is received into association with it in the blood-vessels (p. 370). It denotes gentle aperient medicines (p. 371; cf. Parey, 94).

Indigestion from disorders of the distributive faculty of the chyle, by viscosity of humors. 131. Another disaffection of the intestines, and that none of the least because it concerns the nutrition of the whole body, is when the *distributive faculty of the chyle* is either wholly taken away or much lessened, which may proceed either from the clamminess of the chyle, or from the grossness of pituitous humors, more or less obstructing the orifices of the lacteal vessels seated in the intestines. The cure of this disease may be assisted with a light diet and medicines promoting the digestion (p. 371).

Slowness of excretion from inactiveness of the intestinal nerves. Purgatives stimulate them to activity. 132. The intestines are also incident to divers diseases in reference to their *expulsive faculty*, when the peristaltic motion is too slow, or too quick, or aggrieved with the discomposure of pain. The slowness of the motion of the guts proceeds either from the *torpid indisposition of the nervous coat*, not resenting the irritation by gross excrements, when the nervous fibrils inserted into the inward coat *of the intestines* have their acute sense lessened, proceeding from the want of animal spirits intercepted first in the fibrous parts of the brain, and by consequence in the nerves of the guts, produced by cephalic diseases, compressing or obstructing the fibrils seated in the brain. This disaffection is cured by proper methods and medicines relating to the diseases of the head (p. 371). *In all the diseases of the brain*, Collins recommends *purgatives* to a greater or less extent (pp. 1133, 1134, 1138, 1145, 1153, 1163, 1169, 1181, 1194, 1199; vol. II; cf. Sanctorius, 118).

Torpor of the intestines from narcotics)opium) removed by strong purgation. 133. The slowness of the peristaltic motion, incident to the guts, may be also derived from *narcotic medicines*, dulling the acute sense of the nerves which terminate into the inward tunicle of the intestines, whereupon they are not sensible of their burden, when they are oppressed with excrements. This disease may admit a cure by *strong purgatives* and *sharp clysters* (p. 372).

Hardened faeces are removed by purgatives. 134. The remissness of the expulsive power of the guts may also arise from the viscid and indurated contents, produced by ill concoction; the other from *the heat of the guts*, exhausting the liquid parts of the excrements; the guts being overcharged with excrements, purgatives may be advised (p. 372; cf. Hippocr. 13, 25, 26).

Lientery, Caeliac disease and diarrhea from exalted peristaltic motion. Cure by purgatives. 135. The *over-hasty motion* of the guts is made in a *lientery* and *caeliac disease*, proceeding from the quantity of crude and indigested aliment provoking the nervous and carnous fibrils to excretion. This disaffection of the guts is visible also in diarrhea proceeding from salt phlegm and from bilious and serous excrements discomposing the tender compage of the guts, and irritating them to expulsion. The cure of this disease is performed by lenient and astringent purgatives (p. 372; cf. Sanctorius, 103; Hippocr. 44, 45).

136. Inflammations of the guts producing dysenteries are most commonly seated in the great gut, which, proceeding from a quantity of blood impelled by the mesenteric arteries into the intestines, some part of which is stagnant in the substance of the bowels, and other parts are transmitted sometimes into the small guts, where it seldom makes any long stay, as, being thrown from there into the colon, wherein the blood is long retained; whereupon the tender frame of the coats is corroded by the sharp blood confined in the deep cavities of the colon (p. 372). The vitiated expulsive faculty of the guts coming from inflammations, and from an ill mass of blood, is cured by clysters made of healing medicines and by purgatives (p. 373; cf. Sanctorius,103, 106, 109, 110). *Dysentery from inflammation produced by stagnation of impure blood in the bowels.*

137. The *iliac passion* proceeds from divers causes, sometimes from the small *guts twisted*, other times *entangled and tied in knots*, and also when they *shoot downwards and upwards into one another.* It may be derived from astringents unduly used, and from a stoppage of the intestines by viscious matter from hardened excrements, and from flatulent matter contained in the guts intercepting the passage of the gross feces. . . Now and then the upper shoots into the lower, and sometimes the lower into the upper part of the small intestines, which are much distended in several places, and in other parts contracted for some space both above and below; whereupon the free play of wind being checked, the patient is highly tortured with pain, and, to ease himself, puts his body in divers postures by various agitations and flexures of it. A relaxation is made of some part of the guts adjoining the contracted parts, which, being moved forward by the pressure of wind toward the relaxed intestines, force them into the next expanded parts of the guts, which are afterwards closed up by the duplicature of them, entirely intercepting the passage of excrements. And when in this miserable distemper the lower part of the guts is thrust into the cavity of the upper, the *pressing down of the excrements*, made by art in purgative medicines, discharges the insinuation of the lower gut into the upper (pp. 375, 76). . The iliac passion may arise out of a *gross alimentary liquor or phlegm concreted in the intestines*, wholly shutting up the passage of them; whence ensues a recoiling of the excrements upward, produced by the irregular contraction of the fleshy fibers (p. 377). This disease often happens upon *a long suppression of natural evacuations by stool*, generated by a load of hard excrements, long residing in the guts, productive of intolerable pains (p. 378; cf. Hippocr. 38, 41, 44). *Iliac passion, or pains in the small guts from accumulation of fecal matter generally accompanied with costiveness of the bowels; which is removed by purgative medicines.*

138. The *colic* is near akin to the iliac passion in the situation of the subject and in the cause of the disease, both proceeding from sharp humors productive of vexatious pains, and from the great obstruction and tension of the guts, caused by a *quantity of gross excrements*, and more thin *and flatulent matter* (p. 379). This disease takes up its mansion, if not solely, yet chiefly, in the *colon*. Colic pains are generally felt in the *lower apartment* of the abdomen, accompanied with *nausea, vomiting, suppression of stools, pains in the back*, &c. . . Colic, accompanied with heat and beating pains, arises from blood impelled out of *(Cf. Parey. 83.) Colic: Accumulation of stagnating blood, excrementitious matter, and flatulency,(the cause. Its symptoms.*

the terminations of the capillary mesenteric arteries into the substance of the coats of the colon; piercing and fixed pains come from sharp pancreatic liquor blended with viscid phlegm, or bilious humors lodged within the coats of the guts, which produce pungent and wandering pains (pp. 380, 81)! . This disease denotes purging and alterative medicines (p. 382).

Active, re-peated pur-gation the cure. 139. I conceive the carnous and nervous fibers are much weakened by the inflation of the coats of the intestines, whereupon the irritation of the medicines is not easily felt, and the carnous fibers do not contract; upon this account strong purgatives must be given, or rather gentle, often repeated, assisted with purgative clysters, which excite the peristaltic motion of the guts to discharge the indigested aliment or gross vitreous phlegm, or indurated excrements (p. 384; cf. Hippocr. 55; Coll. 134).

Abscesses and Ulcers of the me-sentery. 140. *Abscesses* and *ulcers of the mesentery* are cured by gentle purgatives and proper drying diet-drinks (p. 393).

Pains of the back and other diseases of the mesente-ry—their causes and cure by pur-gation. 141. Great pains in the back are not the disaffection of the colon only, but of the mesentery, too. . . Mesenteric affections are often derived from the serous feculencies of the blood, impelled out of the capillary arteries into the substance of the mesentery, and from flatulent matter distending the fibers of the mesentery. A cure may be attempted by emollient and discutient *clysters and by purgatives*, gradually increasing their strength, and by fomentations (p. 395).

Diarrhea —full pur-gation. 142. When patients labor under a great diarrhea, I conceive it *very dangerous* to advise powerful astringents until nature has fully discharged herself, or art emptied the guts of gross and more thin excrements (p. 376; cf. Parey, 92, and Hippocr. 2).

Opium the cause of apoplexy. 143. The immoderate use of *opiates* produces *apoplexy*, the drug stupifying and relaxing the nerves, and causing the stagnation of the blood in the cortex (pp. 1128, 1129).

Apoplexy, &c. Cure by strong pur-gation. 144.* The sleepy diseases (apoplexy, carus, coma, lethargy), being akin in their causes, are much alike in their cures, too. . Strong purgatives may be given, and after a purgative has been celebrated, vomitories may be administered (pp. 1131, 1132, 1133).

Vertigo— from irrita-tion of intes-tinal nerves. Purge. 145. *Vertiginous symptoms* arise from irritation of the nervous fibrils of the stomach, intestines, liver, pancreas, spleen and kidneys, proceeding from sharp recrements, which, offending the fibrils of the viscera, taking their origin from the brain, give a lightness to it (p. 1136); and as to the preservatory indication in an ill habit of the body, purgatives may be applied (p. 1138; cf. 132).

Delirium requires evacuation of the bow-els. 146. In *phrenitis* and *paraphrenitis*, produced by an undue effervescence of the blood caused by heterogeneous particles, or by the blood being poisoned with malignant qualities (p. 1140), which is induced by serous recrements vitiating the nervous liquor (p. 1143), clysters are

TO THE DOCTRINE OF PURGATION. 33

very successful to *empty the bowels* of excrements and winds (p. 1145 ; cf. Parey, 94 ; Sanctorius, 109).

147. *Melancholy* being produced by *vitiated blood* and *corrupt humors* in the viscera (pp. 1150, 1151), is cured by vomitories and purgatives, removing the gross phlegm from the stomach and discharging gross, acid, and saline recrements from the blood (p. 1153). *Melancholy. Remove morbid matter from the blood.*

148. *Mania* borrows its first rise from an ill mass of blood, caused by the distemper of the hepatic glands not secreting the bilious from the more laudable parts of the blood (p. 1159). *Strong purgatives* are used with advantage in this stubborn malady, as they purify the blood and nervous liquor (p. 1163). *Mania. Purify the blood by strong purgatives.*

149. Frequent and large doses of opiates incrassate the mass of the blood (p. 1167) and nervous liquor, rendering them effete and vapid, so that the brain cannot accomplish the acts of sense and reason, making men mopes and sots. *To refine the blood,* purging medicines, prepared with cephalics, may be very proper in those diseases (p. 1169). *Opiates produce mopishness & stupidity.*

150. The indication to take away the cause of *epilepsy* is principally founded in *rectifying an ill mass of blood* and nervous liquor, which depends much upon a *laudable state of the viscera,* so that the ill diathesis of the blood and viscera is taken away by vomiting, purging, and bleeding (p. 1181). *Epilepsy from a vitiated state of viscera.*

151. *Palsy.*—The motive faculty is impeded or abolished, because the origins of the nerves are obstructed by the grossness of the nervous liquor, which may arise from a thick, feculent, albuminous part in the blood (p. 1193). A palsy sometimes succeeds severe pains of the stomach and intestines (p. 1194), which are produced by an accumulation of bilious and excrementitious matter and hardened feces and dilatation by flatulency, compressing the beginning of the vertebral nerves and intercepting the current of the circulating fluid (p. 1195). The antecedent cause of palsy is an *ill mass of blood* generated by a bad *diet, hard of digestion* (p. 1196). Vomitories may be advised in a foul stomach, but purgatives and alteratives for a habitual palsy (p. 1199). In a palsy derived from an evident cause—a fall, stroke, or wound—the apertion of a vein may be proper, *after an emollient and discutient clyster* has been administered and rejected (p. 1198; cf. 139; Parey, 83; cf. 136, 137, 138). *Palsy from feculent matters in the blood, produced by imperfect digestion. The first step toward cure: purgation.*

SYDENHAM, THOMAS, *M. D. The whole Works of that excellent practical Physician, written about* 1686. *Transl. Dr. Pechey. London,* 1701. *Sydenham.*

152. Though a purge does for the present raise a greater tumult in the blood and other humors, on the day it is taken, and in the operation, than was before, yet this injury will be sufficiently made up by the advantage that presently follows; for it is found by experience that *purging quells a fever sooner and better* than any other remedy whatever, both as it expels those *filthy humors* from the body, by which, as *the antecedent cause,* the *fever* was *occasioned ;* and if they were not peccant before, yet, at length being heated, concocted and thickened by the fever, *Purgatives quell fevers soonest and best.*

Filthy humors the antecedent cause. do much to render it more lasting (p. 432 ; cf. Hipp. Works, I., 174 ; W. Harvey, 391 ; Sanctorius, 103, 106, 109, 110 ; Collins, 136–138, 151).

Sweating and purging compared. Although nature cures fevers by sweating, man must cure by purgatives.

The reasons given most excellent.

153. *Purging preferable to Sweating.*— . . . On the contrary, as that method which is busied in eliminating the febrile matters through the pores of the skin is less certain, so it is more troublesome and tedious ; for by it the disease is very often protracted many weeks, and the life of the patient thereby endangered. . . . For this reason I insist, upon good grounds, that *purging* is more powerful than any other method for the subduing fevers of most kinds, for though sweating is nature's own method by which she casts out febrile matters, and is more genuine and commodious than the rest, when nature is left to itself it first digests the aforesaid matter, and then, when it is well concocted, gently expels it through the habit of the body.

Yet art, how much soever it may seem to imitate nature, cannot arrogate to itself the privilege that it is able to cure fever certainly by sweating. For, first, art knows not by what means the peccant matter should be fitly prepared to undergo expulsion ; and if it should know this, yet it has no certain signs by which it should be admonished of the due preparation of it ; so that also it is unavoidably ignorant of the fit time for provoking sweat, which it is very dangerous to provoke rashly; while if the physician should, by purging, miss his aim in curing the patient, yet he will not hurt him (pp. 432–34; cf. Gid. Harvey, p. 286; cf. Hipp. 29, 43; Sanctorius, 105; Parey, 69; Hipp. 9.)

☞ *The above a highly important article.*

Humoral Pathology. Diseases various, in proportion to quantity and quality of morbid matters.

154. If the humors are retained longer in the body than they ought, either because nature cannot concoct them and afterwards expel them, or because they have contracted a morbific disposition, they become exalted into a substantial form or species, which discovers itself by this or that disorder, that is agreeable with its own essence.

Like produces like.

The *symptoms of disease*, though to the less wary they may *seem to arise from the nature of the part which the humor possesses, are really disorders arising from this or that specific exaltation or specification of some juice in the body.* For nature is as methodical in producing and ripening these as of plants and animals, unless the order of it be disturbed by some extrinsic thing (as purgation). The species of diseases depend on those humors from whence they were generated. (Preface.)

In Chronic Diseases assist nature.

155. *Chronic Diseases.*—Nature has not an effectual method in these diseases, to eject the morbific matter, as in acute, whereby, we assisting and aiming at the right mark, the disease may be cured. (Preface.)

NOTE.—Purgation usually changes the chronic into an acute disease by assisting nature to expel impurities ; thus the blood becomes endowed with greater vitality.

Disease a natural effort at cure.

156. A disease is nothing but nature's endeavor to thrust forth, with all her might, the morbific matter for the health of the patient, though the cause of it be contrary to nature (p. 1; cf. Hipp. Aph. 2, sect. I; Sanctorius, 106.) •

157. *Impurities* mixed with the blood affect the whole with a mor- Why na-
bific contagion, partly from the various ferments or putrefaction of ture *cannot* expel impu-
humors which are detained in the body beyond their due time, because rities.
it was *not able to digest or evacuate them*, either upon the account of
their bulk being too great, or the *incongruity of their quality* (pp. 1, 2).

158. What is the *Gout* but Nature's contrivance to purify the blood *Gout.*
of old men (p. 2)?

159. *Purification.*—Nature performs this office, sometimes quicker, *Fevers—*
sometimes slower, for when she requires the help of a *fever*, whereby she nature's pro- cess of cure.
may be able to separate the vitiated particles from the blood, and after- When she cannot from
wards expel them, the whole business is done in the mass of the blood, any cause get rid of
and that by violent motion of the parts. . . . When this kind of matter these impu-
is fixed to any part which is unable to exclude it, either upon the ac- rities, Pal- sies, &c , and
count of its conformation, as it is in the morbific matter of a palsy that *Chronic*
the nerves are stuffed with, or upon the account of a continued flux of *Diseases* fol- low. Severe
new matter, wherewith the blood is vitiated, which is only disposed to Purging ne- cessary.
carry it off, does oppress and overwhelm the part. I say in these cases
the matter is very slowly or not at all concocted, and so diseases that
proceed from such unconcocted matters are, and are called, chronic
(pp. 2, 3 ; Cf. p. 432 ; 19.   ; W. Harv. 90, 391 ; Sanctorius, 112).

160. He will not be mistaken much who should affirm that more *Diseases*
diseases arise hence, viz., from the *omission of purging* after autumnal *from want of purga-*
diseases, than from any other cause whatever (p. 21 ; Cf. Hipp. Aph. *tion.*
12, II. ; 43, 56, VI. ; Works, 707, II. ; 728, II. ; Aph. 32, IV).

161. All means to avoid disease or infection are useless, if the *body is* To escape
furnished with humors disposed to receive the infection (p. 59 ; cf. disease, the blood must
Hippoc. W. 102, I). be pure.

162. *Cholera.*—Should I restrain the first effort with *narcotic* medi- *Cholera—*
cines and other *astringents*, whilst I *hindered natural evacuation*, and de- *astringents kill.*
tained the humors *against nature*, the sick would undoubtedly be
destroyed by the intestine war, his enemy being kept in his bowels (p.
115 ; cf. Hipp. Aph. 2, I. ; 21, I; Collins, 142).

163. *Sydenham on Hippocrates, Nature and Disease.*—The excellent Hippo rates'
Hippocrates who arrived at the top of physic, laid this solid foundation axiom : na- ture cures
for building the art of physic upon, viz., NATURE CURES DISEASE, and he disease. His theory sim-
delivered plainly the phenomena of every disease, *without pressing any* ply a descrip-
hypothesis into his service. He also delivered some rules gathered from tion of na- ture. Art of
the observation of that method that nature uses in promoting and medicine : to assist na-
removing diseases, and of these things *consisted the theory of the divine* ture only by remedies few
old man . . . This theory was nothing else but an *exquisite description* and simple.
of nature ; it was reasonable that in practice his only aim should be *to*
relieve her, when she was *oppressed,* by the best means he could ; and
therefore he allowed no other *province for art* than *the succouring of*
nature when she was *weak,* the *restraining* her when she was *outrageous,*

and the *reducing her to order*, and to do all this in that way and manner, *whereby nature endeavours* to expel diseases; for the sagacious man perceived that nature judges diseases, and does in all, being helped by a few simple forms of remedies, and sometimes without any (preface; cf. pp. 432, 2–3; W. Harvey 123).

Scarlet Fever. 164. *Scarlet Fever.*—I reckon this disease is nothing else than a moderate effervescence of the blood, occasioned by the heat of the foregoing summer, or some other way, and therefore I do nothing to hinder the depuration of the blood and the ejecting of the peccant matter through the pores of the skin, which is easily done by the blood itself.

Purgatives cure. Other remedies destroy. 165. But when the scales are gone off and the symptoms ceased, I think it proper to PURGE the sick with some gentle medicine that is agreeable to his age and strength ; and by this simple and plain natural method, this name of a disease, for it is scarce anything more, may be easily and safely removed. Whereas, on the contrary, if we disturb nature by cordials and other needless remedies too learnedly thrust in *secundum artem*, the disease is hightened and the sick dies by the over-officiousness of the physician (pp. 189–90).

Pleurisy : a natural attempt to cure by eliminating morbid matter from the blood. 166. I think pleurisy is a fever originating in a proper and peculiar inflammation of the blood, an inflammation by the means of which nature deposits the peccant matter in the pleurae. Sometimes she lays it on the lung itself, and then there comes a peripneumonia. This differs from the pleurisy only in degree. It exhibits the results of the same cause with greater intensity. (Society's Ed., vol. I., p. 247.)

HARVEY GIDEON, M. D. *The Vanities of Philosophy and Physick. 3d edit. London,* 1702.

Uncertainty in medicine. 167. 1st. Things in philosophy and medicine which we do not know, are beyond all manner of comparison more than those things we do know.
2d. The greatest part of these things in medicine, which we pretend to know, is conjectural and uncertain.
3d. Many if not most of these things which we do peremptorily affirm to be this or that, to be caused by this or that, or to cause and effect this or that, are or may be proved to be false (pp. 7, 8 ; cf. Parey, 66 ; cf. W. Harvey, 124–126).

The blood—source of disease. 168. The antecedent causes of most diseases are the fluid parts of the blood, the fluid *animal lympha*, the *glandulous lympha*, and the *blood* being vitiated (p. 139 ; cf. F. Harvey, p. 391).

Theory of disease. 169. How TRUE.—The weakness of the stomach and its faintly performing its office, is only occasioned by the debility of the stomach-nerves, and their various branches, by being plastered up by too much *fleam, gross and acid dregs, indigestible meals,* or *offensive drinks,* or other matter admitted into the stomach, which, by lodging there too long, assume a corroding quality. . . . (cf. Sydenh., Prof.).

170. This supposed, I do believe, and have experimentally observed, that all those corroborations of the stomach, whose virtue is commonly asserted to consist in a gentle restrictive and warming quality—whereby these slimy humors are more firmly cemented—so far from contributing the least strength to the stomach, being long continued, do carry danger with them (p. 227). *"Strength-eners" do not strengthen.*

171. The only means I have hitherto found to strengthen the stomach are proper abstersive medicines, gently wiping off those clammy substances from the tunic of the stomach, and the terminations of the nervous branches. . . . *Do only keep your stomach clean, you will certainly preserve its strength, and prevent most diseases* (p. 228; cf. Hipp. Aph. 8, sect. II. ; Parey, 87). *Purgatives the only strengtheners.*

172. Herodotus (in Euterpe) who was contemporary with Hippocrates, tells us that the Egyptians, to whom the first invention of physic is ascribed, used to take purging-physic, for three days together every month, for no other purpose than to cleanse their stomachs, knowing they could be subject to no diseases but what the foulness of their stomachs might occasion, in regard their bodies were strong, and their air the most clear and temperate in the world. (p. 232). *Regular purgation among the ancient Egyptians.*

173. It is not to be understood, where a heap and weight of crudities is accumulated, that gently absterging remedies can have power to disengage the stomach, any more than a wet mop can be supposed to rid a room of a heap of rubbish,—in which case something more stimulating is required, that may be used in all seasons of the year, be it sultry or freezing, without the inconvenience of confinement to diet or warmth of air, or without offence to the stomach, or putting the body into any disorder; to which purposes the pill I here now describe, I have experimentally found to be effectively answering in most respects. (p. 228). *Full purgation.*

Brandreth's Pills are superior to the following in all the elements of cleansing physic.

. 174. Take one ounce of the clearest shining aloes; powder it in a mortar, covered over with a brown paper having a hole in the middle for a passage to the pestle. Observe to anoint thinly the bottom of the mortar and pestle with a little Florence oil, to keep it from sticking to the bottom. When it is reduced to a gross powder, by grinding it with the pestle you must bring it to a smooth fineness. Put the powder into a small glazed flat-bottomed earthen pan, that will contain about half a pint, pouring upon it about a quarter of a pint of water, wherein has been dissolved 2 drams of Spanish juice of Liquorish, which is done by slicing it very small and setting the water in a porringer over a gentle heat; place this same earthen pan into one somewhat bigger, having sand in the bottom to the height of an inch, and afterwards filling it up to the brim. Set them over two piles of bricks of three or four bricks laid flat. The piles must stand at such a distance, that they may reach the edges of the bigger pan to support it. Then make a moderate fire of charcoal under it, to heat the same, to cause the superfluous moisture to be evaporated, *The Harvey Pill.*

until the aloes is brought to the thickness of honey. Or you may, by drop-
ping two or three drops on the back-side of a plate, to cool, make a trial
whether it be reduced to the consistence of dough; for if it be over-
done, the mass being rendered brittle, will not only lose most of its
virtue, but also its aptness of being framed into pills; and if it be not
evaporated enough, it will be sticky, and not apt to be brought into a
mass. The lesser pan being taken off, when the evaporation is sufficient,
before it is quite cold, you must with a spatula or slice take out the mass,
and between your fingers, being a little anointed with Florence oil to prevent the sticking, roll it into a round ball, which you may keep in a
sheep's-bladder, being likewise thoroughly wetted over on the inside with
the same oil, for many months, if necessary. A small piece of this mass
being formed into 6, 7, 8, or 9 little pills of the bigness of a pepper-corn,
is a dose sufficient to give two or three motions.

The safeness of this medicine adds much to its character, since the
taking of one pill, or two, more or less, imparts as little hazard, as the
taking it very often, or in any kind of season, be it hot or cold, &c. . . .
By the addition of the use of Liquorish, the aloe is designed to be obtused
in its too purgative qualities, whereby it is apt to raise the piles, and
become somewhat less precipitating, &c.

The same correction may be obtained by taking a large handful of Bug-
loss or Borrage-leaves, and stirring half a pint of warm water with them
in the bruising, and clarified by subsidence in letting it stand in a cellar
for a day or two, and pouring it off the feces or dregs in the bottom.
This evaporated in the same manner, will produce a mass almost equal
in goodness to the former. (pp. 223—5).

The whole of what follows in Paragraph 175 is equally applicable to Brandreth's Pills,
whose virtues far exceed all other cleansing medicines the world has yet seen.

175. I cannot but heretofore observe, that the use of these pills, though
frequently taken, according to the time the stomach, by reason of its
degree of weakness in the digestive faculty, may require, does in anywise
Purgatives debilitate those that may properly use them; but on the contrary, rath-
do not weak- er corroborate their stomach by assisting it, to throw off that heap of rub-
en. bish and crude humors, which those that eat and drink plentifully, and
either live sedentary lives, as many that are educated to professions, or
others that are not used to exercise or labor, are subject to engender,
especially if naturally of a weak constitution or of an advanced age.
(p. 235). (cf. Hipp. Aph. 8. Sect. I). . . For three or four days succeeding the use of these pills, a good *Elixer proprietatis* taken morning and
evening, in a proportionate dose, has, by my observation, ever had the
good effect of preserving health and preventing disease. (p. 235.)
(cf. Sydenh. 153).

176. As *lesser purgatives* do rather *contribute strength* by their con-
Purgatives sequence, so *the greater*, being properly used, *do not carry* that *danger*
strengthen with them people commonly imagine, since I have known many that,
and do not
weaken. for three months successively, have taken strong churlish purging pills, every morning, some few days only omitted. I may say some have swallowed
a bottle of strong purgative pills in a few years, and lived in full health

to a remarkable old age, and not without a libertine mode of eating and drinking. Whence it is apparent, that the toughness of the nerves, upon which the strength and action of the bowels only depend, does suffer as little by the strongest purgatives, as an Indian cane by a thousand times bending, which notwithstanding will recover its former figure and full strength, (p. 236), (cf. p. 223).

Our experience and the experience of all who have used Brandreth's Pills confirm these remarks on bleeding.

177. It were to be wished that bleeding could be admitted with the same safety, of which it may be justly said, that the lancet has, and does in proportion kill more men, than the sword; and it is as commonly observed, *Bleeding.* that those physicians who do so generally practice it, know little else what to do. (p. 236.) . . . It is a consequence an idiot infers, because a person having been bled eight or ten times in a great distemper, does recover his health, he owes the benefit of it to the bleedings, whereas it ought rather to be said, neither the distemper nor the bleeding could kill him. (p. 237).

ON LAUDANUM.

178. I stand amazed at the folly of mankind that is so easily allured, by vain boasting and mendacious encomiums upon *Laudanum liquidum,*   *Laudanum* plainly prepared or disguised; to the frequent and constant use whereof   *—Its evils.* a man being once debauched, under the pretence of ease, and quieting himself of a few gripes, fumes or vapors, he can no more leave it off for a fortnight, a week, or a day, than a laborer his bread and cheese, or a man throw off his coat and waistcoat in a hard winter, or a brandy-drinker forsake his spirits and return to small-beer. Using onesself to such plain or disguised opiates, after some months or a few years, is like making a contract with the devil to live easy and well for a few years, upon condition he shall have his soul to torment afterwards. For certain it is, that the familiar use of opiates, after some months or very few years, does wholly desist from being friendly, by suffering your trouble or distemper to return in a more horrible manner, or create a new one incomparably worse than the former, or strangles you with an apoplexy, ōr some other soporous distemper, which is most amply proved by those that make opium their sacred refuge in every fit of the gout, colic or stone, who seldom or never fail of a speedy exit, by some incurable disease of the brain in very few years. And those that do advise such a lethiferous remedy for a common use to their patients, have a greater title to a halter labelled with an inscription of "Mathews' Pills," or "Pacific Drops," than those that murder a man on the highway. (pp. 237-38.) . . . In short all strong narcotic medicines occasion weakness of the stomach-nerves, numbness, palsies, lethargies, loss of memory and dullness of understanding, diminish and deprave all the offices, actions or operations of the bowels, suppress the appetite, occasion a wildish countenence and paleness, and at last, upon long usage, usher in death (pp. 238-39.) (cf. Collins, 133).   •

Purgation preserves and prevents.

179. To preserve health and prevent disease in valetudinary constitutions—for strong, vigorous bodies stand in no need of other preservations or preventives, than moderation in their *nonnaturals*, the knowledge and sense whereof nature has implanted in all other animals, as well as in man—no better ways and means can be used, than applying at certain intervals to those cleansers and abstersers before mentioned. (p. 239).

Hemorrhoides.

Harvey's Liniment.

180. For those subject to *Hemorrhoides*, the following *Liniment Electuary* is recommended. Four ounces best Cassia Fistularis, newly drawn and evaporated to a consistency—the manner of doing it you may read in a treatise called the " Family Physician and House Apothecary " —Rhubarb, powdered, while Mechoacan, grated and powdered, and clean Rhenish (not cream of) Tartar powdered, of each a quarter of an ounce, Sweet Fennelseeds, powdered, a dram and a half, Syrup of Mash-Mallows, as much as will suffice to make them into an electuary. (pp. 239-40). Take half an ounce or an ounce, dissolved in a quarter of a pint of thin gruel, barley-water, posset, or thin chicken-broth, according to directions given concerning the aloetics. (p. 240).

Harvey's Emetic.

181. In *Headaches from over-eating or drinking*, in *Apoplexies, Palsies, Fevers, &c.*, when purging medicines are too tedious in their transportation through so long a space, as the roundabout of the guts, a vomit that will throw up immediately through the gullet, by a short passage, the whole burden at once and operate kindly, without disturbing any of the other bowels, or raise a mud in the humors—*antimonial* vomits are excluded, as being too long before they operate, too churlish in disturbing all the bowels, and exciting a violent commotion in the humors. *Ipecacuanha*, that new fangle, brought by the French from the West Indies, is the root dried of a mere common *juncas* whereof, in the places where it grows, you may buy a cartload for a two-penny looking-glass, or a penny-worth of bugles, though at Paris they have the confidence of selling it at thirty or forty livres a pound,—which, notwithstanding, our asarum-root does far exceed in the operation—than which there can not be a more unacceptable drug to the taste in the world, &c. . . Take the purest White Vitriol, one and a half ounce, being powdered and ground very fine, put it into a glass bottle-bolt-head, pour upon one and a half pint of springwater, and half a pint of clean English Spirits, once rectified, which they call Double Spirits. Close your bolt-head with a cork and a wet bladder over it, tied with packthread. Place the bolt-head standing upright in a sandbath and let it digest, with a moderate warmth, twenty-four hours. But remember to shake the bolt-head very well, before you place it in the sand. After this digestion decant the liquor gently into a glass funnel, wherein is placed a coffin of cap-paper folded according to art, and so let it filtrate into a glass bottle. When it is almost quite passed through to the quantity of a spoonful, take out the funnel and throw away what is left. If you filtrate it a second time over, it will be the clearer and more depurated. This is a very easy, gentle and safe vomit, operates nimbly, and for cheapness exceeds all others. It may be kept always ready upon every occasion. without making any bustle, and so lasting, that its virtue continues for

many years; and for the most part it will move a stool or two, whereby it carries off those crudities that are remaining in the stomach, or that are escaped into the guts. When you find occasion for using the vomit, you must pour out three, four or five spoonfuls, according to your easiness or difficulty to vomit; but commonly three spoonfuls is enough. This must be mixed with double the proportion of warm small-beer or warm water, wherein a little Carduus has been boiled, or thin gruel; then drink it off. If this do not operate in a quarter of an hour, take a spoonful or two more, or you may load yourself with carduus boiled in water until you vomit. This may be taken safely in the beginning of most distempers without any further consultation. (pp. 244-45).

Gideon makes a grave mistake in respect to Ipecacuanha. It is one of the best and most safe roots ever applied to the use of man, as a vomit or purgative. It is one of the ingredients of Brandreth's Pills. When a vomit is needed take four Pills, and drink hot boneset tea, and your stomach will surely discharge its contents.

182. *About throwing off the febrile matters by sweat.* *Sweats—their use and Purgatives compared.*
. . . Whether diaphoretics ought to be used before the declination of a fever, at which time only they appear to be healthful in assisting nature to throw off, for it must be owned by all experienced practitioners that the *causa febrilis*, be it vicious humors, heterogenous particles, or what other offensive they are pleased to allow, must be first subdued, or digested and separated, before it can be expelled by sweat; and therefore, should you exhibit the largest doses of diaphoretics that nature can possibly bear, and second them by loading the patient with a number of bedclothes, he will scarcely be brought to sweating; and if, peradventure, he should happen to be forced into a sweat at the augment or state of the fever, it must be a very great detriment. . . Supposing, fictitiously, that *diaphoretics* were proper, the *uncertainty* of their operation would often occasion a failure of the effect that is expected from them. *Purgatives* and *vomitories* seldom or never fail in their operation, if justly dosed, but *sudorifics* and *diuretics* very often, though administered in great quantities (p. 286 : cf. Sydenh., pp. 432–434).

The advantage of Brandreth's Pills is that they require no care, and whether taken in large or small doses are sure to be of service. In full doses the beneficial effects in all severe diseases are at once evident. And when the system requires a vomit they usually act on the upper passages of the stomach. But the additional use of hot boneset tea, after a dose of four or six pills, is sure to act as an emetic and without any danger. Some gruel should be ready for the patient to take after the vomiting is over; this is needed, when sleep will follow.

HARVEY, JAMES, M. D. *Præsagium Medicum. London,* 1720.

183. In *delirious distempers* great hopes of recovery are had from all sorts of evacuations, chiefly because they check the velocity of the *Purge in Delirium.* blood, diminishing its quantity, take off its obstruction, and relax the nerves (p. 10).

184. Pains, especially if they be fixed a long time in any of the

Pains and Impurities. noble viscera, impair the strength of the patient, and obstruct the circulation of the blood, concoction, and secretion of the humors. . . But in acute disease it is accounted a sign of recovery when pains invade the legs and feet, and happen upon a crisis or signs of it.

The Crisis. 185. But though such pains speak an impetus of the blood and force of nature to throw off the matter of the disease upon those more ignoble parts, yet, when they go off without any apparent cause, as the administration of medicine, or natural evacuations, *the humors may be justly suspected to have returned into the mass of blood,** by which the case is rendered more dangerous than it was, and a happy event of a crisis in acute distempers, depending upon mere chance, or a favorable turn of nature, is always uncertain and never to be relied on (p. 30 ; cf. Sydenh. 432 : M. Harv. 391 ; G. Harv. 139 ; Collins, 130).

How nature removes impurities, or otherwise disposes of them. 186. In the ordinary and natural motion of fluids that serve either for nutrition or excretion there are necessary passages or channels through which they run easily, but in extraordinary cases, as all diseases are, nature finds out extraordinary ways by which it throws out the noxious matter, or at least puts it in a less dangerous place (p. 43 ; cf. Hippoc., Edinb. ed. Epidem., lib. ii., sect. 5 ; Parey, 69).

Life, Health and Disease. 187. The animal life depends upon many and different causes, and an integrity of all the parts of the body, especially those that are principal, as the head, heart, arteries, and veins, and the liquors that run in them, namely, the blood, chyle, &c. But because our bodies cannot always continue in the same state, its parts, both solid and fluid, being worn, consumed, and dissipated by continued motion, there must be a continual supply of food for its reparation, as well as proper instruments and vessels, in which it may be prepared and made fit for that purpose.

The Stomach. 188. Nature, therefore, has contrived the *stomach, intestines,* and *glands,* in which, by a wonderful mechanism, our food is pounded and concocted, and its grosser parts separated from those that are more fine and subtle, the one for the preservation of life, and the other as the useless, to be thrown out by emunctories ordained for that end. But when those instruments are defective—which often happens—and the muscular force of the stomach is insufficient to grind the food and make a chyle of fine parts, *that which we receive for nourishment and reparation of our bodies not being duly prepared, is so far from being useful that it is rather hurtful to us. For this unconcocted food or crudity entering into the mass of blood,* renders it *viscious, tough,* and of a *clary substance,* unfit for motion and circulation, and *the cause of most diseases* (cf. Collins, 137 ; Sanctorius, 109, 101*). . .

189. Whatever, therefore, is useless to the body, or *inconsistent with the blood, must be separated from it,* that it may be preserved in a per-

---

* At these times an extra dose of Brandreth's Pills should be administered.

fect state. Hence the *endeavors of nature*, and the contrivance of *the intestines, cuticular glands*, and other emunctories appropriated indeed to *their peculiar excrements, but sometimes common to all or most of them* (p. 92; G. Harvey, 163). *The Intestines, and their various office.*

190. Evacuations by sweat are to be attempted with the greatest caution, not indiscriminately by all persons nor at all times. For if medicines to procure it be given when the blood is of a texture not open enough—which it cannot be near the beginning of most feverish disturbances—or when too heterogeneous substances abound in it, *forced sweats* oftener dispose the blood to stagnate in the tender vessels of the brain and nerves than to separate its noxious particles at the designed secretory parts (p. 129; cf. Sydenh., pp. 432–434; Gid. Harv., p. 286) *Forced Sweats—their danger.*

191. *Nature*—by which I mean the effects of matter and motion. according to the laws and constitution of animal economy—is indeed the great physician and cure of disease; so that now-a-days several disturbances are happily taken off by the slightest remedies, or by a mere abstinence from them. But, in *acute diseases*, the die is cast for life or death, and in this case nature is not to be altogether relied on; neither must we, as the advocates for the doctrine of crisis, patiently wait for the issue of the conflict between nature and the disease, the peccant humors of some fevers being sometimes so stubborn, that *art must interpose to promote their evacuation some other way.* (pp. 207–8.) (Cf. p. 92 Sydenham, 163, 166.) *Assist nature by promoting evacuations.*

WILLAN, J., M. D., *An Essay on the King's Evil.* London, 1735.

192. The diminution of the morbific matter, *both in the primae viæ and whole body*, is to be effected by cleansing that canal, and evacuating the morbific matter out of it; and by this means we cannot fail of *lessening its quantity in every other part of the body.* (p. 21.) (Cf. J. Hamilton, 218.) *Diminish the morbid matter, and you lessen the cause of disease.*

Purging with Brandreth's Pills infallibly lessens the quantity of impurities; and as they are harmless to the most tender age, or the weakest or most feeble, they can be used every or every other day, reducing the sum of unhealthy matters contained in the body, and thus taking an extinguisher or weight from the blood, whose vitality becomes thereby increased, and all the parts of the body be duly nourished into a renewed life and vigor.

PRINGLE, SIR JOHN, M. D., on the *Diseases of the Armies.* London, 1753. 3d Ed., 1761.

193. *Early Sweats.*—It has been usual to give the *theriaca*, or some other hot medicine for this purpose; but *all such increase the fever*, if they fail in bringing out the sweat (p. 131). *About sweats.*

194. The *bilious* or *remitting fever* of the camp begins with chilliness, lassitude, pains of the head and bones, and a disorder at the stomach. At night the fever runs high, the heat and thirst are great, the *Bilious and remittent fevers—symptoms.*

tongue is parched, the head aches violently, the patient gets no better and often becomes delirious, but generally in the morning a perfect sweat brings on a remission of all the symptoms; in the evening the paroxysm returns. These periods go on daily, till the fever changes insensibly either into a continued, or into an intermitting form. *Some-* Nature's *times loose stools carry of the fit and supply the sweats.* Although the effort at cure fever most frequently appears in the form of a quotidian, yet sometimes complete when evacu- it is to be seen in a tertian shape.....*I remember of no natural evacua-* ations are powerful. *tions making a complete cure, unless when a* VIOLENT DISCHARGE *super-vened of the corrupted bile, or other humors which seemed to be the cause of the disease* (pp. 165–67). (Cf. J. Harvey, 190.)

Sweat.   195. When the sweat is abundant, the putrid parts of the blood are, either wholly or in some degree, expelled, after which the fever is either entirely cured, abated or brought to intermit. (p. 183,) (cf. 194.)

Evacua-tions pre-vent many forms of disease.   196. On *bilious fevers in Britain.*—Instead of *evacuating* or correct-ing what is amiss, we often neglect it, till it ends in *obstructions of the viscera.* So that hence may proceed *nervous complaints* without fever, or *fevers of a nervous kind,* instead of *fluxes, intermitting or remitting fevers,* the common consequences of a more sudden and thorough cor-ruption of the humors. (p. 200.) (Cf. Collins, 132, 135.)

Why the Spring is the fittest season to purge.   197. We may observe that the fibres are more relaxed in the spring than in the winter; hence that the body becoming more plethoric, the humors will then be apter to corrupt, upon any suppression of perspira-tion. And this may perhaps be forwarded by the *effluvia* arising from all putrid substances which, being locked up during the cold of winter, are then set at liberty by the greater heat of the sun. (p. 201.)

Dysentery. Excellent ob-servations concerning the use of purgatives.   198. *Dysentery.*—We must at all times *attend less to the dose than to the effects,* which are never to be judged of by the *frequency* but by the *largeness of the stools,* and *the relief* the patient finds *from the gripes and tenesmus after* the operation. The *motions* are generally more fre-quent *from the disease* alone than from the *purgation.* As on the one hand, the physician must avoid all the rough and stimulating purges, so on the other hand, he is not to spare those of a lenient kind. (p. 240.) *Opiates and astrin-gents are most danger-ous pallia-tives.* The necessity of continuing the physic is to be determined more by the obstinacy of the gripes and tenesmus, than by blood in the stools. *Without such frequent evacuations, it is in vain to attempt a cure; as all opiates and astringents by themselves only palliate and render the disease more fatal in the end.* (p. 241.) (Cf. Sydenham, 162; Hippocr. 8. G. Harvey, 175, 176.)

Opiates "fix the cause" of the disease.   199. As to *opiates,* it were better they were never used at all, than given before the first passages were thoroughly cleansed; for *though they afford some ease, yet by penning up the wind and corrupted humors,* THEY FIX THE CAUSE. This I presume to affirm from *repeated experience.* I am well assured, that the fluxes I have seen in the army, are *never to be cured without evacuations.* (p. 241-42.) (Cf. J. Harvey, 191.)

200. In some cases the patient would seem likely to recover, but would relapse upon voiding hard scybala which, coming away in small parcels for several days together, made a constant irritation. These, therefore, were to be speedily removed by a full dose of rhubarb with manna, or by some other lenient physic. (pp. 245-46.) (Cf. Collins, 134, 139, 151.)

Hardened fœces the cause of disease, to be removed before convalescence ensues.

201. *Palsy.*—Of purgatives the most active should be selected, and such as influence most energetically the principal secreting viscera ; as calomel, colocynth, jalap, scammony, &c. In *paraplegia*, and even in *hemiplegia*, the bowels are very torpid, and require *repeated and full doses of those*, and even of still more energetic cathartics, as croton-oil, or elaterium, in some obstinate cases. In many cases recourse should *also* be had to *purgative enemata.* It is not merely necessary regularly to evacuate fecal matters by means of these, but to employ them so, as to derive from the cerebro-spinal axis any increased flow of blood to it, which may have occasioned, or prolonged the attack. Indeed, with these conjoined objects, they are advised by *Halle, Dalberg, Brodie*, and others, who have insisted on their use. (p. 242.) (Cf. J. Harvey, 183 ; J. Harvey, 171, 175, 179.)

Palsy— ACTIVE PUR-GATIONS. Paraplegia —Hemiplegia.

I have advertised the above sentiments for forty years, at an outlay of more than a million of dollars, and long before I saw the above able remarks.

I now insert the following testimony, which applies well to Sir John's remarks.

The following was published in 1863. It tells its own story :

SANITARY COMMISSION.

" What is it doing to economize the Life and Health of our Soldiers ?"

" Is it using all the means Providence has placed within its reach, or is it stiff-necked, and determined that so *great* a *remedy* as BRANDRETH'S PILLS shall not be used to economize the life and health of our Soldiers ?"

Sagacious men believe that the administration of BRANDRETH'S PILLS, in its " Homes " and as " Special Relief" would more than quadruple the present value to the " Life and Health of our Soldiers."

Let the following testimony from *sixty returned volunteers* be studied by members of the United States Sanitary Commission. If the statements be true, can they be doing their duty as *Christian Men* in not using the means Providence has placed within their reach ?

FRIENDS OF SOLDIERS—READ !

Brandreth's Pills protect from the arrows of disease, usually as fatal to soldiers as the bullets of the foe.

Sing Sing, October 26, 1863.

We, the undersigned, surviving members of Company F, Seventeenth N. Y. Volunteers, hereby certify that we have used Brandreth's Pills during our two years' service, and to them we attribute the fact that our constitutions are uninjured by the necessary hardships and privations of a soldier's life in the field. In costiveness, colds, chills, diarrhœa, dysentery, and typhoid fever, their prompt use cured us in a few days. Our health was often restored without having been entered on the sick list ; in fact, a single dose of four or five pills usually cured what, under the regular treatment, would have been a serious sickness. Others, who appeared to be sick in no way different to us, but who used the remedies prescribed by the regimental surgeon, either died or were sick for weeks in the hospital.

When we left Sing Sing, in June, 1861, you gave us a supply of these Pills, and we feel sure, from our experience, that if every soldier was supplied with this medicine, the general health of the army would be greatly improved. For ourselves, it is our sole remedy, answering all our wants in the way of physic, and we have known and tested it from our childhood, and our parents before us.

John Vickars, *Captain ;* J. J. Smith, 1st *Lieutenant ;* William See, 1st *Sergeant ;* G. H. Dearing, 2d *Sergeant ;* Dennis Shay, 3d *Sergeant ;* Patrick Cullen, 4th *Sergeant ;* Benj. F. Brown, 1st *Corporal ;* Wm. Mathers, 2d *Corporal ;* Noah W. Miller, 3d *Corporal ;* Theodore Crofut, *Drummer ;* Geo. B. Coe, *Drummer.*
Francis J. Jenning, William W. Campbell, William J. Charlton, Albert Wesley, John W. Griffin, William Holmes, William W. Rider, Martin See, George Ackerly, Hiram Seagle, Alfred Wilkins, William Griffin, George Ayles, William J. P. Hewett, John L. Branden-burgh, Thomas A. Barlow, Henry Hannah, William Waldron, John Conover, Jacob Baker, Lewis B. Coy, Albert Lane, Ellis Jones, Wm. Van Wert, James B. Crofut, Roscoe K. Wat-son, Frederick Hunt, William Tuttle, Jotham Carpenter, Charles Wright, Sanford Olmstead, Fuller Carpenter, James Bentley, Robert W. Westcott, Jacob H. Dyckman, John M. Bodine, James N. Hines, Edward Waldron, Warren Wright, David Baker.
T. B. Lane, 1st *Lieut.* 36th N. Y. Vols. ; M. C. Larle, 1st *Sergt.* Co. D, 17th N. Y. Vols.; Wm. Knight, Co. I, 6th N. Y. Artillery ; Millard F. Lanning, *Musician,* 1st N. Y. Vols.; Wm. Kenney, Co. R. Berdan's Sharpshooters ; Cassius Bishop, Co. E, 38th N. Y. Vols.; Elliot See, Co. B, 38th N. Y. Vols. ; Daniel Gillis, *Sergt.* Co. B, 3d N. Y. Vols. ; Caleb S. Frisbie, Co. B, 5th N. Y. Vols.

STATE OF NEW YORK, Westchester Co., *ss.* :
I, William M. Skinner, a Notary Public, duly commissioned and sworn, residing in the village of Sing Sing, County and State aforesaid, do hereby certify that the names of the sixty persons subscribed to the Certificate hereto annexed, dated October 26, 1863, concern-the value and efficacy of Brandreth's Pills, beginning with Capt. John Vickars and ending with Caleb S. Frisbie, were signed in my presence, and that I, at their request, witnessed their signatures to said Certificate.
I further certify that I am well acquainted with all who signed said Certificate, and know them, individually, to be men of truth and veracity.
In witness whereof, I have hereunto subscribed my name and affixed my official seal, this eleventh day of January, one thousand eight hundred and sixty-four.
WM. M. SKINNER, *Notary Public.*

STATE OF NEW YORK, County of Westchester, *ss.* :
I, Hiram P. Rowell, Clerk of the County aforesaid, and also Clerk of the Courts in and for said County, do hereby certify that *Wm. M. Skinner, Esq.,* whose name is subscribed to the Certificate of the Proof or acknowledgment of the annexed Instrument, and indorsed thereon, was, on the day of the date of the said Certificate, a Notary Public, in and for said County, residing in the said County, appointed and sworn, and duly authorized to take the same according to the laws of the said State. And further, that I am well acquainted with the handwriting of the said Notary Public, and verily believe that the signature to the said Certificate is genuine.
In testimony whereof, I have hereunto set my hand, and affixed the seal of the said Courts and County, the 12th day of January, 1864.
HIRAM P. ROWELL, *Clerk.*

CULLEN, WILLIAM, *M. D., First principles of medicine, London,* 1777.

Fevers. Sweating often dan-gerous. 202. *Fevers.—Sweating* employed to prevent intermittent fevers, has often changed them into *continued fever,* which is always dangerous. (p. 164.)

Urging the sweat, may produce hurtful *determination to* some of the *internal parts,* and may be *attended with very great danger.* (p. 166. †.)

ROBERTSON, ROBERT, *M. D., An essay on fevers, &c. &c. Robinson,* 1790.

203. *Idiopathic fever.*—Whenever men complain of being seized with chilliness, or alternate chills and heats, headaches, sickness at stom-

ach, universal pains, or as the sick express themselves "pains all over
them; or pains in all their bones, or joints, especially in their loins and
back, with less or more debility;" and if their countenance is at the same
time obviously diseased, whatever the other symptoms accompanying
these are, I can, from experience, assure the reader, that a most virulent
infection is present (p. 59).

Fever. Its general character.

204. Whatever has a tendency to *debilitate the system*, may either
be *a remote or a proximate cause of fever*, according to the constitution of
the patients. A sufficient reason may be assigned for many people being
seized with fever at the same time; which is, their being exposed to the
same debilitating powers of heat, cold, draught, or wet, or sudden
changes of these (p. 88).

Cause of fever is all that debili-tates the sys-tem.

MILLER, EDWARD, *M. D., Inquiry concerning cutaneous perspiration
and the operation and uses of sudorific remedies. New York*, 1798.
MEDICAL REPOSITORY, 1798, *Vol. II.; See Med. & Phys. Journ.* 1799,
Vol. I.

205. That *sudorifics can not be usefully employed* as a general remedy
in *fevers*, is apparent from the fatal course pursued by many of these
diseases, notwithstanding the most copious, universal, and continued
sweats, spontaneously taking place. The memorable sweating sickness,
which first appeared in England, towards the close of the fifteenth century, and was one of the most fatal epidemics on medical record, affords
ample proof of this position (Journ. p. 288).

Fevers are not cured by sweats.

206. On the whole it may be concluded, that much of the use of
sudorifics has arisen from mistaken doctrines, concerning the nature of
perspiration and of fever, particularly from the erroneous opinions, that
the matter of perspiration is excrementitious; that its occasional obstruction is noxious; that it ought as much as possible to be eliminated from
the system; and that it is only carried off, in considerable quantity, when
discoverable by sight or touch (ibid).

Errors about sweat-ing.

207. It may be also concluded, that *sudorific remedies*, especially
those of the more powerful kind, are, in general, *highly unsafe*, and calculated to *augment the violence of inflammatory and malignant fevers ;*
and, that though they may succeed in some cases of less violence, or by
a favorable concurrence of circumstances, yet they are so constantly
liable to produce mischief, and exasperate the disease, that the abuse, on
the whole, must be pronounced greatly to overbalance the use (ibid).

Sudorifics unsafe and injurious.

SELLE, H., *M. D., Professor in the University of Berlin ; new contributions to physical and medical knowledge, Berlin*, 1798. *See* MED.
& PHYS. JOURN. 1799, *Vol. I.*

208. *Puerperal fever.*—This disease originates in an accumulation of
corrupted humors in the abdomen, which humors have either been already separated in the form of milk, or intended by nature to be so.

Puerperal fever, from accumula-tion of mor-bid matter in the abdo-men.

The causes of this accumulation may be various, but are principally an epidemic miasma, passions, sudden cold, and inflammation (Part III. p. 92).

In corroboration of Professor Selle's theory, Dr. Hermbsteadt has proved by chemical experiments, that the fluid matter found in the cavities of the abdomen was *virtually milk.* It deserves, however, to be remarked, that the fat of the omentum and the mesentery, being dissolved by the febrile heat, may combine with the extravasated lymph, so as to produce a fluid of a more or less viscid consistence, and resembling milk in its external characters (Journ. p. 387).

BACHE, WILLIAM, *M. D.. On a successful case of Asthma, Birmingham,* 1799. *See* MED. & PHYS. JOURN. 1799, *Vol. II.*

Asthma. Acidity of the secretion the cause. 209. I became convinced that an *acid* pervaded the whole of the circulating system, and I presumed that it existed in a morbid degree, either as to quantity or strength, and was the *exciting cause of the spasmodic affections observable in the lungs,* and other membranous parts, to which it might occasionally be applied, probably sometimes in a gaseous state, and at others in a more dense and concentrated one, and perhaps variously combined. The indications of cure suggested to my mind were *to restrain its influence,* and my attention was principally directed to the *state of the stomach, the bowels, the expectorations, the kidneys and the skin* (p. 141).

CONRADI, D. G. C., *M. D., Resident · Physician at Northeim, Germany. Practical remarks on the most prevailing species of cramp in the stomach. See* MED. & PHYS. JOURN. 1799, *Vol. 1.*

Cramp in the stomach. Its cause: neglect of purgation; the cure indicated by the cause. 210. The affection is not violent in the beginning, but a pressure, and stricture, and griping, rather than an acute pain, is felt in the region of the stomach. The patient has an oppressive sensation, as if something, not unlike a nail, were fixed behind the stomach : if the attack increases in violence, he complains of stitches in the breast and towards the back, and endeavors to procure relief by shifting his posture. The principal paroxysms are observed to take place generally in the afternoon, in consequence of bodily exercise immediately after dinner, the use of acid food and drink—and particularly after giving way to gusts of passion, such as terror, anger, grief, and anxiety.

This affection is often contracted by persons subject to passionate emotions, on their neglecting to take an *emetic occasionally;* it is not, in general, attended with acidity, but rather and most frequently is produced by a bilious acrimony ; and it at length almost invariably degenerates into a nervous habit (Jour. p. 49).

Denman, Thomas, *M. D.*, *On a case of dropsy in the ovarium.* See Med. & Phys. Journ. 1799, *Vol. II.*

211. After giving the history of a female patient, who had suffered *Dropsy of the ovarium from consti- pation.* from violent pains in her bowels, tension of the abdomen, and much soreness on pressure, accompanied with vomiting, constipation, and frequent fainting, symptoms which were chiefly relieved by clysters and gentle purgatives, hemorrhages from the uterus, violent pain in the lowest part of the back, and, on pressure upon the sacrum or hip, in the neighboring parts, Dr. Denman says : There was great tension and pain above the " ossa pubis," and the whole hypogastric region was full and hard. She discovered a large hard tumor, extending to the right side of the navel, the increase of which was so rapid that in the course of a few days it occupied the whole abdomen. She was then freed from a pain in all the parts contained in the pelvis, could lie on either side, and walk much better. She frequently after this had slight shivering fits, and a sense of coldness down her back, followed by restlessness and feverish heat, especially in her hands and feet in the evening, which went off with a free perspiration toward morning. Her pulse was at all times very quick. *Though one or more stools had been regularly procured every day, an immense quantity of hardened fæces, of a large volume, were now discharged for three or four successive days*, by which her size was much lessened. She had been treated for sciatica. When I first *Regular and daily evacuation prevents not fecal accu- mulation.* visited her, the whole abdomen was distended by a circumscribed tumor springing from the right side, near the groin, thence extending across, and high up in the abdomen, and I thought I could feel an obscure fluctuation in it. I could also feel an angle of the tumor in the posterior part of the pelvis, by which the " os uteri " was projected so high and so far forwards as to be almost beyond my reach, as is the case in the retroversion of the uterus. She was not pregnant. I did not therefore hesitate in the opinion that it was a dropsy of the ovarium ; and by supposing this, early in the disease, to have dropped low down in the pelvis, and afterwards to have risen according to its increase, all the symptoms which had occurred could be satisfactorily explained. I directed *only a strong purging draught.* On the following day, she informed me that after suffering considerable pain in the bowels, she had four or five copious motions, and that after every motion she was sensible of her size decreasing. The *motions were unusually offensive*, and, before they came away, the desire to expel them was unnaturally urgent and painful. On examining them, I found that they almost wholly consisted of *Powerful and contin- ued purga- tion the cure.* a gelatinous fluid, with many streaks of blood, and with little or no mixture of fæces. Instead of feeling weakened by the evacuation, the patient felt herself very much relieved. The medicine was continued for two days more, producing the same number of motions ; the swelling of the abdomen had gone, the *os uteri* had descended into its proper position, and no tumor whatever remained in the cavity of the pelvis. I concluded that, in consequence of preceding inflammation, an adhesion had taken place between the cyst of the tumor and some part of the intestine, probably the rectum, the adhering portion of the bowels had given way, and, by that opening, the contents of the tumor had been evacuated. She was perfectly restored to health (pp. 20, 22).

Let the reader examine the Van Wart case at the end of these quotations.

50 THE DOCTRINE OF PURGATION.

HENDERSON, STEWART, *Surg. Practical remarks on the diseases which occurred on board of H. M. Ship Astrea, on the Jamaica station, &c. See* MED. & PHYS. JOURN. 1799, *Vol. I.*

Remittent fever from marsh effluvia.

"THERE IS BUT ONE FEVER," but under different modifications.

212. *Remittent* or *Marsh-fever.*—This fever, the legitimate offspring of all hot climates, especially where marshes abound, is the *autumnal disease* of most parts of Europe, only appearing *in a milder degree.* It has been described under various names—*bilious, yellow, Jamaica, Senegal,* and in Bengal, *pucka*—but multiplying distinctions which do not exist only serves to perplex and mislead, for *it will be found to be the same individual disease, under different modifications,* depending on constitution, season of the year, and local situation. The cause of this fever, in all its varieties, is marsh effluvia. We find that in some places at the Cape of Good Hope, where no such cause exists, this fever is unknown. We likewise find that strangers are more liable to be affected by this noxious effluvia, and have the disease in a more formidable degree, than the natives of the country, whose constitutions acquire a certain power of resisting it from habitual exposure : at the same time, its effects on them are obvious, by shortening the duration of life. I do not think that the original disease produced by this miasma is infectious, but that it may alter its type and become highly contagious from concurrent causes; as from too many diseased bodies being crowded together, without paying sufficient attention to ventilation and cleanliness. (p. 141.) This noxious exhalation enters the system either by the lungs, the skin, or stomach ; but the manner in which it produces those symptoms of disease which characterize the fever does not appear to be well understood. We can only perceive its general effects on the system; and that it may lurk for a certain time in the habit before morbid movements take place (ibid).

Miasmata increase the bilious secretion; purgatives carry it away.

213. In men not below nor above the common standard of health, although there were marks of irritation and inflammatory diathesis, it seemed not sufficient to justify blood-letting; which I considered would have diminished the vital power. Antimonial emetics were not used, having always observed that they increased the irritability of the stomach, which is the most troublesome symptom attending this form of the fever. I, therefore, thought it more advisable to employ mercurial *purgatives,* which had a very good effect in *carrying off the bilious sordes collected in the first passages;* emetics were sometimes given ; James' powder with camphor, to promote perspiration, and effect a complete remission (p. 143).

Dysentery —from cold and wet obstructing the perspiration and increasing the flow of fluids to the intestines.

214. *Dysentery.* This disease is not limited or peculiar to any climate, nor is there any natural cause known to produce it : if it were occasioned by any particular quality in the air, the natives, as well as seamen and soldiers, would be attacked with it, but we find this is not the case. For, when the dysentery was raging among the British troops at the Cape of Good Hope, not one of the inhabitants were seized with it, nor is it a disease known among them. Whenever it becomes epidemic among the inhabitants of any country, it may always be traced to infection introduced; it being the constant attendant on camps, and the scourge of an army more destructive than any other enemy. I, therefore, consider it an artificial disease. *Cold and dampness,* when the body is not sufficiently covered, by obstructing perspiration, and increas-

The cure by evacuation by the mouth and anus.

ing the determination of the fluids to the intestines, sometimes combined with febrile miasma, produce the whole phenomena of dysentery. In the treatment of this disease, I generally began with an emetic of ipecacuanha; bleeding was never employed, unless the patient was of a strong plethoric habit; purges of salts or rhubarb with calomel were frequently repeated; emollient injections and fomentations were of use, when the pains were wandering, and large blisters in every instance removed the pain where it was fixed (p. 237).

215. *Diarrhœa* generally arose from relaxation brought on by eating unripe fruits, and committing other irregularities. It was easily removed by lenient purgatives (ibid).

Diarrhœa —purgation cures.

216. *Hepatic complaints* were brought on by violent exercise in the sun, joined to the abuse of spirits. Symptoms: pain in the side, some difficulty in respiration, pulse full and frequent, sometimes pain in the shoulder, and about the region of the liver, which, when pressed, was attended with a catching and troublesome cough. Bleeding, calomel purges, a blister to the side, sometimes mercury in small doses, were alternately resorted to, until health was perfectly restored (ibid).

Liver Complaint. Cure by evacuation.

217. *Spasmodic affections* were mostly confined to the *abdominal viscera*, and brought on by lying on the deck in the night. The patients complained of excruciating pain and stricture, commonly about the umbilical region, nausea, and sometimes vomiting. If fomentations did not cure the pain, a large blister was applied; calomel with jalap taken internally and clysters given, until stools were procured, which removed the complaint (p. 238).

Cramp of the stomach. Strong purges the remedy.

HUGGAN, A., *M. D.*, *On the Croup, Plymouth*, 1799. *See* MED. & PHYS. JOURN. 1800 *Vol. III.*

218. In a manuscript copy of the late *Dr. Gregory's Lectures*, I found a *caution respecting bleeding in children*, even with leeches, as apt to bring on fits. Now, if the learned professor's admonition was the result of experience—and a case which I myself once saw, leaves me little room to doubt it—what have we not to dread from taking blood away in a large stream from infants? (p. 57.) . . . With regard to blood-letting in general, as a means of cure in *inflammation, synocha, &c.*, let me ask, *whence the necessity of diminishing the quantity of blood in such diseases?* or *what proof have we that the quantity of blood being increased,*—allowing, however, that it actually is so,—*is the increase of it the cause of evil?* By taking blood away we undoubtedly lessen the quantity of it, but *do we really diminish the bulk of the circulating fluids, and contract the size of the bloodvessels?* This is but doubtful; for, it is more than probable that from the loss of blood the secretions are diminished, and absorption of moisture from the atmosphere increased. (p. 58.) . . From the prevalence of bleeding in inflammatory diseases, some have, either from prejudice in its favor, or from want of proper discrimination, used it copiously in genuine *typhus*, accompanied, as it sometimes is, with *thoracic pains*, &c. The result of such practice will be obvious (p. 59).

Croup.

Blood-letting dangerous in children, is altogether an injudicious and useless practice, in inflammation as well as in typhus.

Bleeding is NEVER NECESSARY, SELDOM SAFE, OFTEN HURTFUL, SOMETIMES FATAL.

Upon the whole I think that I am *sufficiently warranted, from experience*, to draw the following conclusions respecting the use of venesection in the practice of medicine, viz. : *That it is* NEVER NECESSARY, SELDOM SAFE, OFTEN HURTFUL, AND SOMETIMES FATAL (p. 60).

MILLER, E., *M. D., On the effects of Abstinence on the approach of Acute Diseases. See* MEDICAL & PHYSICAL JOURN. *London,* 1799, *Vol. I.*

Moderate habits of life prevent disease and preserve health.

219. If the art of preserving health and prolonging life chiefly consist in a *frugal and sparing use of stimuli*, and adapting them with caution and skill to the fluctuating circumstances of the vital principle, we shall surely find still stronger motives to apply this doctrine at the approach and in the treatment of diseases, when noxious powers of such preternatural violence invade the body, baffle every remedy, and stimulate it to death. The regulations of this vital principle, here denominated excitability, the preservation of it when present, and its restoration when deficient, the restraint of the excitement within the bounds of moderation, the prohibition of all wasteful and undermining excesses, will probably hereafter, at some more enlightened era of medicine, form a system of rules for the management of health and the prevention of disease, for the enjoyment of sense and the refinement of intellect, which, instead of the present feverish dream of human life, will present a consummation of improvement and happiness which we now ascribe to superior beings (Journ. p. 45).

Abstinence of all aliment interrupts the advance of disease.

220. If I do not mistake, it has been proved, that abstinence will be often a complete, generally a useful, and *almost always a safe means of obviating the approach of acute diseases.* And, in a word, if it were possible to offer to mankind a maxim of universal application to the treatment of incipient fevers, in all their variations and circumstances, I should be inclined to hazard the following aphorism : *When symptoms denoting the approach of acute diseases are discovered, abstain, for a proper length of time, from all aliment* (ibid).

In the place of abstinence from all aliment, purgation is the method which experience has proved safe and effectual, both as a preventive and cure for acute or chronic or incipient affections. Brandreth's Pills and weak oat-meal gruel for a few days will do more good than abstaining from food, or half starving for weeks. And purging with these pills never weakens the vital forces, which cannot be said of the other plan. I think that the starving method is next in evil effects to bleeding. One takes the life out, the other prevents its renewal. It is effete matters, impure humors, floating in the blood or settling upon some organ, that cause all general or local disease. Purging takes these out, and, being done, the health is often restored at once. If you have poisonous matters about you, get rid of them as soon as possible. This is the sensible way. Starving does not get rid of them, it only reduces your life, your power to feel, that is all; places you nearer the grave. While every dose of Brandreth's Pills takes the death principle away, and places a greater distance between the sick and the grave.

NOOTH, J., *M. D., Superintendent-General of the hospitals in British America. Letter on the treatment of dysenteries and other autumnal diseases, to Dr. Mitchell, Quebec, Jan.* 24, 1799. *See* MEDICAL REPOSITORY, *Vol. II. p.* 437, *quoted in* MED. & PHYS. JOURN. 1799, *Vol. II.*

221. Having seen, in the course of my practice, a great number of

dysenteric cases, and having experienced the inefficacy, in general, of the usual mode of practice, I was induced to try the effects of the *several purgatives* now in use, with the view of ascertaining how far any one was preferable to the others, *in the treatment of dysenteric patients.* Experience soon taught me that the neutralized tartarit of potass was the most salutary in its effects; and of course I have always, since that discovery, had recourse to it in dysenteries and other autumnal diseases, *with the greatest success, both in children and adults* (Journ. p. 181). Dysentery and other autumnal diseases— purgation the cure.

SKRIMSHIRE, J., *M. D.*, *Cases of Fractured Skull, Wisbeach,* 1799. *See* MED. & PHYS. JOURN. 1800, *Vol. III.*

222. A boy four years of age had fallen from a height of ten feet upon a brick pavement. He *vomited* soon after he was taken up, and complained of a bruise on his head, but seemed otherwise quite well. There was a very evident depression of the right temporal bone, and fracture of the right parietal bone. Merely a spirituous embrocation and *a gentle laxative* was given. On the next day the depression was considerably less. *No one bad symptom* had come on, but as the physic had not operated, I ordered an *enema*, took six ounces of blood from the arm, and ordered a strictly antiphlogistic regimen for three weeks; in a few days the depressed bone had risen to its natural situation, and in a few weeks every trace of it had disappeared (Journ. p. 28). Fractured skull. Purgatives, as soon as they operate on the bowels, remove the bad symptoms attending fractures and bruises.

Another boy, nine years of age, fell from a cart-horse upon a stone pavement and the wheel of the cart passed over his head. I found the whole left side of his head very much flattened, the temporal and great part of the parietal bone being very much depressed; besides, there was a fracture of both bones, which crossed the squamose suture. The boy was comatose, but roused for a moment when spoken to. His breathing was laborious, pupils dilated, pulse of natural velocity, but intermitting. He *had vomited* several times, *had bled* much from the nose, and likewise from the right ear. Trepanning was proposed, but the parents objecting, the antiphlogistic plan was all that was left us. He, accordingly, was bled and an enema administered. The clyster had not operated, neither a purgative given on the second day; the depression kept on lessening, but the boy remained comatose; another aperient was given, and on the third day a purgative enema produced a copious stool; the symptoms abated, and disappeared after a repetition of the enema, the bowels now being opened (Journ. pp. 28-29).

SUTTON, T., M. D., *Considerations Regarding Pulmonary Consumption.* *London,* 1799. *See* MED. AND PHYS. JOURN., 1801, *vol. VI.*

223. The *first symptoms* of disease were *in the bowels,* and by degrees the disorder became a confirmed phthisis pulmonalis. Hence I was led to suspect *the emaciation and debility to be induced by some disease of the abdominal viscera,* which, however, I could not account for in any other way except by supposing the mesenteric glands to be obstructed, as the symptoms led to no suspicions of any other cause or causes that could be considered as adequate to produce such effects. I have seen several cases where *affections of the bowels preceded the pulmonic symp-* Consumption proceeds by sympathy from a disorder of the bowels, especially from disease of the mesentery.

toms. It is a very common thing for patients, in *protracted dysenteries, to have pulmonic affections before death;* and it frequently happens that diseases of the abdominal viscera are, in their latter stages, accompanied by pulmonary consumption. By writers on this disease the."tabes mesenterica" is mentioned as sometimes accompanying it. . . . Hence, it appears to me that *phthisis pulmonalis is caused by a disease in the mesenteric glands,* and that the tubercles in the lungs, and some other of its symptoms, are excited by sympathy (Journ., pp. 89, 90).

Purgatives and emetics cure.

224. For, an increased action may be produced by exciting an increased motion in the contiguous parts, which may be effected by the use of *emetics and purgatives,* which *promote a greater motion in the intestinal canal,* and, *from their contiguity,* in all probability, communicate some of it to the mesenteric glands (Journ., p. 90).

WHITE, W., Surg., *Remarks on Hydrocephalus Internus. Bath,* 1799. *See* MED. AND PHYS. JOURN., 1800, *vol. III.*

Hydrocephalus, like all dropsies caused by an abundance of fluid which cannot be absorbed.

225. Case of *hydrocephalus* given. He took small doses of calomel combined with digitalis. As purgatives produced no effect in stimulating the intestines, clysters were resorted to for that purpose. After a fortnight, evident symptoms of amendment took place, and he soon recovered (Journ., p. 113). *Dr. Whytt,* to whom we are greatly indebted for a very minute description of the symptoms usually attendant on the disease, observes: " *The immediate cause of every kind of dropsy is the same,* viz., such a state of the parts as makes *the exhalent arteries throw out a greater quantity of fluids than the absorbents can take up.*" Which

Purgatives remove the cause of disease.

state, from what he afterwards mentions, he evidently considered as consisting in debility (p. 117). *Purging is necessary,* not only on account of lessening the determination to the head, but particularly as the symptoms, which proceed merely from fullness in the stomach and bowels, have been frequently soon removed by evacuating the bowels (p. 119).

CARSON, WILLIAM, M. D., *Letter on the Applicability of Mercurial Preparations in Children's Diseases. Birmingham,* 1800. *See* MED. AND PHYS. JOURN., 1800, *vol. IV.·*

Infantile diseases. Calomel never safe, in minute doses always a poison.

226. For several years I have been dissatisfied with the general and indiscriminate use of *calomel in the diseases of children;* I am not more certain of any one fact that pertains to medicine than that I have seen many children who have fallen a sacrifice to the improper application of this medicine. Calomel, when mixed with sugar, forms a medicine agreeable to the palate of the child; its exhibition is easy to the mother or nurse, and it may *with safety be given as a purge,* when a purge is indicated. When given as a purge, its action is confined to the first passages; but when the dose is *frequently repeated,* either for the purpose of obviating habitual costiveness, or with any other intention, *it is absorbed by the lymphatics,* and enters the system, by the action of which it is decomposed, . . . and that state of the system produced which is called *mercurial fever.* Although mercury does not appear to have so powerful an action on the salivary glands of children as it has on adults, yet I apprehend its general effects upon the system are greater. The mercurial fever *in adults* soon runs into *indirect debility.*

227. The injurious consequences likely to flow to children from the high degree of excitation and extreme succeeding debility produced by a mercurial course I wish to impress upon your readers. Mercury has been erroneously held forth as a specific in *hydrocephalus*, and is often given as a preventive of that fatal malady. Hydrocephalus appears to be the result of debility succeeding too high an action of the vessels of the brain. If so, can any medicine more powerfully produce hydrocephalus than mercurial calces? (Journ., p. 411.)

Hydrocephalus is rather induced than cured or prevented by mercury.

CHAPMAN, JOHN, Sur., *Cases of Injuries of the Head, with Observations.*
Ampthill, 1800. *See* MED. AND PHYS. JOURN., 1800, *vol. III.*

228. The fondness for trepanning, so much inculcated by Mr. Pott, and so very anxiously supported by Mr. Benjamin Bell, has justly met with two very able antagonists in *Mr. John Bell* and *Mr. Abernethy* (p. 31, Journ). Every man, previous to applying the trepan, ought to ask himself for what he is going to trepan? " To think that a fractured skull is a chief cause, or even an absolute sign of danger, is a very erroneous notion; it is not the damage done to the skull, but the injury to the brain, that is the cause of danger; and the fracture of the skull is but a faint, uncertain mark of the harm done to the brain" (*J. Bell's Discourses on Wounds of the Head,* p. 137). Again: "There is still but one motive for applying the trephine, viz., to relieve the brain from compression " (ibid., p. 144).

In injuries of the head, chirurgical operation must be postponed, the safer way being to purge, and thereby determine the blood from the head.

Now, I am speaking of affections of the brain, I cannot forbear observing that I have long been dissatisfied with the Edinburgh treatment of concussions of the brain, viz., with cordials, wine, and stimulants. My ideas on this subject are so exactly consonant to what has been said by *Mr. Abernethy* (*Surgical Essays, vol. III., pp.* 59, 60), that I shall therefore refer my readers to his Essays (Journ., pp. 33, 34). *N. B. Abernethy employs purgatives,* bleeding, and antiphlogistic regimen.

FOWLE, WILLIAM, M. D., *A Practical Treatise on the Different Fevers of the West Indies, and their Diagnostic Symptoms. London,* 1800. *See* MED. AND PHYS. JOURN., 1800, *vol. IV.*

229. Very early after my arrival in the country I observed that *persons attacked with fevers, in almost any situation, very generally became* YELLOW. This soon led me to conceive it *merely a concomitant symptom,* and by no means such as could be sufficiently characteristic of any one fever to give it a particular denomination; it also led me to discover the cause of the variety of symptoms attributed by different authors to the *yellow fever,* and to account for successful methods of cure which were often diametrically opposite to each other. The longer I remained in the country the more I was convinced of the danger attendant on giving a name to one disease from a symptom common to so many (Journ., p. 355).

Yellow fever a denomination without particular meaning—the disease a common fever.

Dr. Fowle divides the fevers of the West Indies according to their appearances into intermittents, remittents, ardent fever, and the malignant or jail fever.

GEOGHEGAN, EDWARD, Surg., *On Strangulated Hernia.* *Dublin,* 1800. *See* MED. AND PHYS. JOURN., 1800, *vol. IV.*

Strangulated hernia.
A plain view of the case indicating cause of cucuation.

230. Let us for a moment consider the state of the parts: A portion of the intestine lies without an aperture, through which it is too large to pass; the question then arises, what occasions its bulk? Surely, the nature of the part, the touch, and all the circumstances of the case, clearly *evince it to be flatus,* and sometimes *together with excrement and an inflamed intestine,* whose *functions* are so far *deranged* that *it cannot act upon its natural contents,* so as to move them in their ordinary course. . . Nothing can be more obvious than that every effort should be made to *lessen the bulk* of the hernia, and none to push it through the ring; it will pass in of itself after the air has been extracted (Journ., p. 318).

Purging with Brandreth's Pills is what is needed.

MAGENNIS, J., M. D., *On Epilepsy.* *Birmingham,* 1800. *See* MED. AND PHYS. JOURN., 1800, *vol. IV.*

Epilepsy.
The torpor of the stomach and intestines requires powerful purges.

231. I observed in these patients, and in most others who have long labored under this untoward disease, a dullness of apprehension, a particular stare and vacuum of countenance, a dilated pupil, and an inability of the iris to contract on the admission of light, accompanied with stupor and a general irritability of the muscular fiber. This *torpor extends to the stomach and intestinal canal,* as those people subject to the disorder usually *require the most active cathartics* and emetics *to excite* the primæ viæ into action (Journ., p. 419).

REEVE, R., Surg., *On a Successful Case of Hydrocephalus.* *See* MED. AND PHYS. JOURN., 1800, *vol. III.*

Case of hydrocephalus proving the necessity of full, continued, powerful purgation of the intestinal canal.

232. *Hydrocephalus internus.*—The author's own child, at the age of eight months, in December, 1798, could stand alone, and had every appearance of a healthy, forward child. His temper was unusually placid, and his spirits invariably good. Towards the end of the month he became extremely costive, and though medicine for a time relieved him, he was frequently and violently seized with pain in the abdomen, which was generally mitigated by a clyster. . . He ceased to grow, except the head, which, towards the end of January, 1799, was perceptibly increased in size, and his costiveness was become so obstinate as scarcely to yield to the most active purgatives. It was this singular state of the alimentary canal, which had existed upwards of six weeks, that first led me to suspect some material derangement in the state of the brain. On the 12th of February he was convulsed in the night, took antimon tartaris in small doses, with little or no effect, and on the following day castor oil, which was repeated a second time, before any motion was produced; the abdomen was very hard, and of an extraordinary size; the stools of a clay color, and of such an adhesive nature that they could not easily be separated from his napkins; his urine high-colored, secreted in large quantities, and gave a yellow tinge to his linen. James' powders were given, but fever and delirium set in, with a voracious appetite, and all the symptoms of hydrocephalus. Calomel given as purgative in the be-

ginning of March was charged with mercurial friction, but all hope of
his recovery was lost; he cried much, had much pain in his bowels,
which were distended by flatus to an alarming degree, and the only relief
that could be obtained was by clysters. A blister that was applied to
the anterior fontanelle was kept open and discharged copiously, and in
April he commenced slowly to recover. . . Now his bowels are quite
restored, and he has left off all medicine (Journ., pp. 61–64).

Brandreth's Pills could have saved all this pain and suffering.

UNWINS, DAVID, Surg., *On Febrifuge Medicines.* *See* MED. AND PHYS.
JOURN., 1800, *vol. IV.*

233. A derangement of the nervous system, occasioning *general de-*   *Fever.*
bility, is an invariable attendant on *fevers of every denomination,* and to " THERE IS
this single cause, debility, are all the symptoms which occur under differ- YER," one
ent circumstances of constitution, situation, habit, &c., of the patients *different*
to be referred; for, notwithstanding the minute division and extensive *manifesta-*
classification which have been adopted by nosological and systematic *tions.*
writers on febrile affections, there appears to be *no specific or abstract*
difference in the diseases themselves, the variety of appearance which they
assume being totally dependent upon the state of the constitution receiving the affection. Thus, *the same causes* operating upon a person of a
sanguine temperament and plethoric habit will occasion the disease
which has obtained the appellation of *inflammatory fever,* with symptoms
of vascular excitement, which, on a patient of a contrary description,
will be productive of a *typhus* or *nervous fever* (p. 54).

234. When the quickness, smallness, and irregularity of arterial pul- *Debility,*
sation, distressing pains in the head, extreme oppression of the mind, ly attending
and other symptoms are present, denoting the highest state of nervous moved,
debility, a dose of powdered antimony, in such quantity as to create a sympathy,
slight nausea of the stomach, will often reduce the pulse to its proper by stimula-
standard, and, by inducing a regularity and due proportion between the *stomach.*
action and reaction of the system, will effectually arrest the further progress of the disease.

WOODWARD, W., Surg., *On Infantile Diseases.* *See* MED. & PHYS.
JOURN. 1800, *Vol. IV.*

235. There is a liquor in the bowels of infants and many other ani- *Infantile*
mals, when they are born, which is necessary to be carried off; *the medi-* *diseases.*
cine which nature has provided for that purpose *is the mother's first* The moth-
milk; this, indeed, answers every purpose, and effectually; but we er's milk
think some drugs forced down the child's throat will do much better— *medicine.*
the composition of which varies, according to the fancy of the good
woman who presides at the birth. . . . We see that notwithstanding the
many moving calls of natural instinct in the child to suck the mother's
breast, yet the usual practice is to deny that indulgence till the third day
after the birth; by that time, *the suppression of the natural evacuation*

The natural eracuation prevents and cures milk-fever. *of the milk* usually *brings on a fever*, the consequence of *which is often fatal to the mother*, or puts it out of her power to suckle the child at that time. The sudden swelling of the breasts, which commonly happens about the third day, is another bad consequence of this delay. When the breasts become thus suddenly and greatly distended, a child is not only utterly unable to suck, but, by its cries and struggling, fatigues and heats both itself and the mother; this is another cause which prevents nursing. . . . The gentlemen of the Lying-in-Hospital in London ordered the children to be put to the mother's breast as soon as they showed a desire for it, which was generally within ten or twelve hours after birth; this rendered the usual dose of physic unnecessary; the milk-fever was prevented; the milk flowed gradually and easily into the breasts, which before were apparently empty, and things went on in the natural way. If a mother is determined not to nurse her own infant, she should, for her own sake, suckle it at least three or four weeks, and then wean it by degrees from her own breast. In this way the more immediate danger arising from repelling the milk is prevented (pp. 43-44).

The vital energy in children higher than in adults. Bleeding alone injurious to it, purgation never. 236. There is, in truth, a greater luxuriancy of life and health in infancy than in any other period of life. Infants, we acknowledge, are more delicately sensible to injury than those in advanced life; but to compensate this, their fibres and vessels are more capable of distension, their whole system is more flexible, their fluids are less acrid, and less disposed to putrescence; *they bear all evacuations more easily, except that of blood;* and, which is an important circumstance in their favor, they never suffer from the terrors of a distracted imagination. . . . Children recover from diseases under such circumstances as are never survived by adults; if they waste more quickly under sickness, their recovery is quick in proportion and more complete than in older people; in short, a physician ought never to despair of a child's life while it continues to breathe (p. 43).

MOORE, JAMES, *Surg., A case of Synocha, London,* 1801. *See* MED. & PHYS. JOURN., 1801, *Vol. V.*

Synocha is a common fever, only of high degree of irritation and longer duration. 237. *Synocha,* or *pure inflammatory fever,* is a disease so rare in this country that many experienced practitioners have doubted its existence. Here follows a case:—*The treatment* employed during the five days he was under my charge *consisted simply of two purgatives,* and a draught of one-fourth of a grain of tartar emetic, and two drachms of the acetate Purgation. ammonia water, which was exhibited regularly every six hours. (Journ. p. 233.)
Synocha certainly very much resembles the symptomatic fever attendant upon phlegmon; the common ephemera is undoubtedly of the same species, and the synocha seems to be precisely the same malady, in a more violent degree, and running on for a longer period. (ibid. p. 234.)

PRICARDS, J., *Surg.*, *On Hydrocephalus, Brentford,* 1801. *See* MED. & PHYS. JOURN., 1801, *Vol. V.*

238. Case of a boy, 8 years of age, *strong purgatives* given: This produced *very brisk evacuations* at each time of repeating it (every other morning); *after each repetition,* however, *he appeared better and more lively.* The plan was *continued for several weeks,* during which every symptom of the disease gradually subsided, until his pristine state of health was completely renewed. (Journ. p. 344.)
Therefore it appears to me, that *drastic purgatives, frequently administered,* have a much fairer chance of *success by increasing very powerfully the action of the absorbents,* while they *do not produce that debility of the system* which is the consequence of mercury (ibid. p. 345).

Hydrocephalus. Brisk. continued pur- gation r - stores health and ri a . Mercury weakens the system.

SAVARESI, ANTONIO, M. D., *Physician to the French Army in Egypt, on the Cure and Prevention of the Endemic Ophthalmia of that Country. Transl. by G. Blane, M. D., London,* 1801. *See* MED. AND PHYS. JOURN., 1801, *vol. VI.*

239. *Dr. Savaresi* first divides this complaint into the sthenic and asthenic; the one depending on an excess, the other on a defect, of tone. The former effects the bulb of the eye; the latter sometimes the "sarsus," sometimes the "tunica conjunctiva."
In the beginning I purge in all the three species, without distinction, with an ounce of magnesia vitrolata, otherwise called Epsom salts. The sthenic ophthalmia requires very close and strict attention, inasmuch as the cure depends on the efficiency of the first remedies. After this, topical remedies, as emollient collyria, are employed, and low diet.
As preventive, he recommends avoiding exposure to the sun with the head uncovered, and to the night dew, abstaining from salted food, avoiding cold after being heated, and attention to the intestinal evacuations (Journ., pp. 357–359).

Ophthalmia of three va- rieties, purging the first remedy upon which the cure de- pends.

TAINSH, W., Surg., *Account of Some Cases of the Plague, which occurred on board of a British ship-of-war on the coast of Syria. See* MED. AND PHYS. JOURN, 1801, *vol. V.*

240. *Plague.—Mr.* Tainsh employed, after removing all clothes from the patients, and washing them with soap over the whole body, powerful repeated evacuations of the bowels by *emetics and laxative clysters.* The sick used to discharge "*an enormous quantity of bile, viscid sordes, and tough phlegm,*" and the stools gave the sick evidently much relief; when a bitter taste and nausea continued, emetics were repeated, which cleared the stomach of a large quantity of disagreeable matter, which gave great ease. After thus removing the cause of the disease, a strengthening treatment was pursued, and the buboes treated by poultices (Journ., pp. 539–541).

Plague. Powerful and repeat- ed evacua- tion removes the cause.

VAGE, T., M. D., *Criticisms on the Treatment of Venereal Diseases.* *London*, 1801. *See* MED. AND PHYS. JOURN., 1802, *vol. VIII.*

241. *Opiates* are usually and properly given, in the intention of mitigating severe pains in the venereal disease; but, notwithstanding their utility, a free and frequent use of them *always induces a relaxation of the system,* and *debilitates the chylific organs,* which are primary things to guard against in mercurial courses. Although both these effects of opium appear to spring from one common source, by producing a nervous, sedative stupefaction, yet some observation in practice inclined me to suppose that ease may be procured without any concomitant debility (Journ., p. 8).

[margin: Opium relaxes the nervous system, and diminishes chylification.]

242. *Mercury,* however, with all its anti-venereal properties, *is naturally inimical to the nervous system,* and exerts its injurious effects, in some degree or other, *in the most judicious use of it.* When it is exhibited too copiously, and suddenly, it is apt to produce violent effects, as great *swelling of the head and tongue, apoplexy,* &c., because *it breaks down the blood* before any outlet is prepared for its evacuation. When its use is gradual, these effects will be moderate, but they will accumulate in time to considerable injuries of the same nature. *The most violent and mildest effects of remedies are produced upon the same principle,* and the former are frequently the only index to explain the latter, which would otherwise be too minute for observation (Journ., p. 9).

[margin: Mercury breaks down the blood.]
[margin: Axiom.]

243. *The infirmities* which arise *from the use of mercury* appear to originate *from two principal sources: one* is its *dissolution of the blood,* by which a redundance of serum is forced into the interstices of the cellular substance of the muscular, vascular, and nervous systems; in consequence of which the gluten, which gives strength and stability to the solids, becomes relaxed, and the different functions of the animal economy so debilitated as to be incapable to be properly actuated by the nervous influence, while the nervous system itself may remain in a tolerable condition. *The other source* of infirmity, on the contrary, is *when the nervous system has been left impaired* and cannot invigorate these functions, which may not have suffered any considerable detriment. For, it is experimentally ascertained, that if the nerves of any part are injured, either at their origin or in their course, that part will become proportionally inert in its office (Journ., p. 9).

The effects of mercury are somewhat similar to those of lead; both have power to produce paralytic affections; both, in a weaker degree, abate inflammations and mitigate pain; and *the imbecility of both remain after they have been quite expelled from the habit* (Journ., p. 10).

[margin: The two causes of mercurial disease.]
[margin: Parallel between lead and mercury.]

244. In considering the *dyspeptic symptoms* of this or any other disease, it appears to be generally conceived that the cause of them is the weakness of the stomach alone. This opinion has probably led to some important mistakes in practice; for this organ is not less subject to be affected by causes, and the condition of parts remote from itself, than it is capable of affecting the whole system. Thus an *indolence of the in-*

[margin: Dyspeptic symptoms from sympathy between the intestines and the whole system.]

testines, or *a diminution of their action in any part*, from the pylorus to the rectum, will produce *nausea and indigestion*, even when the stomach itself may be in a good condition; and hence it is that often a cathartic will remove these symptoms by giving an additional irritation to the obstructed and enervated parts. In general, however, here *the stomach participates of the mercurial debility*, and corroborating aperients become requisite. In regard to the inertness of the intestinal action, it may be further noted that it frequently proceeds from a *deficiency of the bile*, which a cathartic stimulus is likely to prevent, for undoubtedly this secretion depends much upon the proper action of the duodenum. But the chief utility of the bile results from its chylific property, which appears to consist, in a great measure, of mixing the oily and aqueous parts of the aliment, and assimilating them into a uniform liquid. This great importance of *the hepatic secretion, whenever it appears defective, demands immediate assistance by active purgative medicine* (p. 172).

Purgatives remove the symptoms and invigorate intestinal action, promoting the elaboration of good bile and the chylification.

AULD, ISAAC, M. D., *of Edisto, S. C., Case of Acute Bilious Fever read before the Medical Society of South Carolina*, 1802. *See* MED. AND PHYS. JOURN., 1808, *Vol. XIX.*

245. *Case.*—A young man who had spent a month in the country, on the morning after his return complained of slight *chilliness* and a dull *pain at the pit of his stomach*, which soon after terminated in excessive *vomiting, violent fever*, and intense *pain in his head*. These symptoms continued without abatement until about three o'clock in the afternoon, when they suffered considerable remission. At this time I saw him. I found that so general a *suffusion of bile* through the system had taken place as to resemble a person laboring under jaundice, with the exception of the eyes, which were slightly inflamed. His bowels were obstinately bound, having been in a state of constipation for the two or three previous days. His tongue was moist, the edges inflamed, the top white, excepting the middle, down which ran a yellow streak (Journ., p. 106).

Acute bilious fever (vulgo yellow fever), symptoms: costiveness preceding and attending, fever and pains in the head and stomach, vomiting, yellowness.

246. *Treatment.*—As his pulse, which was slow and irregular, seemed now to forbid the lancet, though there was still some pain in the head, and *costiveness and debility* appeared to be the principal inconveniences under which he labored, I contented myself with leaving for him *two smart purges* of calomel and jalap, with directions to take one immediately, and the other in four hours, if the first did not procure eight or ten copious stools. On visiting him again, about nine o'clock, I found that he had taken both his purges with the happiest effect; they were then operating briskly, and had already produced several *large evacuations of hard, dark, and very fœtid fœces*. The pain had entirely left his head, his pulse had become regular and more full, a gentle moisture had overspread his skin; his stomach had recovered much of its usual tone, and this was accompanied with desire for food. On the next morning he had left his bed with an assurance that he felt himself quite free from indisposition. The discharges from his bowels were still kept up, but had entirely lost their fœtor, and appeared to consist chiefly of healthy-look-

Cure: Powerful purgation, removing the cause, i. e. accumulation of hard, dark and fœtid fœces.

Natural stools succeeding morbid evacuations do not absolutely indicate cessation of the purgative treatment.

ing bile. His skin had become much clearer, as had his urine, which before was of a deep bilious hue.

I suggested the propriety of his taking *gentle purgatives for a day or two longer;* but *this advice,* from the comfortable state of his feelings, he declined, and I, of course, left him. On the third morning after this I was sent for to attend in all possible haste, as the patient was supposed to be dying. I found him speechless, his jaws were fixed, as also were his eyes, which were nearly closed; he had no pulse at the wrists, his feet, legs, and knees were perfectly cold, and his stools, which were black and very offensive, came from him involuntarily; his breathing had been very laborious, but now it appeared to be free from anxiety. I was informed that the day I left him the pain in his head and the fever had returned with its former violence, and had continued without any diminution until this morning, when it terminated in the comatose state described. The cure was hereafter effected by nitric acid and blisters, which restored the vitality of the patient, and by a continued application of that acid and strong purgatives, which carried off large masses of very fœtid, hardened fæces (Journ., pp. 106–109).

Aurful consequences of imperfect purgation.

BADGER, JOHN, Surg., *On a singular kind of Eruptive Disease.* See MED. AND PHYS. JOURN., 1802, *Vol. VIII.*

247. The first opportunity of witnessing this disease was at Putney, in the month of July, 1801; it seemed to be confined to children only of a certain age, having never seen a child affected with it before seven nor after fifteen years, though equally exposed, as it was evidently infectious to them. It commences with a slight fever, which continues three or four days; it then increases; nausea, and sometimes vomiting, attend (in one or two instances I have observed the patients to complain of violent sickness after they were put to bed), with pain in the head and loins; it is then succeeded by an eruption containing a well-matured pus; the pustules are large and very thick about the head, resembling those of small-pox; and in every case I have seen they have been confined to the head, particularly to the scalp. The *bowels during the progress of the disease* were *unusually constipated,* and, in one or two instances, not only the body but the face likewise was much swelled. The first two or three cases I had not an opportunity of seeing till after the eruption had taken place to a great extent, covering almost the whole of the scalp. •

Eruptive disease of the head.

Physiology.

248. The hair was shaved off as close as possible, tar ointment and a mild purgative applied; but this treatment produced no amendments, the ointment rather increasing the number of pustules. I ordered, therefore, the head to be kept clean with warm soap and water, the patient to use a spare diet, and the bowels kept open with an active purgative once or twice a week, or "pro re nata," and a few drops of antimonial wine given once in four or six hours, till the feverish symptoms had subsided. This plan was pursued for several days without having at all mitigated the complaint, though it seemed, under every circumstance, to be the best mode of treatment that could be adopted. Accordingly it was continued for a few days longer, at which period the pulse became regular, the pain in the head and loins was removed, the pustules began

Treatment by cleanliness, with spare diet and purgation.

to dry off, and in about a week the complaint entirely ceased (Journ., pp. 106, 107).

CURRIE, WILLIAM, M. D., *Observations on the Treatment of the Malignant Yellow Fever which prevailed partially in the City and Liberties of Philadelphia in the summer and autumn of* 1802. *Philadelphia,* 1802. *See* MED. AND PHYS. JOURN., 1803, *Vol. IX.*

249. *Mercury* was generally employed both internally and externally for the purpose of exciting salivation as speedily as possible, both at the hospital and in private practice; but, if I can trust my observations, *seldom with success,* excepting where employed at the very commencement of the disease, and so conducted as to affect the mouth before the dangerous symptoms of the second stage had time to make their appearance. *Yellow fever.*

Mercury seldom useful in the first stage, absolutely injurious in the second stage.

When employed in the *second stage* of the disease, at which time the predominant *symptoms* are generally *disordered stomach, restlessness, oppression,* and *deep sighing,* and a countenance that denotes great misery, *it constantly aggravated the disease,* and *hurried on the fatal* symptoms of *black vomiting.*

In this stage of the disease, when the recited symptoms predominated, the frequent exhibition of *mild laxatives in small doses,* particularly Rochelle salts, soda phosphorata, soluble tartar, castor oil, senna, and cream of tartar, and when these could not be obtained, laxatives and clysters, were *the most successful remedies,* especially when aided by blisters to the stomach, wrists and ankles, at the same time. *Purgatives and laxative drinks remove the worst symptoms.*

A solution of carbonate of soda in water, which is much more palatable than the vegetable alkali, followed immediately by a tablespoonful of diluted lemon juice, or cream of tartar in water, had also sometimes the effect of allaying the distressing propensity to puke. But these, as well as every other means that I have seen tried, too frequently failed of affording relief (pp. 98, 99 Journ.)

[If *mild laxatives* were *frequently* apt to allay the worst symptoms, · it is reasonable to expect *complete success* from *active purges.*]

250. In this state of the stomach the internal use of mercury, either alone or when combined with opium, always increased the distressing propensity to puke ; and, *when it failed to operate by stool, it aggravated* every symptom of the disease (Journ., p. 100). *Mercury and opium aggravate the symptoms.*

251. In cases where the disease began with *strong action of the arteries, severe pain in the head, back and limbs,* with little or no sickness at stomach, bleeding, *purging with active medicines,* and the strict observance of every part of the antiphlogistic regimen, generally occasioned a partial solution of the fever on the third, and a complete solution on the fifth, day from the attack (Journ., p. 101). *Active purgation combined with depletion cures.*

HEBERDEN, WILLIAM, M. D., *Commentaries on the History and Cure of Diseases.* London, 1802.

252. A *diarrhœa* arises from a variety of causes, most of which are void of all danger, and are easily removed. *It is often brought on by that* *Diarrhœa.* *power which is exerted in every part of the body of freeing itself from* *Nature's way* *anything painful and oppressive.* Not only the mischief from the nox-*of cure.* ious qualities and improper quantities of what has been taken, and immediately offends the stomach, *are carried off by means of a diarrhœa,* *but likewise many disorders of remote parts or of the whole body are,* *by the self-correcting powers of an animal body, determined to the bowels,* *and thence discharged by diarrhœa.* It is frequently useful to coöperate *Co-operate* with nature in promoting this evacuation. (Chap. XXVII.) (Cf. Coll. *with nature.* 136, 143 ; Pringle, 200.)

253. *Dysentery.*—The *usual methods* of treating this malady, with *Dysentery* which I was acquainted, *often failed of procuring ease,* and of preventing *cured only* *by remov-* its ending fatally. It appeared that in a dysentery *some hurtful humors* *ing mor-* *bific mat-* *had been deposited in the intestines, which threw them into such disor-* *ters.* *derly agitation as to hinder the expulsion of what had offended them....* *Purgatives* were administered with the *double good effect, both of afford-* *ing present ease,* and *afterwards of entirely removing,* by effectual evac- uations, *the cause* of the disorder. (Chap. XXXI.)

254. *Icterus (Jaundice).*—Good effects may with reason be expected from purging medicines, by their increasing the natural motions of the *Jaundice.* intestines and soliciting a greater flow of bile as well as of all the other *Avoid mer-* humors which are poured into them. Mercurial purges have been pre-*cury, but* *use other and* ferred by some practitioners, but *there appears nothing in the known* *safe purga-* *powers of mercury peculiarly useful in dislodging a biliary concretion,* *tives.* *and the preference should be given to those purges wich act with the most* *ease, and may be continued with the greatest safety.* (Chap. L.) (Cf. 254.)

Colic. 255. *Ileus (Colic).*—The peculiar and *distinguishing symptom* which characterizes the *inflammatory colic* in the very beginning is *cos-* *Purgatives* *tiveness,* which it is always extremely difficult, and too often impossible, *cure.* to conquer. As soon as a *discharge downwards* can be procured in a copious manner, *the patient perceives a quick abatement of all his mis-* *Evacua-* *tions must* *ery, and is often restored to health.* But it is *not from one or two small* *be contin-* *ued and co-* *evacuations* that we can entertain much hope of the distemper beginning *pious to in-* to give way. This has happened on the first or second day, from the *sure recov-* *ery.* excrement which was lodged in or near the rectum, far below the seat of mischief. And later in the distemper, a very small portion of that liquid matter with which the bowels are deluged has seemed to have been forced downwards, while the disease was every hour growing worse. Such *inefficacious evacutions* have been observed more than once or twice in the course of this illness, without saving the patient's life.....Warm baths, fomentations, &c., are *serviceable helps in dis-* *posing the bowels to yield to the power of cathartic medicines, by the fail-* *ure or success of which the life or death of the patient must at last be* *determined.* (Chap. LI.) (Cf. Hipp. 12, 38, 41, 45, 57. Parep, 85, 87.)

* TYRO.—*On Apoplexy. See* MED. & PHYS. JOURN., 1802. *Vol. VIII. (Controversy between Mr. Crowfoot and Dr. Langslow on the question whether emetics or bleeding be applicable in apoplexy ?*

256. In addition to the testimonies adduced by *Pyrrho* (one of the writers participating in the controversy), I shall only add, that *Baglivi*, who divides apoplexy into sanguineous and pituitous, observes: " Arcanum in sanguineis est phlebotomia. In pituitosis contra *emeticum, aut purgans vehimens.* Sunt qui apoplexia (pituistosa scilicet) liberati sunt, hausto singulis mensibus vomitivo ex infuso prædicto (infus. croc. metal cum vino)." [a] .... *Aretaeus* does not recommend emetics, but observes : " if the *sacred purge* should excite vomiting, it is not to be restrained, because it evacuates pituita, the cause of the disease, and rouses the patient by imparting a degree of vigor." *Bœrhaave,* among the general evacuants to be used in this disease, mentions *vomits and strong purges*; though he adds, there is something uncertain in their action. *Vanswieten,* also, in his Commentaries upon this Aphorism (1026), observes, that emetics ought not to be condemned in this disease, and are often useful, because they evacuate pituita ; though he afterwards thinks *purgatives less objectionable.* (Journ., pp. 68–69.)

Apoplexy. Evacuation of the bowels by purgation and vomiting is the cure and preventive.

BARDSLEY, SAMUEL ARGENT, M. D., *Physician to the Manchester Infirmary, Dispensary and Lunatic Hospital. An Account of the Epidemic Catarrhal Fever or Influenza in Manchester, &c. See* MED. AND PHYS. JOURN., 1803, *Vol. IX.*

257. *Emetics* were found highly beneficial on the first attack; indeed, the frequent occurrence of spontaneous nausea and sickness pointed out their use. They scarcely ever failed to relieve the urgent symptoms of pain in the head and stricture of the chest. To obviate costiveness, and at the same time to cleanse the primæ viæ, *moderate doses of calomel, with rhubarb and antimonial powders combined,* were exhibited with excellent effects. . . *Opiates* were seldom employed during the first stage of the disorder, as they had a tendency to *exasperate* the complaints of the head and chest, and *increase* restlessness and feverish heat (Journ., pp. 525, 526).

Influenza. Evacuation of stomach and bowels relieve the symptoms; Opium increases them.

KINGLAKE, ROBERT, M. D., *On Influenza. See* MED. AND PHYS. JOURN., 1803, *Vol. IX.*

258. My experience authorizes me to say that the benefit of abstracting heat, by atmospheric exposure, light bed-clothes, copious dilution with cold water, and avoiding stimulants of every description, will almost certainly rescue the patient from danger, and leave *nothing more for medicine to do than gently to move the bowels* in case of costiveness, and, at most, to aid the refrigerant plan by the milder sudorifics (Journ., p. 520).

Influenza. Purgatives the only medicine required.

---

a In the sanguineous, phlebotomy is the arcanum. In the pituitous, on the contrary, *emetics or strong purgatives.* Some people remain free from apoplexy by taking every month a draught of aforesaid vomitive infusions. (Inf. croc. metal. c. vino.)

The *refrig-*
eration plan
contended
for.
259. It is an erroneous notion that occasional refrigeration and abstinence in disease weaken more than a heating and stimulating treatment. The native energy of healthy power is certainly reduced both
by the abstraction and increase of excitement, but by its due diminution
vital force may be said to be nursed, while undue stimulant agency tends
to dissipate it even to extinction; hence a moderate negation of excitement debilitates much less *directly* than its excessive employ does *indirectly* (Journ., pp. 519, 520; Remark).

Our method for the cure of Influenza is to purge very freely with Brandreth's Pills, six
pills every twelve hours the first day. Keeping in bed as much as possible; oatmeal gruel
or light broth; if the head is very painful, feet in hot water with mustard or wood ashes;
if throat is sore, gargle with weak alum-water; outward applications are the Allcock Plaster, mustard poultice, red pepper, or any stimulating liniment. When the skin of the
throat becomes a little red, the outward applications dispensed with. Should a choking
sensation be felt, or the breathing be difficult, four Brandreth's Pills must be taken every
four hours, or even oftener, until relief is experienced.

O'BERNE, P., Surg., *Observations on the Fevers in Hot Climates.* London, 1803. *See* MED. AND PHYS. JOURN., 1803, *Vol. X.*

*Yellow fe-
ver.*
260. The more severe in symptoms, and dangerous in effect, any disease is, the more necessary the investigation of, and researches after,
methods of cure must be fully impressive on every mind; it is scarcely
necessary to add that perhaps none comes more strongly under this description than that generally termed *yellow fever;* none, therefore, more
Its com-
mencement,
symptoms
and *general
course.* interesting claims our attention.
In the commencement, generally nausea, pain in the head, loins and
hams, succeed; dry surface, increased pulse, but not to be depended on,
varying from 80 to 140, chills, anxiety, sighing, prostration of strength;
vomiting soon takes place, and not unfrequently is the first indication of
the disease. The vessels of the tunica conjunctiva become turgid, and
a yellow tinge of that membrane takes place, frequently extending over
the body. Notwithstanding this circumstance gives rise to the name
usually given this complaint, it is by no means a constant attendant, and
in many totally wanting. Watchfulness and desire to sleep, without
being able to effect it; whilst in others constant dozing, pain and sensation of heat in the stomach, great thirst; vomited matter gradually
changes from yellow to dark green, and at length perfect black. Clammy
skin, sometimes petechiæ, but unfrequent; stupor or violent delirium
succeed; paroxysms of vomiting become more rapid, and many expire in
one of those paroxysms too shocking to describe, whilst others placidly
resign exhausted nature (Journ., pp. 36, 37).

Anomalies
and *sudden
changes.*
261. No disease perhaps exhibits a greater variety of symptoms, and
often less to be depended on, than this; sometimes it goes on with every
favorable appearance, suddenly changes to the worst, and patients, apparently almost in a state of convalescence, expire in an hour or two.
This is a melancholy fact (Journ., p. 37).

The *favor-
able symp-
toms.*
262. The symptoms that we may call favorable are, settled state of
the stomach, lessened headache, eyes lively, formation of pustules over
the surface, or that eruption known in tropical climes by the name of
prickly heat, I have ever remarked as almost a certain indication of recovery; bilious flux, copious and high-colored urine, free perspiration,
and sound sleep (ibid.)

263. The dangerous, and, I am sorry to add, most common, symptoms, are severe headache, frequent vomiting, heat increasing to a burning sensation, extending down the trachea and alimentary canal; matter vomited and fæces becoming dark, frequent sighing, dull or glassy eye, pale and little urine, dark fur on the tongue, muscular and nervous debility, intermittent pulse, clammy feet, cold sweats, stupor or violent delirium, singultus, coma (ibid.) *The dangerous symptoms.*

264. That dark matter vomited, termed *black vomit,* it may be necessary to remark, although laid down by most authorities as a certain fatal sign, is by no means so, as I have seen many recover after it; it is also said "that a diarrhœa almost precludes any hopes of recovery." *If by diarrhœa is understood a simple (or bilious) flux,* I have ever observed it a decided fortunate event; certainly a flux of *putrid dark fæces is extremely bad, and yet even that* I have many times seen *prove salutary* (ibid.) *The black vomit and diarrhœa NOT AT ALL fatal symptoms.*

265. *Our first and principal attention* should be directed to *clearing the first passages,* and to *keep them free* during the disease *being of the greatest importance.* *The TREATMENT.*
Emetics are by many laid entirely aside, on the principle of increasing the already irritable state of the stomach. That a great deal of caution and discrimination in their use is extremely necessary must be allowed; but I am decidedly of opinion much benefit is to be obtained by them. Where nausea or slight vomiting occurs, ipecacuanha is the best; but if the vomiting be more severe, an infusion of chamomile will answer every intention. *In the first stage: PURGATION AT ALL EVENTS; emetics admissible with caution.*
Cathartics.—Calomel, combined with powder of jalap, is perhaps one of the best; the irritating quality of the neutral salts seldom makes them advisable.

266. *Blood-letting* has been advised by some of the most respectable authorities; I shall therefore only observe that *I never saw it used with advantage;* on the contrary, *I always thought it of disservice* (Journ., p. 38). *Bleeding never useful, always hurtful.*

267. Our next intentions must be directed towards lessening the irritable state of the stomach, supporting the strength, and resisting that tendency to putrescency that exists in this disorder. *In the second stage, besides the peculiar treatment, the bowels must be kept constantly free.*
Notwithstanding the great variety of opinions that have been, and still are, on this subject, calomel will still perhaps be found the most successful medicine hitherto employed, and, in general, I have but little doubt its want of success in many instances may be attributed to the manner of giving it, or want of *atten ion to the state of the bowels.* Calomel if not given in large quantities quickly repeated had better not be given at all. I have used from five to eight grains every two hours, and sometimes every hour, combined with three grains of the antimonial powder, until a diaphoresis was induced, when the latter was omitted, and the calomel continued until the effect was evident, as metallic taste, foetid breath, or sore mouth. When a gentle salivation is raised, desist

in frequency, yet continue so as to keep up the effect of the mercury; the criterion of its success may be determined by its action or non-action. When a speedy and copious salivation comes on, the most happy effects may be looked for; while the contrary prove the reverse. And here *External remedies.* again let me observe that *the most minute attention must be paid to keep the bowels free,* for which purpose enemas are the best (Journ., pp. 38, 39).

268. *Blisters,* although uncertain, are of great utility both in preventing delirium and lessening vomiting, applied to the region of the *Enemas.* stomach. *General warm bath* is of the utmost service, or, where that cannot be conveniently had, *washing all over with warm water* (Journ., p. 39).

269. Of all remedies in use for this disease, excepting calomel, perhaps none are of more real service than *enemas,* and the more simple the better—such as warm water, oil and vinegar; but on the increased vascular action and heat subsiding, enemas composed of orchis, sago, or *Opium* portable broth; this last I have found of such uncommon service as *and bark* makes me wish most strongly to impress the use of it; in many cases, *useless.* where animation seemed nearly exhausted, recovery was the unexpected and welcome effect of this salutary practice (ibid.)

270. *Opium* I have found of little, if any, service, in any stage. *Cinchona* appears to me evidently of disservice until the patient is in a convalescent state (ibid.)

Brandreth's Pills are in every respect superior to calomel as a purge, and they leave no evil after effects.

POTTER, NATHANIEL, *M. D. Letter on the Epidemic Distempers of the year* 1802. *Baltimore,* 1803. *See* MED. AND PHYS. JOURN., 1804, *vol. XI.*

271. The cure of *measles* this year may be almost reduced to two *Measles.* simple remedies, *blood-letting* and *purging.* For, when these were used *Purging* in time, and carried to a sufficient extent, little or nothing remained to *actively em-* *ployed cures* be done. These remedies were no less efficacious in removing the im- *and pre-* *vents bad* mediate symptoms than in removing the consequences of the disease. *conse-* *quences.* This will be sufficiently apparent when we enumerate the deplorable train of consequences that followed their neglect (Journ., 7, 312).

272. *Purging* was *a very useful remedy,* and required to be *repeated* *Purgatives* *every second day,* or oftener, as there was a constant *reaccumulation of* *cure by car-* *that green and acrid matter* that was sometimes ejected from the stom- *rying off* *the morbid* ach on the first attack; and this disposition commonly lasted four or *matter.* five days. *Where purging was neglected* in the commencement, *the evacuations* from the intestines *were often of a dark green, brown or black complexion,* just as it happens in other malignant fevers (Journ., p. 313).

273. *Antimonials* were certainly improper remedies in this disease; they depressed the pulse, and seemed to act too much like the causes of the disease. Are not antimonials equally unfit remedies in all malignant

fevers, where the tendency to indirect debility is great, and more especially in those called contagious, where the "vis nocens" is so prone to
induce the same state of the system? *Antimonials altogether injurious; blisters and opiates applicable only conditionally.*

Blisters were equally inapplicable in the first state of the disease,
but co-operate powerfully with emetics in arresting the progress of indirect debility in the advanced state of measles, and sometimes called
forth dormant excitement to great advantage.

Opium was also inadmissible in all its forms, unless toward the latter
state, when fever did not contraindicate its prescription for the cough,
which was often the last troublesome symptom, and seemingly occasioned by the action of a small portion of the pulmonary vessels (Journ.
p. 314.)

POWER, GEORGE, *Surg., Assistant Surgeon to the Twenty-third Regiment
of Foot, Royal Welsh Fusileers. Attempt to investigate the cause of
the Egyptian Ophthalmia, &c.* See MED. and PHYS. JOURN., 1803,
vol. IX.

274. The next local cause of *Ophthalmia in Egypt* is the custom of
sleeping at night in the open air, imbibing with every inspiration, and
absorbing at every pore, the putrid virus contained in the descending
dews. . . . Thus in a system peculiarly debilitated, and unable to resist
all its powers combined, it produces that *highly putrid fever* called
plague. In a patient less relaxed, as the habit of the body determines
the disease either to the surface of the skin or to the intestines, an *eruptive fever* or *dysentery* is produced; and when the putrid virus is but
partially applied, to the eyes for instance, or to the mouth, or even on
the surface of the body, *ophthalmia, ulcerated fauces,* or *ichorous blotches*
on the skin ensue (Journ., p. 78). *Ophthalmia. Influence of night-dew in hot climates producing different diseases, according to predisposition.*

275. As the author frequently refers to a treatise of the French Surgeon Bruant, it will be of interest to know what this writer says on the
cure: "This disease is frequently cured by the *simple operation of nature,* and without any assistance from art; and indeed we may affirm
with truth that *nothing so much opposes the cure as too great a profusion
of remedies,* especially topical. Some patients have been relieved by an
eruption coming on at the temples; others, and the greater number, by
a slight diarrhœa; and hence, to act conformably to the views of nature,
I have encouraged a discharge from the bowels during the whole duration of the disease, by employing tamarinds or other laxative titans
(Desgenettes Histoire Médicale de l'armée de l'Orient.—Journ. p. 580). *Nature indicates the cure by evacuation.*

WADLEY, T. W., *Surg., on the Prevailing Epidemic Influenza. Stow on
the Wold* 1803. *See* MED. and PHYS. JOURN., 1803, *vol. IX.*

276. First, the exhibition of *an emetic was always promised,* which
seldom failed of evacuating the stomach of a *dark colored, greenish, and
most offensive fluid.* Aperients were always rejected when given before

Influenza from bilious accumulations of fœtid dark-colored excrements.

Cure by purging off the cause.

an emetic, and an enema was found of no service. The pain in the head was constantly lessened and frequently removed by the vomit, and a freer expectoration sometimes relieved the cough. When *costiveness* was a very urgent symptom *an active purgative* was given, which never failed of being *followed by stools of a peculiar fœtor and black color*, and this state of the alvine discharge often accompanied the disease throughout (Journ. p. 516).

MEDICUS, *Practical Observations on the Treatment of the Scarlet Fever and Sore Throat. See* MED. and PHYS. JOURN., 1804, *vol. XII.*

Scarlet fever, when mild, requires but little medical assistance.

277. It is well known that many pass very safely through the *scarlet fever*, in its mild state, with *little or no medical assistance.* But when in that state medicines are administered, I fear the cure is, by the ingenious *theoretical* practitioner, ascribed too often to their effects and not to the mildness of the disease, especially if some fashionable medicine has been prescribed. Hence remedies undeservedly creep into practice, and, I fear, in serious cases frequently supersede the use of those which have long stood the test of sound practical experience.

The cause —morbid matter in the bowels— must be removed by purgatives.

I pretend not to account for the *source or origin* of the scarlet fever and sore throat, but am well satisfied that the "fomes morbi" of the disease, however generated, *lurk in the bowels.* Under this conviction I enjoin them *to be well cleared, in whatever stage or however violent the disease may be*, when I first see the patient, if I suspect that such necessary treatment has not been before observed. The *very fœtid smell of the* evacuation, and *the relief such evacuation immediately procures, strongly prove to me the necessity of purgatives*, and I may add, from reiterated observations, that the longer they are delayed the more severe proves

Brisk purgation does not hurt, but strengthens the vital power.

the disease. Many practitioners, alarmed at apparent debility, are deterred from exhibiting brisk cathartics lest their operation should irrecoverably sink the patient. Such apprehensions would be justly founded if purgatives were administered without due discriminating attention to age, constitution, and immediate state of the patient. But where such attention is paid, I have never seen any mischief arise; on the contrary, the most salutary effects have taken place merely from *the bowels being relieved from the contained accumulated fœtid fæces*, and hence *every febrile symptom becomes milder, and the vital powers invigorated, not debilitated* (Journ., pp. 25, 26).

PATTERSON, W., M. D., *Case of Brainular Affection from an Internal Cause. Londonderry*, 1804. *See* MED. AND PHYS. JOURN., 1804, *Vol. XII.*

Apoplexy. Case of erysipelatous character.

278. A gentleman, aged above sixty years, was suddenly attacked with a severe pain in his forehead, accompanied with so much megrim and stomach sickness as would have caused him to fall had he not received support; to these symptoms was added coldness. He was put to bed; blood-letting pretty largely in the arm; purging, and blistering the back, legs and head, in succession, were employed. Four days after the seizure, when I was called, I found him in bed complaining grievously

of a violent pain in the forehead, together with an irksome stricture in the eyeballs and surrounding teguments. The functions of the brain were impaired by a degree of stupor, attended frequently with incoherent mutterings. His pulse was unequal, laboring, and accelerated with a tenseness in the vessel ; the temporal arteries throbbed considerably, but were uniform in their action. The countenance was sometimes pale, sometimes reddish, and at other times suffused with a bluish tinge ; the eyes were languid, and the sense of vision much diminished, at periods almost lost. The temperature of the skin was sometimes pretty high, more frequently below the medium warmth, and generally felt languid and flaccid. There was sometimes an urgent thirst, but for solids little or no appetite. His stomach, indeed, continued to have a loathing, and so retrograde a disposition as to approach vomiting, which he himself considered to proceed from vitiated bile. His bowels were sluggish, and had not emptied themselves since the operation of the laxative medicine, which was a space of thirty-six hours before I saw him. He was rest-less, and when he seemed to sleep it was a morbid comatose state rather than a salutary repose. The organs of respiration did not appear par-ticularly engaged, and the urinary organs were equally unaffected.

Cure by purgation driving the blood from the head and restoring the equilib-rium of circulation.

From the preceding phenomena I concluded that there existed a de-termination of blood to the head, with increased tension of the arteries of the part. Under this impression, I ordered local evacuations, by means of numerous leeches to the temples, and *a brisk cathartic* to excite and empty the bowels, as well as to promote an equilibrium in the gen-eral circulation. The first application of leeches procured a sensible relief, and therefore it was repeated. The *cathartic was not active enough* in its operation, and *accordingly a stronger one*, composed of calomel and aloes, was given, and with manifest advantage. The stupor in a short time decreased, and was succeeded by a loud talkative raving, accom-panied with unconsciousness of persons and things around him, of which inattentive state a remnant continued for several days. The delirious condition lasted for some hours, and was followed by a profound sleep, attended with a stertor resembling that of apoplexy, but distinguishable from it by softness and equable movement in the pulse. This change was the harbinger of convalescence, which gradually but slowly took place.

Considering the phenomena of this case, I am led to conceive that we would be justifiable in setting it down as a decided instance of apo-plexy ; but certainly it was rather of an anomalous description, as it assumed many of the features of a species of erysipelas which takes place in the membranes and vessels of the brain in the evening of life (Journ., pp. 109–111).

PEARSON, A., Surg., *in the service of the East India Company. Some Observations on the Pathology and Prevailing Diseases of Warm Climates. London*, 1804. *See* MED. AND PHYS. JOURN., 1804, *Vol. XI.*

279. *On Acclimation.*—In the first change from a cold to a hot cli-mate it was formerly the practice to bleed indiscriminately ; it is now per

haps too generally omitted, as it might be often employed to obviate or remove disease arising from inflammatory congestion. *Purging* has also been *recommended for universal adoption;* and when we reflect that *the constitution both admits and requires this evacuation more frequently in warm than in cold climates, and bears it better,* its utility will be found · as probable as experience proves it to be. The neutral salts have been generally prescribed, and these are certainly of the most universal application and use; but vegetable purgatives will be best for frequent use. (Inf. sennæ et temarind, p. rhei. et kali tartar, separately or combined; of the former ℈j. to ℥i., and ℥j.to ℥ii. of the latter.) Occasionally four or five grains of calomel may be taken with much advantage, from its effect in stimulating the mucous or biliary excretories, when some of the laxatives above specified ought to be given next morning. The day on which any of these remedies are given ought to be one of peculiar moderation, and dilution with barley-water or rice gruel attended to. With regard to the use of tonics, or antiseptics, the indications for employing them, and their utility, are much less than is generally supposed. The *feeling of debility* is often fallacious, and *produced by the organs being overloaded,* or *a biliary absorption* (Journ., pp. 161, 162).

Purgation is safest and most relative prevention of all diseases.

Debility from irregularity of excretion.

280. In the warm climates the attacks of *febrile disease* are generally accompanied with symptoms of *bilious absorption,* and *torpor of the intestinal canal,* and with a greater or less *tendency to remission.* The treatment recommended by authors is very contradictory; some advising a continued and severe evacuant plan, while others administer bark on every appearance of remission, and even without waiting for it. If *purging* with calomel and neutral salts is *assiduously practiced* in the first days, giving intermediately mild diaphoretic and antimonial medicine, the use of bark will be found unnecessary (Journ., p. 201).

Fevers. The symptoms indicate purgation from beginning.

281. I am doubtful if the genuine remittent fever appears without a previous exposure to the *exhalation of marshes,* or that from rank vegetation; and the distinct remissions and exacerbations described in books are not frequently to be met with. . . It is frequently *some time after the application of the remote causes before the disease comes on.* . . The debilitating effect of the marsh-miasmata is generally recognized, and it is probable that the *nervous energy and muscular irritability are much and suddenly impaired* by their impression upon the sensorium; the powers of circulating the mass of blood are for a time diminished; from that, irregular actions of the vessels of different viscera, a relative degree of plethora and inflammation takes place, while, from the excretories being similarly affected, the power which the economy possesses to rid itself of an excess of heat is abated. In such a state it is not surprising that *congestions* should take place *in the brain and glandular viscera* (Journ., pp. 201, 202).

Miasmata the cause, and how they act upon the system, depressing the nervous and muscular activity.

BENNION, THOMAS, *Surg.,* on the *Gibraltar Fever. Gibraltar,* 1805. *See* MED. AND PHYS. JOURN., 1805, *vol. XIV.*

282. In the first the patient is seized, without any previous notice, with giddiness, pain of the head, slight sickness at stomach, darting pains from the head to the back, and spasmodic affections of the calves of the legs. The breathing was very hot, incessant sighing, the greatest dejection of spirits. The tongue was in the beginning white; a bad

The Gibraltar-fever a species of fever partaking of the character of plague, yellow fever and typhus.

taste was complained of; the sense of smelling was imperfect or depraved; the visage extremely distressed, and unwillingness to speak. The countenance on the first attack became suddenly sallow; in a very short time, however, it became red, full and bloated, with the exact appearances of intoxication. Drowsiness and sleep followed in a few hours, when a little moisture came out on the skin. This appearance, however, at this stage was delusive; it suddenly left the patient, and was succeeded by the most intense heat, that gave a smarting sensation to the fingers when applied to the skin. There was at this time a most uncommon and offensive smell from the whole body. The eyes were now much inflamed; there was violent pain in the temples and over the arches of the eyebrows, darting to the orbits. The pulse from first to last was greatly increased, but never so strong and firm as in inflammatory diseases; the thirst less than generally in acute diseases. There was strong pulsation in the carotid arteries, and an evident enlargement of the jugular vein. The color of the skin approximated that of the lilac, cocklicoque, violet or poppy, and changed as the disease advanced to a deep yellow. By the early administration of *strong emetics and purgatives on the first attack*, the yellowness seldom appeared, and *every other bad symptom was averted* (Journ., pp. 137–138). *Symptoms of the first stage averted by emetics and strong purges.*

283. When these had not been exhibited, and in cases where the disease from first appeared in a more aggravated form, the second set of symptoms soon appeared; the patient was very comatose, much tremor of the limbs, frequently an incessant vomiting of black matter, with convulsive hiccough; the eyes were drawn in a direction alternately from the nose to the temples in a frightful manner, with nearly total blindness. The skin was now parched with burning heat, or covered with a clammy offensive sweat. The body was covered with petechiæ and vibices, swellings appeared in the armpits and groins, often degenerating into abscesses; foul gangrenous sores on the back, and carbuncles on different parts of the body. There were hemorrhages from the nose, ears, mouth, and pores of the body, with every appearance of a total dissolution of the blood-vessels. Then the fæces and urine were passed involuntarily, and the other usual symptoms indicated speedy dissolution (Journ., p. 138). *The symptoms of the second stage and the close.*

284. My first step was invariably to put the patient into a warm bath, then to rub the body well with soaped flannel, and put him to bed. If the powers of life were strong a solution of *tartar emetic and glauber salts* was given, which generally operated smartly both on stomach and bowels, so that I frequently had little more to do but remove the debility, the patients being often well on the third day. If the solution, persevered in, did not operate, the stomach and bowels being very insensible, I gave *calomel either alone or combined with jalap and the compound extract of colocynth.* I endeavored *by all means to keep up the alvine discharge*; when obtained, the patient was perfectly relieved and free from fever; if not, the fourth or fifth day put an end to all enquiry. *The treatment by full evacuation, of stomach and bowels.*

After procuring evacuation, I prescribed saline medicines, when little fever remained; but when the disease continued after the third day, it turned out to be the severest typhus. *Opium* or *bark* did not succeed; *when liberally given,* I perceived them *evidently doing mischief* (Journ., p. 139).

74 THE DOCTRINE OF PURGATION.

CLARK, THOMAS, Surg., *Observations on the Nature and Cure of Fevers and Diseases of the West and East Indies, and of America, &c.* Edinburgh, 1805. See MED. AND PHYS. JOURN., 1806, *Vol. XV.*

285. *Dysentery.*—Having, in violent cases, often found the remedies now described, or any others that I had tried, ineffectual, I at last had recourse to the use of emetic substances in the way of injections. I did not adopt these, however, till I had reflected very seriously and reasoned very fully on the subject. The other remedies already mentioned, except injections, were administered at the same time. From much experience I do not hesitate to assert that they have been, and, I believe I may venture to say, will be, found extremely beneficial in *dysentery.* It appears to me more than probable that they will also prove useful in cases of *piles,* and, in short, in *all kinds of inflammation affecting the rectum and parts adjoining.* When given early in the disease they generally afford immediate relief, and sometimes one or two injections effect a cure. When they have not been used until the advanced stages the patients experience more uneasiness from them, particularly on their first being thrown up; but if they can be prevailed upon to keep them for a minute or two, the uneasiness in a great measure ceases, and they are often able to retain them for a considerable length of time. The manner in which these injections operate is for the most part as follows:

In the incipient stages of the disease, even when attended with violent pain and tenesmus, and all the more violent symptoms of this disease, immediate relief is almost constantly experienced from them; and they are commonly retained for a considerable length of time with little or no uneasiness. At length an effort to go to stool comes on, and *several copious natural evacuations, mixed with mucous,* are procured; and *in the more violent cases* several *evacuations of slime, or mucous alone, or intermixed with blood, succeed to the natural stools,* accompanied with little or no straining. After this, the patient commonly remains for a number of hours without any symptoms of disease, and in some instances it does not return.

Those injections do not appear to occasion vomiting, or even to increase the irritability of stomach that may have previously existed. They probably assist in increasing perspiration, however. I do not believe that they operate very powerfully in that way; at least, in some cases, I have found it impossible to produce a copious perspiration by ipecacuanha, both in the form of injection, and also at the same time given by the mouth, in considerable quantities.

The salutary effects of these injections appear to me to depend chiefly upon their exciting *a copious secretion of mucous* from the internal coat of the great guts, and thereby removing the inflammation affecting them.

I have known a few ounces of this injection give immediate and permanent relief in several instances of very painful inflammatory affections about the extremity of the rectum; a copious secretion of mucous, resembling the white of eggs, being produced.

I generally have given two, and sometimes three, in the course of twenty-four hours. The best general rule, I believe, is to administer injections whenever the more violent symptoms of dysentery return, or threaten to do so.

Marginal notes: DYSENTERY. Enemas of emetic substances. Also in piles and inflammation of the rectum, &c. — The manner how they operate. — They increase the secretion of mucous and carry it off per anum, without producing vomiting, and remove the inflammation from the intestinal canal and rectum. — Their application.

Strangury, which frequently accompanies violent cases of dysentery, will be found very seldom troublesome when these injections are used; the reason why it is not so must appear obvious to every one. *Strangury removed by this injection.*

The form of injection which I have found to answer best has been about three drachms of ipecacuanha root, bruised, and boiled down in a quart of water to one pint, and given at once as a clyster. From ten to twenty grains of tartar emetic, dissolved in a pint of warm water, will produce nearly similar effects (Journ., pp. 85–87). *The preparation of the enema.*

Dysentery and Diarrhœa.—These affections of the bowels are Nature's efforts to expel diseased matters from the blood, and must never be suppressed; but nature must be assisted by a free use of Brandreth's Pills, which are absolutely certain to cure if used before the powers of life are exhausted.

Dr. Clark's method is vastly superior to opium or any of the astringent remedies so readily prescribed by the generality of medical men. But Brandreth's Pills are certain and commit no mistakes. If convenient, an ejection of pure water, about summer heat, will be found to comfort the bowels, but the cure depends upon purging the humors from the blood.

HAMILTON, JAMES, M. D., *Physician to the Royal Infirmary and various Hospitals in Edinburgh. Observations on the Utility and Administration of Purgative Medicines in Various Diseases. Edinburgh,* 1805, 8th edit., 1833.

2∙6. The history of medicine clearly shows that theory or reasoning has contributed in no small degree to impede its progress. *Theory RETARDS,*

Let it be our endeavor, by circumspect induction from facts, to establish sound principles which may lead to the discovery of other facts, and these again to the introduction of more general doctrines, or a comprehensive and connected theory of medicine (p. 21). *facts ADVANCE true medicine.*

2∙7. The nutritious part of our food is prepared and separated by the changes which it undergoes in the mouth, œsophagus, stomach, and, with the assistance of fluids secreted from the liver, pancreas, and spleen, is perfected in the smaller intestines; while the lacteal vessels, opening on their internal surface, absorb and convey the nutrimental fluid into the circulating system. The residue of the food, which is not adapted to afford nourishment, constitutes part of the fecal evacuation which is made directly from the intestinal canal (p. 21). *The mode of digestion. Functions of the stomach and intestines.*

288. This fecal residue is discharged into the more capacious colon, where the ilium enters it by a lateral opening, so contrived that the contents of the colon cannot be returned. This circumstance makes a distinction between the functions of the smaller and larger intestines, which is not commonly noticed. The former complete the preparation of the nourishment, and afford opportunity of its being absorbed; while the latter receive and detain the fecal part till after it has accumulated, and, perhaps, undergone certain changes, when it is voided in a given quantity and at stated intervals (p. 22). *The colon.* *The big and small intestines.*

289. *Besides, the intestines exhale and throw off fluids which have become noxious in consequence of changes which they undergo in the body.* The intestinal canal, therefore, serves the double purpose *of repairing waste and of preventing decay.* In this latter function, which I am solely to consider, the intestines co-operate with the other secretory *Double function of the intestines.*

organs, the skin, the lungs and kidney. All these organs have, in respect of this their common relation to the system, a dependence upon one another, and any of them will compensate, to a certain extent and for a limited time, the interrupted action of the others. Nevertheless, their full activity is necessary to the enjoyment of perfect health, and the continuance of life; and the regularity of the intestinal evacuation is connected in a particular manner with the well-being and healthy state of the stomach and intestines themselves. The urine and perspirable matter pass off immediately after being secreted, and do not load the organs which separate them. The unnatural detention of these excretions has indeed a more or less remote, and often fatal, effect upon the general system, but the skin and the kidney remain uninjured. It is otherwise with the intestines : secluded from that communication with the atmosphere by which the perspirable matter is carried off, and unprovided with an appendage resembling the urinary bladder connected with the kidneys, they are the reservoirs of fecal matter as it is poured out, which they retain till the accustomed period of evacuation comes round. Different circumstances are apt to induce irregularity in this evacuation; these, together with the facility with which the larger intestines admit of distension without uneasiness being excited, give frequent opportunity for a progressive accumulation of fæces, whence arise interrupted action of the stomach and smaller intestines, and consequent dangerous and fatal ailments (p. 22).

Vicarious function of organs.

Pretention of fecal matter causes disease; regulation necessary for health.

290. In infancy, the alvine evacuation is frequent, and the fæces are abundant and fluid. In mature years the body is generally moved once in twenty-four hours, and the fæces, although soft, preserve a form too well known to require description; they are of a yellow color, and they emit a peculiar odor. When, therefore, the fæces are evacuated less frequently than the age of a person demands; when they are indurated; when they change their natural color and odor, derangement of the stomach and bowels is indicated, and the approach of disease, if disease be not already formed, is to be apprehended. For it is not to be imagined that organs of so great importance in the animal economy as the stomach and bowels are, can be long in a state of inaction, and the general health remain unimpaired (p. 23).

Evacuations.— Their appearance indicative of either health or derangement of the bowels.

291. The *propulsion* of the contents of the intestines is effected by means of a vermicular, or, as it has been called, a peristaltic motion of the bowels from above downwards; hence torpor, or loss of tone in the muscular coat of the intestines, by which this motion is thought to be interrupted, is understood to be the cause of much distress, and tonic or stimulant medicines are employed to remedy this torpid state. I use this language, and speak of torpor of the bowels, although my ideas respecting it do not correspond with those of others. I am inclined to think that the symptoms referred to loss of tone proceed, in many occasions, more directly from the impeded peristaltic motion, the consequence of constipation. In this situation we may easily understand that the distended colon cannot, for want of space, receive the contents of the smaller intestines, which will of course stagnate throughout the whole canal; the action of which being thus interrupted, will soon altogether cease, and be at last inverted. The various ailments which

Peristaltic motion of the bowels, if interrupted by constipation, causes excrementitious accumulations producing disease. Its cure by purgation.

thence ensue, are daily before our eyes ; and the relief which, under these circumstances, we observe to follow soon after the exhibition of a purgative, and the cessation of complaint which takes place upon its operating freely by stool, are in proof that this opinion is well founded. *If, again, we farther consider that the greater part of the exhalations made into the cavity of the intestines is excrementitious, and will, if retained beyond the usual period, undergo changes and acquire injurious acrimony :* and if, moreover, we advert to the sympathy which many of the organs of the complicated animal frame have with the stomach and intestines, we cannot but recognize the great influence which these must possess over the comfort, the health, and the life of the individual (p. 24).

292. These are weighty considerations, and ought to excite our *attention to any irregularity of the alvine evacuation.* The necessity of this will farther appear when we reflect that many circumstances, unavoidable in social life, expose mankind in a peculiar manner to constipation ; *Constipation—its causes* such as improper food, intemperance, sedentary occupations in confined or otherwise tainted air. Besides, in a therapeutic view, we are encouraged to exercise this attention. It is admitted that diaphoretic and *Constant attention to the state of the digestion recommendable.* diuretic medicines employed to remedy interrupted secretion by the skin and kidney, operate circuitously, often possess deleterious qualities, or are uncertain and irregular in their effects ; while the means of removing constipation act directly on the seat of disease, are safe, and seldom disappoint us in the attainment of our object (p. 25).

293. In the dawn of physic, *purgatives* were employed. But, although they have been *recommended by the earlier as well as by later writers,* and although the indications they are meant to fulfill have been *The purgative method, however, ancient, not sufficiently appreciated.* an object of attention to the practitioners in all ages, yet I do not think that the extent of their utility has been always clearly perceived, or that their administration has been always properly directed (p. 27).

294. Another objection to the use of purgatives is urged with a force that seems to carry conviction along with it. It is observed that the *How to regulate the application of purgative medicines.* constant application of stimulating articles creates a habit not only of using them, but entails also the necessity of occasionally increasing their stimulating power. Habit or custom will indeed reconcile us to the impression produced by unusual stimuli, and will counteract their effect in such a manner, that if the stimulus be suddenly withdrawn, or, which is the same thing, be not gradually increased, the functions of the organ to which it had been applied will become languid and irregular. This law of the economy no doubt extends to the promiscuous use of purgatives given unnecessarily during the enjoyment of perfect health. In many instances, however, of disease, constipation and accumulation of fæces demand this stimulus to restore the healthy state of the intestines, and to promote the expulsion of their indurated contents. In proportion as these objects are accomplished, the stimulus from the same purgative becomes more and more powerful ; and so little is the necessity for continuing it, or for increasing its dose, that, on the contrary, were

not the activity of the purgative diminished, or were it not withdrawn altogether, as convalescence advances, we should be in danger of inducing weakness by an excess of purging (p. 29). (Cf. Hipp. 16.)

Purgation removes debility.

295. *Purgative medicines*, properly administered, *will not induce debility ; on the contrary*, the bowels being excited to propel their contents, their functions are restored, appetite and digestion improved, and the patient, so far from being weakened, is nourished, supported, and strengthened. (29.)

How excrementitious accumulated on are produced without much food, and purgation justified.

296. Purgative medicines have also been thought unnecessary on this account, that in many diseases little food is taken ; and, therefore, regular alvine evacuations are neither requisite nor to be expected. *The residue of food unfit for the purpose of nutrition contributes, no doubt, its share of feculent matter ; yet the abundant secretion from different organs, and the exhalation of excrementitious fluids made into the cavity of the intestines, constitute the bulk of the fæces collected within them.* So long, therefore, as fluid is supplied, and so long as the circulation is supported, it is equally easy to understand how fæces are produced, independently of much solid food, as to perceive the necessity of their daily evacuation during the course of fever, and of other diseases of long continuance (p. 30).

Typhus fever. Purgation cures, and why consonant to nature.

297. I refer the superior utility of *purgative medicines in typhus fever* to the circumstance of their *operating throughout the whole extent of the intestinal canal*, the healthy functions of which are essential to the recovery, in a manner that is consonant to the course of nature, by propelling its contents from above downwards, and to their moving and completely evacuating the feculent matter, which in this case becomes offensive and irritating (p. 35).

Purgation from begin-ning to end.

298. More extended experience confirmed these conjectures ; and I was gradually encouraged to give purgative medicines during the course of typhus from the commencement to the termination of the disease (ibid.)

Full purgation ; its beneficial effects.

299. I have directed a strict attention to this practice for a long time, and I am now thoroughly persuaded *that the full and regular evacuation of the bowels relieves the oppression of the stomach, cleans the louded and parched tongue, and mitigates thirst, restlessness, and heat of surface*, and that thus the later and more formidable impression on the nervous system is prevented, recovery more certainly and speedily promoted, and the danger of relapsing into fever much diminished (ibid.)

Purgation supersedes wine in re-moving de-bility.

300. For many years past I have found wine to be less necessary (in typhus fever) than I formerly thought. . . This chiefly attributed to the purgative medicines which I employed with freedom, obviating and removing symptoms of debility. This doctrine is at variance with that

which is commonly entertained, but I am confident it is consonant to the fact (p. 36).

301. The complete and regular evacuation of the bowels, in the course of *fever*, is the object to be obtained (ibid.)

Purgation the thing needful in fever.

302. The *early exhibition of purgatives* relieves the first symptoms, prevents the accession of more formidable ones, and thus *cuts short the disease* (p. 37).

Early purgation an axiom.

303. I had learned that *the symptoms of debility* which take place *in typhus fever*, so far from being increased, *were obviously relieved by the evacuation of the bowels*. I have never in *scarlatina*, in a long course of experience, witnessed sickness and fainting, which some authors have so much dreaded; neither have I observed revulsion from the surface of the body and premature fading, or, in common language, "striking in" of the efflorescence, to follow the exhibition of purgatives (p. 45).

Accordingly no variety of the disease has hitherto prevented me from following out this practice to the extent which I have found necessary (p. 46).

Purgation relieves debility in typhus; cures scarlet fever, and causes no striking in.

304. Purgative medicines are useful in removing *dropsical swellings* the consequence of scarlatina, when the weakness of the patient is often very great. Purgatives also afford a means of preventing this swelling, and other derangements of health (ibid.)

Dropsical swelling prevented and removed by purgation.

305. When I consider the languor and lassitude which precede *marasmus*, instead of adopting the common opinion of its being occasioned by worms, I am more disposed to think that a *torpid state*, or *weakened action of the alimentary canal*, is *the immediate cause* of the disease. From this proceed *costiveness, distention of the bowels, and a peculiar irritation, the consequence of remora of the fæces;* and I have accordingly been long in the habit of employing *purgative medicines for the cure of marasmus;* the object is to remove indurated and fœtid fæces, the accumulation perhaps of months, and as this object is accomplishing, the gradual return of appetite and vigor mark the progress of recovery (p. 59).

Marasmus from torpid bowels, consequent diseases and their cure by purgatives.

306. *Epilepsy*, than which no disease is so afflicting to the patient, is frequently the effect of particular irritation of the mind or body. Practitioners enumerate worms in the intestines, or marasmus, among the causes of epilepsy. Surely this will induce us, *on the first attack* of epilepsy in children, arising from an uncertain cause, to *set on foot the most decided and active course of purgative medicines*, lest we peradventure allow the disease to strike root, while we are idly employed in the exhibition of inert and useless vermifuge medicines, or are groping in the dark in quest of other causes of the disease, or of uncertain remedies for their removal (pp. 63, 64).

Epilepsy.

Purging the first step to be taken.

Chlorosis.

Fearful results of costiveness.

307. *Chlorosis.*—The slightest attention to the history of the disease evinces that *costiveness precedes and accompanies* the other symptoms. *Costiveness induces the feculent odor of the breath, disordered stomach, loss of appetite, and impaired digestion.* These preclude a sufficient supply of nourishment at a period of growth when it is most wanted; *hence paleness, laxity, flaccidity, the nervous symptoms, wasting of the muscular flesh, languor, debility, the retention of the menses, the suspension of other secretions, serous effusions, dropsy, and death* (p. 71).

Women require full purgation more than men.

308. The *greater capacity* of the female pelvis gives more room for that part of the intestinal canal which is contained within it to dilate, and, of course, *to admit of greater accumulation of feculent matter,* which, *in proportion to its remora,* becomes more and more abundant, and more impacted. Hence *costiveness is more obstinate,* and *chlorosis and other diseases originating in costiveness,* are more severe and are *of more difficult cure in the female* than the male (p. 72).

To escape failure purge freely and fearlessly.

INSPECT THE STOOLS.

309. Great attention and assiduity is requisite in the exhibition of purgative medicines in *chlorosis,* and the frequency of its repetition must be varied according to circumstances, which can only be ascertained by the *inspection of the " alvine egesta."* The practitioner who is not aware of this, and who, yielding to the importunity of his patients, or the caprice of their relations, does not steadily pursue his plan of cure, will be disappointed, his abilities will be called in question, and his practice vilified and neglected (p. 73).

Hysteria and all its symptoms removed by purgation.

The purgative irritation soon subsides.

310. The symptoms (of hysteria) undoubtedly denote a preternatural *affection of the stomach and alimentary canal.* In my opinion they afford conclusive evidence that this affection is primary, and that the other multifarious symptoms of hysteria depend upon it (p. 87). The first purgatives that we use may seem on some occasions to aggravate the symptoms, but the practice must not be deserted on that account. The *additional irritation which purgatives may give in the first instance soon passes away, and perseverance in the use of them removes* that irritation which gave rise to *the disease,* which, of course, *disappears in proportion as the bowels are relieved* of the oppressive mass of accumulated fæces (p. 88).

St. Vitus' dance.

Let the purgation be a continued action.

Small doses dangerous; large doses and perseverance successful.

311. *St. Vitus' Dance.*—*Powerful purgatives must be given in successive doses,* in such manner *that the latter doses may support the effect of the former,* till the movement and expulsion of the accumulated matter are effected, when symptoms of returning health appear. Whoever undertakes the cure of chorea by purgative medicines must be decided and firm to his purpose. The confidence which he assumes is necessary to carry home to the friends of the patient conviction of ultimate success. Their prejudices will otherwise throw insurmountable obstacles in his way. Half measures in instances of this kind will prove unsuccessful, and were it not for *perseverance in unloading the alimentary canal,* the disease would be prolonged, would place the patient in danger, and thus bring into discredit a practice which promises certain safety (p. 97).

312. The agonizing spasms, the prominent symptoms of *tetanus*, have arrested the notice of every one. *To resolve the spasm and to cure the disease* have been conceived to be *one and the same thing.* Accordingly, opium, musk, warm bathing, cold bathing, and mercury, have been employed in tetanus. But have they mitigated the severity of tetanus or obviated its fatal tendency? " The records of physic bear a sad testimony in the negative." However just these observations may be, I should yet have been sorry to have advanced anything to shake the tottering fabric of medical practice in tetanus unless I thought it had been in my power to substitute one more efficacious, originating in other views of the disease. These views, I apprehend, will warrant the expectation of *considerable benefit from the full and free exhibition of purgative medicines* (pp. 107, 108).

Tetanus cannot be cured by " antispasmodics," but by free and full purgation.

" The tottering fabric of medical practice."

313. Under the impression which I entertain of the utility of purgative medicines, and of the *inefficiency of the tonic plan* of treatment in tetanus, no doubt remains with me respecting the mode of attempting the cure of *hydrophobia*, which has *hardly* in any instance *yielded to the most powerful antispasmodics. Purgatives* are proposed to *remove a cause which frequently induces, and which may always aggravate spasmodic affections* (p. 123).

Hydrophobia. Antispasmodics useless—PURGE.

314. *Palpitation of the heart* merits particular notice in this place. I have witnessed the *efficacy of purgative medicines* in the most forbidding and apparently desperate instances of the ailment, in so much, that I am not now disposed to despair of any case, till I am satisfied that purgative medicines have been fully employed, and employed in vain (p. 122).

Palpitation of the heart. The worst cases cured.

315. I am persuaded that *the preservation of regularity in the alvine evacuation*, will at all times *prevent the accession of* those *diseases* (previously enumerated). If these expectations be not too sanguine, it is likely that the marasmus and chlorosis, the vomiting of blood, chorea, and hysteria, of which I have spoken, will rarely, if ever, appear. It is fitting, therefore, that this observation should be widely spread, that it should be conveyed to mothers and nurses, to superintendents of nurseries, of manufactories, and of boarding-schools, and to all instructors and protectors of children and young people, and strongly impressed on their minds, by such of their medical advisers as think with me, and who will acknowledge that to *prevent disease is the paramount duty* (p. 125). (Cf. Sanctorius, Aph. 1., Sect. I.)

AN APPEAL TO ALL CLASSES: " Keep the bowels regular and thus prevent all forms of disease.

316. The practice which leads to this conclusion (the free use of purgatives in the case of diseases), is presented in a simple form. It is neither disguised by hypothesis, nor obscured by the simultaneous employment of various remedies. At the same time it is supported by proofs of unquestionable authenticity, which are not surpassed by any in the records of medicine. On these accounts, the truth or fallacy of my opinions may be easily investigated, and an adequate judgment of them

The purgative plan justified— the proofs irrefragable.

readily formed (p. 114). Here follow upwards of fifty cases of cure in various diseases, extracted from the records of the Royal Infirmary.

317. The *steady exhibition of purgative medicines* is absolutely necessary to the success of the practice *in chronic diseases.* The puny state of the sufferer may on some occasions excite alarm in the breast of the practitioner; and the caprice of his patient, and the whims of relatives, may oppose obstacles to his conducting the cure in the most advantageous manner. But these he must disregard; for unless he can suppress his own improper feelings, and overcome the unreasonable objections of others, he had better not adopt *measures* which, *to prove successful, must be conducted with firmness.* A contrary conduct will necessarily terminate in the vexation of the practitioners, in the disappointment of the patient and of his relatives, and in the discredit of that practice which it has been my wish and study to recommend (pp. 124, 125).

(margin note: Chronic diseases require the fullest purgation.)
(margin note: Half measures bring discredit on the cause.)

318. Diseased actions depend on the nature of the impressions, the parts on which they are made, and on the constitution of the patient. The same impression applied to different parts of the body may produce different actions; cold to the extremities producing chilblains, or gangrene; to the head catarrh; to the chest cough or pleurisy (p. 125).

(margin note: Location determines the nature of the disease.)

319. To conclude, the reader must have observed the beneficial effects of purgative medicines, in diseases apparently different, and incident to people at various periods of life. The facts are undeniable, and serve to prove the extent and importance of the subject; but of these I do not feel it to be incumbent on me to give any explanation at present. Such an attempt might be premature. I am satisfied to have established certain leading facts, and to have opened views which, if properly prosecuted, must give an opportunity to extend our knowledge respecting the utility and administration of purgative medicines. It will then be time to generalize the facts, and to form a system of medical doctrines at once clear and comprehensive, and thence to deduce practical precepts useful in proportion as they will be simple and precise. WHEN THESE EXPECTATIONS ARE FULFILLED, OUR POSTERITY MAY SEE DECEPTIVE REASONING, HOW INGENIOUS SOEVER, BANISHED FROM THE SCHOOLS OF MEDICINE, AND FROM THE PRACTICE OF THE HEALING ART A MULTIFARIOUS PRESCRIPTION OF INERT AND NAUSEOUS MEDICINES (pp. 125, 126).

(margin note: Facts alone establish reliable science.)
(margin note: Practical experience must supersede theoretical schemes, and simple remedies the rubbish of the materia medica.)

IMPORTANT SERIES.

McMULLIN, JOAN, M. D., *On the treatment of Chorea Sti. Viti, by purgatives. See* EDINB. MED. AND SURG. JOURN., 1805, *Vol. I.*

320. Many *diseases of symptomatic debility*, which have *resisted* the use of *tonics*, have either been considered as incurable, or our failure has been ascribed, not to our pursuing an erroneous method of treatment, but to our means having been too feeble, or employed too late; and obstinately persisting in the tonic plan, on each succeeding occasion,

(margin note: The tonic plan a failure.)

we push it with greater vigor and with the same want of success. There are, however, fortunately, practitioners who act more philosophically, and regarding with distrust theories which do not stand the test of experience, endeavour to advance the science of medicine by the slow but sure method of observation and induction. It is in this way that we sometimes find a disease yielding to a plan of treatment diametrically opposite to that which the established opinions concerning its nature would have suggested (p. 25).

321. With the view of alleviating the sufferings of those laboring under similar complaints, and of correcting the erroneous ideas entertained of the nature of the disease, I am induced to publish some observations which occurred to me in consequence of having witnessed the cure of some cases of *Chorea Sancti Viti* in the Royal Infirmary of this place (Edinburgh). In these cases, a mode of treatment was adopted which no opinion of the disease hitherto published seemed to authorize ; although *in every instance* it was attended with the *most marked advantages.* This treatment consisted in the *repeated frequent exhibition of drastic purgatives,* which will appear on perusing the following cases *not to have had the effect of debilitating still more* an apparently debilitated system ; but on the contrary, *during their employment the patient recovered strength,* the involuntary motions gradually abated, and *by persisting in this treatment* for a short time, *a perfect cure was effected.* What is particularly worthy of observation, is *the appearance of the alvine discharges,* which *in every instance was black and fetid* (p. 26). Here follow five cases.

St. Vitus' dance.

Cure by drastic purgatives;— they do not debilitate, but strengthen.

322. From these cases, the following facts seem to be established :
1. From the exhibition of *even two or three cathartics,* the *involuntary motions* and other symptoms were *much abated.*
2. Although the *cathartics were continued daily for a considerable length of time,* the patient, instead of becoming more debilitated, *became stronger* and walked with a firmer pace.
3. During the progress of the cure, *if* at any time *the cathartics did not produce* an evacuation, the involuntary motions *recurred,* and all the symptoms were *aggravated.*
4. The fæces *before* the exhibition of the cathartics, were *small in quantity,* required a *large dose* of the purgatives, and *in every instance were black and fetid.* And lastly,
5. When the disease was *cured,* the appearance of the *fæces became natural* (p. 30).

General advantages from purgation.

323. Upon the whole, the connection of the disease with the state of the intestinal discharges seems evident ; and as in all the five cases *fetid, dark-colored evacuations preceded the cure,* it would appear that, *with them, the cause* of the disease was *removed.* We may, therefore, legitimately conclude that the *involuntary motions, debility,* and other symptoms,, were in these cases *produced by local irritation in the bowels,* which was *afterwards communicated to the whole system,* through the medium of the nerves (p. 31).

Disease from intestinal impurities.

324. All systematic writers have considered *chorea* as *a disease of debility,* and the same opinion has been almost universally adopted by practical physicians, who, seeing their patients laboring under evident debility, have ransacked the whole materia medica for *tonics and antispasmodics.* *Under this treatment,* chorea has always been considered *very difficult to cure.* Now, when we compare the frequent failures of the tonic plan of cure with the invariable success of the purgative, we must conclude, in direct opposition to the hypothetical dogma of *Brown,* that the *symptoms of chorea do not depend primarily on debility,* but that the *debility is merely symptomatic of the disease.* But in whatever manner the phenomena of these cases may affect the theory of the disease, they establish incontrovertibly a much more important conclusion —*that it yields readily to the repeated and continued use of drastic purgatives* (pp. 33, 34).

[margin: The tonic and purgative plans compared. •]

ABERNETHY, JOHN, M. D., *Surgical Observations on the Constitutional Origin and Treatment of Local Diseases.* London, 1806. *Eighth Edit.,* 1826.

325. That *the stomach and bowels are disordered by injuries and diseases of the parts of the body* has been remarked by various persons; but the subject has never been extensively surveyed, nor viewed with that accuracy of observation which its high importance merits. It has been observed that sprains of tendinous or ligamentous parts produce sudden sickness; and *Mr. Hunter* has attributed that shivering which is consequent to accidents, and attendant on some diseases, to the state of the stomach. It is known that in some local injuries from accident or operations, the stomach has appeared to be the part principally affected. But remarks on the affections thus induced in the digestive organs have been made only in a cursory manner. . . . It also appears to me, that *the connection of local diseases with* the state of *the constitution in general* is either *not sufficiently understood,* or *not duly regarded by the generality of practitioners* (p. 5).

[margin: Sympathy between the viscera and other parts of the body.]

326. The operation for *hernia* (in a certain case) was followed by general disorder of the system, manifested by a full and strong pulse, furred tongue, great anxiety, restlessness, and total want of sleep. The stomach was particularly affected, being distended, uneasy on compression, and rejecting everything that was swallowed. He was bled largely in the evening, and took saline medicines, but could not be prevailed upon to swallow anything else except some toast and water. The sickness had in some degree abated on the next day, a solution of sulphate of magnesia in mint-water was prescribed, in small doses, given at regular intervals, in order to relieve the disorder and distension of the stomach by procuring discharges from the bowels. In the course of the day the salts were administered which were not rejected by the stomach; yet he could scarcely be prevailed upon to take anything else. The tongue was still covered with a thick yellow fur; the skin was hot and dry, and the pulse frequent. As there was no particular tenderness about the epigastric region, he was not again bled. The second night was passed without sleep. As the salts had produced no effect, the same

[margin: Hernia from accumulation of fetid matter—advantage of perseverance in the purgative plan.]

medicine was ordered in an infusion of senna, with the addition of some of its tincture, which by being given in very small doses, was retained. When, however, it seemed likely that no effect would result from this medicine, a grain of calomel was given at night, and repeated on the following morning. Still the loathing of food continued. The third night passed like the former ones without sleep, and in great anxiety. On the next morning two pills, containing five grains of the pil. colocynth and the same quantity of the pil. aloes cum myrrha, were given every fourth hour. They procured no stool, nor produced any sensation which inclined the patient to believe they would operate. Again he passed a sleepless night, but toward the morning he felt his bowels apparently filling, to use his own expression, and a profuse discharge ensued. *A dozen copious, fetid and black evacuations took place between five and ten o'clock, and he had several others in the course of the day;* after which *his appetite returned,* his *tongue became clean,* and a *sound and pleasant sleep succeeded,* from which he awoke apparently well (pp. 7–10).

327. It is most probably the *disorder of the brain first affects the stomach;* but the reaction of the latter affection is liable to increase and maintain the former, by which it had itself been produced. The effects that result from the *sympathy of the whole constitution with local disorder* vary greatly both in nature and degree (p. 8). I could relate numerous cases in support of the inference, that local irritation acting on the nervous system may affect the digestive organs in a very serious manner, and thereby create great disorder of the whole constitution, which is afterward alleviated in proportion to the amendment that ensues in the state of those viscera. Such cases of great local irritation must frequently occur to every. one; it is, therefore, unnecessary to adduce more instances to support the opinions here delivered (p. 12). *The whole system sympathizes with its every part.*

328. With respect to the *treatment* of cases of this description, it may be right to add, that *the primary object* should be *to produce secretion from the irritable organs.* In the case which has been related, and in many others recorded in this volume, the effect of secretions from the disordered organs in relieving their irritable state is very manifest. In many instances *opium will not prevent the continual efforts to vomit,* yet *when* by sulphate of magnesia, or *purgatives administered in the form of pills and clysters, stools are procured,* the *vomiting ceases,* the stomach retains both food and medicine, and general tranquillity of constitution is as suddenly restored (p. 13). *Spontaneous vomiting not to be cured by opium but by purgatives.*

329. A slighter degree of disorder occurs in the advanced stages of *lumbar abscesses, diseased joints, compound fractures,* and all kinds of local disease, which impart considerable and continued irritation to the whole constitution. We also find a less important disease, as, for instance, a *fretful ulcer,* keep up a disorder of the system in general, and of the digestive organs in particular, which subsides as the irritable state of the ulcer diminishes (p. 17). *Every external disease in connection with the digestive organs.*

330. If the *brain and nervous system* should be disordered, *without* any apparent *local disease,* similar derangements may be expected to take place in the functions of the digestive organs (p. 18). *The nervous system and the digestive organs.*

Thorough examination of the patient necessary.
"Restlessness and nervousness" from disordered digestion.

331. *Patients commonly declare* that they are in good health, except that they feel disturbed by their local complaints; yet they are found, on inquiry, to have all the symptoms which characterize a disordered state of the digestive organs. The mind is frequently irritable and despondent; anxiety and languor are expressed in the countenance. The pulse is frequent or feeble, and slight exercise produces considerable fatigue and perspiration. The patients are sometimes restless at night, but when they sleep soundly they awaken unrefreshed, with lassitude, and sometimes a sensation as if they were incapable of moving. Slight noises generally cause them to start, and they are, to use their own expression, "very nervous." These circumstances seem to indicate weakness and irritability of the nervous and muscular systems, which, in addition to the disorder of the digestive organs, are the chief circumstances observable relative to the general health. *By correcting the obvious errors in the state of the digestive organs*, by the judicious administration of purgatives, *local diseases*, which had baffled all attempts at cure by local means, *have speedily been removed*, and the patient has acknowledged that such an alteration has taken place in his general health as greatly excited his surprise (pp. 21, 22).

Imperfect digestion—various effects: produces gas; impoverishes the blood; disorders the brain, the muscular system, &c.; i. e. causes local diseases.

332. When *digestion is imperfect, gaseous fluids* are extricated from the alimentary matters. Vegetable food becomes acid, and oils become rancid. *Uneasy sensations* are also felt, and undigested aliment may be found in the fæces (p. 24).

Imperfect digestion *must influence the qualities of the blood*, and all parts of the body may be affected from this source (p. 65).

Disorders of the digestive organs may produce, in the nervous system, a diminution of the functions of the brain, even so as to produce *apoplexy* and *hemiplegia* (p. 70). It may produce, in the muscular system, *weakness, tremors, and palsy*, or the contrary affection of *spasms and convulsions*. It may excite *fever*, by disturbing the action of the sanguiferous system, and cause various *local diseases*, by the nervous irritation which it produces, and by the weakness which is consequent on nervous disorders or imperfect chylification (pp. 71, 72).

Indigestion or constipation—further effects of.

333. Being in a warm and moist place, the undigested food will undergo those chemical changes natural to dead vegetable and animal matter; the *vegetable food will ferment and become acid, the animal will grow rancid and putrid*. . . These effects must continually take place, *unless*, by the digestive power of the stomach, *the food is converted into a new substance* which is not liable to these chemical changes. Such irritating compounds cannot fail to be detrimental to the whole tract of the alimentary canal. Part of the food thus changed will be absorbed from the bowels and render the blood impure, from which there is no outlet for various kinds of matter but through the kidneys, and this may prove a cause of foul urine, as well as of the presence of many substances in that fluid not natural to it (pp. 74, 75).

All purgatives are not equally efficient.

334. Persons may be *purged without having their bowels cleared* of the fecal matter which may be detained in them. We should therefore endeavor to ascertain what kind or combination of purgative medicine will excite a healthy action of the bowels (p. 89).

335. The *principle* that should govern our conduct in the adminis- *How to re-gulate the administra-tion of pur-gatives.* tration of purgatives may be briefly stated ; *the excitement is to be repeated till the requisite action is induced,* yet no single excitement being such as may prove an irritant to the organs (ibid.)

336. I am aware that laxative medicines may relieve irritation merely by augmenting the natural secretions of the viscera, and thus unloading *Laxative medicines—their effect.* their vessels ; and also by determining the fluids from the head, when the nervous symptoms are aggravated by a plenitude of the vessels of the brain. As I have found *the lenient plan of treatment*—that of ex- *The lenient plan.* citing the peristaltic action of the bowels, so as to induce them to clear out the whole of their contents, without irritating them (so as to produce what is ordinarily called purging), particularly successful—I have rarely deviated from it. I am not, therefore, warranted from experience in speaking decisively respecting the more free use of purgative medicines (pp. 90, 91).

337. The most judicious treatment will not remedy the disease if the *Disease cannot be cured while its cause continues.* exciting causes continue to operate—*such as improprieties of diet, agitation of mind, sedentary habits, or impure air* (p. 96).

338. It is necessary to the cure of disorder, *first,* that the stomach should thoroughly digest all the food that is put into it; *secondly,* that *What is necessary for cure?* the residue of the food should be daily discharged from the bowels (pp. 99, 100).

339. The profuse discharges which sometimes follow the continued exhibition of purgatives consist of morbid secretions from the bowels *Character of evacua-tions.* themselves, and not of the residue of alimentary matter detained in those organs (p. 35).
The *stools, which resemble pitch,* are principally composed of diseased secretions *from the internal surface* of the intestines (p. 36).

340. All the experience which I have had relative to the treatment *Tetanus from consti-pation.* of *tetanus* (locked-jaw) has convinced me that *more benefit is obtained by correcting the errors of the digestive organs than by any other means.* It *Purgation necessary in all external lesions.* may be useful to mention one case as a striking proof of this fact : A man who had been wounded in the foot, was brought about ten days after the accident to the hospital, and so violent and general were the spasms that it was scarcely expected he could be taken to his bed alive. The jaw was fast clenched, and the muscles of his back and belly rigid ; convulsive actions came on frequently, and then all his limbs were violently affected. His bowels had not been relieved for many days. When, after twenty hours, his bowels were purged, the discharges were not like faeces, and so extremely offensive that the patient could not stay in the ward. From this time, however, there was a complete subsidence of the spasm, and the *patient recovered* seemingly *in proportion as the digestive organs regained their healthy functions* (p. 130).

341. A female patient, about twenty-seven years of age, was lately *Paralysis from neg-lected sta 6* admitted into the hospital for *paralysis of the arm,* which had come on *of the bow-els; cure by* suddenly. She complained of much pain when pressure was made along

the outer margin of the scalene muscles, where the nerves emerge that

cont'nued purgation. form the axillary plexus. Her *digestive organs were greatly disordered,* and, in one week, *by means that could only operate directly on those organs,* she regained the use of her arm (p. 132).

A gentleman of the medical profession, whose digestive organs had been long disordered, suddenly lost the use of his right arm, without any apparent disturbance of the cerebrum. A professional friend asserting that the *paralysis* was *a consequence of the disorder of the digestive organs,* the patient promised strictly to adhere to any course of medicine that his friend would prescribe. The only medicines ordered were pills, containing two grains of calomel, at night, and purges on the following morning, for one week. The bowels were cleared daily. On the sixth day, however, *several copious, dark-colored and offensive discharges* took place, and *the patient immediately regained the use of his arm* (p. 132).

BLEGBOROUGH, HENRY, Surg., *On Chronic Croup. London,* 1806. *See* MED. AND PHYS. JOURN., 1806, *Vol. XV.*   •

Chronic croup Purge re-move the cause. 342. When the disease has subsided some days there is generally thick and short breathing, with heat of skin and frequent pulse; but as these symptoms are always relieved by a calomel purge, I conclude they are produced by loaden bowels. Being removed, they always in a few days return, and are, by the same means, again and again relieved (Journ., p. 509).

BRADLEY, JAMES, Surg., *On Hernia. Huddersfield,* 1806. *See* MED. AND PHYS. JOURN., 1806, *Vol. XVI.*

Hernia. Purgatives useful as cooling sed-atives, re-moving the irritation in the primæ viæ, and pro-moting the reduction. 343. *Mr. Bradley* gives seven cases of hernia in patients of different ages, sexes and constitutions, demonstrating his method of employing the taxis in inguinal or scrotal hernia. Generally costiveness precedes the hernia, and vomiting accompanies it. On the employment of pur-gative medicines he says:

In case seventh, the *cathartic solution* was administered from evident symptoms of enteritis; and here, as well as in case first, where this medicine was administered, *I could not perceive* any of those *unpleasant effects* ascribed to purgatives in general. The small quantity taken into the stomach not proving sufficient to increase the disorder of that organ, and the position in which the patients were placed, might tend, perhaps, in some measure to obviate any increased distress arising in that quarter. I gave this medicine, not with a view of obtaining any laxative effects, but as *a cooling sedative,* calculated *to abate irritation in the first pas-sages, under the circumstances of a quick pulse, considerable thirst, and great pain in the abdomen.* I was led to adopt this remedy in prefer-ence, from observing its good effects in enteritis, and in obstinate con-stipations of the bowels attended with *colic,* which *I have seen it fre-quently remove,* BEFORE ANY LAXATIVE EFFECTS *have been produced* Journ., p. 48).

MORGAN, CHARLES, M. D., *On the Use of Purgative Medicines. See* EDINB. MED. AND. SURG. JOURN., *Vol. II.,* 1806.

Purgation removes de-bility. 344. *Debility* is itself *an effect of disease,* and, *when the disease is removed, the strength and vigor* of the system will *return.* Have we not often seen the debility which attends some of the complaints of infancy removed, as well as the disease of which it was a symptom, by *evacuating the bowels ;* and *nausea,* and *anorexia,* with all the depressing symptoms of *dyspepsia,* how often *alleviated by a brisk purgative ?* (p. 100).

345. If we would follow out this practice on general principles, we must ⬤late the whole effect of our remedies. Sometimes we empty the bowels simply; at others we promote an increased secretion of fluids by purgative medicines. In some cases it appears sufficient to unload the bowels of their contents accumulated by long retention, and thereby relieve the system from the effects of this local irritation ; but in others, and especially in those in which a freer and more continued purging becomes necessary before the symptoms yield, we *bring off not only the contents of the bowels* which are out of the course of circulation, we eliminate also the secretory organs which terminate in the *intestinal canal—the obstruction, torpor, or deranged actions of which may have been a chief cause of the morbid actions of other parts of the system* (ibid.) *Effects of various degrees of purgation.*

346. We are surely authorized to make this inference from cases in which the purging is continued for weeks, to the exhibition of three or four stools daily, with *progressive relief* of the morbid symptoms, with improved looks and strength, and at length followed by the perfect cure of a complicated disease. In other cases we find the *cure advancing with the discharge of fetid stools of a bilious appearance, or black and greenish color* (p. 101). *In proportion as the morbid matters are discharged, so health is restored.*

347. Having been an eye-witness of *Dr. Hamilton's* practice, I could not avoid being struck with its *simplicity and success,* and adopting it as my own. Much dissatisfaction may have arisen among practitioners, from the unwillingness of patients to submit to a repetition of purgatives, who all esteem purging a debilitating operation, and think themselves " far too nervous " to undergo it with impunity. Many too, I believe, are disappointed in their hopes of cure, by stopping short of the wished-for point (ibid 1807, vol. III. p. 144). *The danger is in not purging sufficiently.*

348. Both these evils may arise from a neglect on the part of the medical adviser. I mean, not inspecting the stools. If the practitioner be too much an " emunctæ nariæ homo " to submit to such a drudgery, let him go on trusting to remedies that have long failed, or rather let him lay aside the practice of medicine altogether. It is *only by daily inspection of the stools* that *the purging can be regulated ;* for, *as long as they exhibit* MORBID APPEARANCES, SO LONG ARE PURGATIVES NECESSARY, *and no longer.* *Always examine the stools.*
When the stools are not seen, *the patient conceives that he is discharging far more* than you are aware of, and more than his constitution can bear. By an earnest inquiry after them and a strict injunction that the whole may be saved, together with an occasional appeal to the patient, whether such matters can remain in the body with impunity, I have never failed in inducing a cheerful submission to the plan, and the pa-

tient at last looks for the repetition of the doses as a sure relief from the misery he is suffering. Having premised these remarks, which arise from the objections of several medical friends, I proceed to the relation of two cases, not picked out as proving more than others, but as exhibiting the obstinacy of the disease, and the ultimate advantages derived from a steady perseverance in the purgative plan (p. 145). Here follow the cases:

WALSH, E., M. D. *An account of a malignant fever, which appeared in the Garrison of Quebec during the Autumn of* 1805, *with some preliminary observations on the diseases of the Canadas.* London, 1806. *See* MED. AND PHYS. JOURN. 1806, *vol. XV.*

Lake fever. Emetic and brisk purges. 349. *Lake Fever.*—The cure of this fever is not less easy and certain at its commencement, than difficult in its advanced stages. An antimonial emetic, followed by a brisk purge, with attention to regimen for two or three days, seldom failed of curing it on the access. But if this was neglected, and the disease far advanced, such a torpor of the system was induced as frequently rendered ineffectual the most active medicines (Journ., p. 448).

Dr. Walsh characterizes the malignant fever at Quebec exactly like Mr. Bennion describes the fever at Gibraltar, and has employed the same remedies against it; confer, therefore, Bennion on the Gibraltar Fever (Journ., pp. 451-453).

CHEYNE, J., M. D. *Observations on the Effect of Purgative Medicines.* London, 1808. *See* EDINB. MED. AND SURG. JOURN., 1808, *vol. IV.*

Fits and inability to walk cured by purgatives. 350. *Case of a youth who, in consequence of a fall, was subject for a year to most distressing fits, intense pains, etc., and who, in consequence, had lost the power of walking.* (Case given.) This boy in about two months was restored to health. During this period he used a great quantity of strong cathartic medicine. A scruple of aloes and ten grains of gamboge were given daily for several weeks before his stools became natural; and as his stools became large, loose and natural, the fits left him and he recovered the use of his limbs. About the end of my attendance, when his bowels were acting more naturally, one pill of the same kind, of which it before required sometimes ten to produce the desired effect, was a sufficient dose (pp. 310, 311).

In this case our practice is supported by analogies drawn from the successful treatment of other diseases where, along with *convulsions* or *spasmodic affections*, we have also been able to detect a great degree of foulness in the bowels. It is in compliance with a common idiom that I use the expression of foulness of the bowels. I am persuaded that such a state cannot, with any propriety, be said to exist. Take the *slow infantile remittent* of *Dr. Batter*, or the *marasmus* of *Dr. Hamilton*—we have a train of symptoms supposed to be induced by foulness of the bowels; and the appellation seems to be countenanced by what is observed during the cure, the effects of the *purging medicines* employed. *By these medicines stools are procured, at first dark, slimy*

Spasmodic affections.

Infantile remittent, marasmus.

Fetid stools.

and fetid, which perhaps, for a considerable time, have nothing of the appearance of natural fæces; the evacuations seem merely a collection of vitiated secretions, but *at last, by pursuing the purgative plan, large* natural *stools* are evacuated, and it is generally supposed that these stools have been all the while lodged in the intestines, *and that our medicines were not powerful enough at once to expel them—that the disease was solely from an accumulation of fecal matter* (p. 312).

Powerful purgation.

351. But the fact is, that *these critical stools are produced by the restoration of the viscera to a healthy condition.* The purgative medicine employed is useful, not so much by *removing the accumulations,* but that *it stimulates the bowels.* By the steady application of this stimulus *the visceral functions are restored.* The bilious and slimy stools are expelled, the light food is concocted, and from the fecal residuum, with the increased supply of gall, of gastric and pancreatic fluids, and the secretions from the large intestines, in consequence of the *renovation of the organs* supplying these fluids, the large natural stools are produced and the disease resolved. Were the bowels in a healthy condition, they would be acted upon by what at all other times is their natural stimulus, and, consequently, they would not admit of this supposed accumulation. If there be accumulation, the torpid state of the intestines is the cause of it; but the disease may exist without any accumulation whatever (p. 312).

Critical evacuations by stool.

Critical or fetid stools indicate removal of disease and return of healthy action.

352. In *dysentery,* where hardened fæces are lodged in the bowels, we see a constant succession of unsatisfactory stools, and of these stools the hard fæces or scybala would seem often to be the cause. For, it is observed by every practical writer, that when, by proper purgatives, the scybala are evacuated, there is immediately a remission of the most urgent symptoms, in particular of the tenesmus, and frequent mucous stools (p. 313).

Dysentery from scybala.

353. *Hydrocephalus.*—The cure. The *exhibition of the largest dose* which can be safely prescribed *of some powerful cathartic medicine,* two, three, or four times a day; and *this* continued for several days, or until natural stools are produced. The advantage of keeping *the intestinal canal under the continual influence of a stimulus,* I have, in various instances, found to be so great, that I am induced to repeat the declaration of my belief, that the happiest result may be expected from this measure. (*Essay on Hydrocephalus Acutus,* Edinb., 1808; ibid., p. 346.)

Water in the brain— cure by the fullest purgation.

GAY, M., M. D., *An Essay on the Nature and Treatment of Apoplexy. Paris,* 1808. *Translated by Ed. Copeman, Surg., with an Appendix. London,* 1843. *See* BRIT. AND FOR. MED. REV., 1843, *Vol. XVI.*

354. This treatise proves that *bleeding is injurious in all cases of apoplexy,* and that the primary cause is always to be found in the primæ viæ; that *purgatives are indicated in every case,* except when the attack follows a full meal, when emetics should be first administered (Rev., 272).

Apoplexy. Never bleed, but purge.

HALLIDAY, ANDREW, M. D., *On Epilepsy. Blandford*, 1808. *See* MED.
AND PHYS. JOURN., 1808, *Vol. XIX.*

Epilepsy from worms.

355. Case given of a girl of five years old who was subject to fits with violent contraction of the limbs, had an unnaturally voracious and depraved appetite, and could articulate but very few words, however she understood what was said to her.

Continued purgation removes the cause by carrying off accumulation of morbid matter in the intestines.

Upon an attentive consideration of this case, it occurred to me that purgatives were likely to be of service, and from my intimate acquaintance with the practice of that justly-celebrated physician, *Dr. Hamilton*, of Edinburgh, I entered upon the treatment with great confidence, and did not hesitate to promise success to the parents of the girl if they would faithfully and implicitly follow my directions. I confess that I had my fears lest there should be some organic disease; yet the pulse, though rather slow, was regular. The bowels, I was told, were very irregular, but generally costive; I felt the abdomen very tumid; and notwithstanding the feebleness and emaciated state of the patient, I felt convinced that no time was to be lost; I therefore ordered an active purgative. The fits recurring and no stool being procured, infusion of senna was given, one ounce every half hour, which produced several *scanty, fluid motions, of a greenish color, and highly fetid.* Both medicines were continued for four days, without alteration in the state of the patient or her bowels, several lumbrici were voided, the fits had rather increased in violence; on the fifth day she had two motions, the last *very copious, consisting chiefly of hardened scybala*, and containing two worms; fits returned only during the night. Three days more brought more large evacuations of the same kind, diminished voraciousness, and less severity of fits which occurred during the nights. From this time (the 6th of January) to the 20th, I continued the exhibition of calomel and rhubarb, and the senna occasionally, never intermitting more than one day. The quantity of feculent matter which she passed during that period is beyond conception. Her appetite began to flag about the 14th, and on the 16th her mother informed me that she had not had a fit for twenty-four hours; on the 17th she had one very severe fit, but remained free from them again till the 20th, when she had one which did not continue above ten minutes. During this period she had voided three lumbrici. The fits gradually abated, the appetite became natural, while purging pills were continued so as to secure a regular alvine discharge (Journ., pp. 305–308).

Large doses and perseverance secure cure.
SUCCESS.

356. Thus far the purgatives have fully answered my expectations. The child appears to be cured of her fits, but I am afraid she will remain an idiot while she lives. The *doses* of medicine that were necessary to move her bowels *were very large, and also the length of time* which elapsed *before the bowels* could be said to *be properly moved*, for I conceive that she had no proper motion till the seventh day. The large doses of medicine which were necessary may be accounted for, perhaps, from the state of the sensorium; and the difficulty which there was in moving the bowels was, no doubt, owing to the great accumulation which had taken place (p. 308).

357. Though the fits are removed at present, I fear they will be apt to return, unless *great care* is taken *to keep her bowels open for some considerable time, until the predisposition from habit is overcome, and the bowels are restored to their natural tone;* but if this is attended to, I am certain the cure will be complete. This case, then, I would say, tends to corroborate the very valuable observations of *Dr. James Hamilton*, but indeed those observations stand in no need of any such testimony; for *Dr. Hamilton* has proved every position which he has advanced by facts that never can be controverted. The *novelty, the simplicity, and the efficacy of Dr. Hamilton's practice* attracted much notice on the first appearance of his invaluable work; and as the doctor did not venture to give his discoveries to the world till experience had most fully confirmed them, he was able to speak with certainty; and I will venture to affirm that *if purgatives have failed in any instance to pr̃o-duce the effects which Dr. Hamilton's observations have so incontestibly proved them capable of producing, that that failure is to be attributed more to the prescriber than to the medicine prescribed* (Journ p. 309).

It is necessary to establish regularity of alvine evacuations in order to secure health.

The purgative plan of treatment and Hamilton's doctrine vindicated.

358. I have often heard it argued, by those who were unwilling to give too much credit to Dr. Hamilton, as was generally allowed, that though no doubt the cases which he had related seemed to prove the good effects of purgatives, yet that many of those cases—for example, his cases of *typhus fever*—were so trifling that any other remedy would have done as well as purgatives. And, moreover, it has been often hinted that though this practice may do very well in the north, and in the Royal Infirmary of Edinburgh, yet that it is by no means calculated for the delicate constitutions of this country. I shall only say, that those who have witnessed *Dr. Hamilton's* practice have been fully convinced of the good effects of purgatives in severe as well as slight cases of fever; and, indeed, had the doctor felt any anxiety about this, he might have filled the second number of his appendix with cases more severe than any he has given. With regard to the second hint, I can add my testimony to that of *Dr. Morgan*, of Dover. (See Edinb. M. and S. Journ., 1807, April 1.)

Typhus.

Further vindication of the purgative plan and Hamilton's practice.

I have prescribed purgatives in different diseases since my residence in England, and have found their effects uniformly the same as in the north. While I resided at Halesworth, in Suffolk, I attended Robert White, of Walpole, with Mr. Walker, surgeon, in one of the worst cases of typhus I ever saw. The disease was speedily subdued by purgatives. The bolus jalapæ compositus had the same good effect in Suffolk as in the Royal Infirmary of Edinburgh (Journ., pp. 309, 310).

WATT, ROBERT, M. D., *Cases of Diabetes, Consumption, &c., with Observations on the History and Treatment of Disease in general. Paisley*, 1808. *See* EDINB. MED. & SURG. JOUR., 1809, *Vol. V.*

359. The *functions of the lungs* are twofold: *to assimilate* the new *materials supplied by the digestive organs*, and *to preserve the blood* in a healthy state. In health there must be a due balance between the digestive and assimilative organs. If this balance be disturbed, disease ensues (p. 93).

The lungs; —health and disease.

Chyle.   360. If more *chyle* be thrown upon the lungs than they can assimilate, it must remain an incumbrance upon the system, or *be discharged by* one or other of the excretories (p. 94).

The blood.   361. The *blood may be deteriorated,* and yet support life, in an imperfect manner. The vessels which increase and repair the solids may be in want of proper materials, though the system were overcharged *The nerves.* with blood. The *nervous system* being deprived of its natural support from these vessels, acquires a depraved sensibility, and all the phenomena follow which we have described as attending a diseased habit. The *Secreting organs.* greatest number of *secreting organs* are idle for the want of *arterial* *The liver.* blood, *the only stimulus which can call them into action.* The *liver* *" Bilious complaints,"* receiving its stimulus from venous blood, *has more to do* than in health; *debility.* hence arise " bilious complaints " which, with low spirits, prostration of strength, &c., generally mark the first stage of disease (p. 94).

Reaction.   362. If the system possesses sufficient vigor, reaction takes place, and goes on to a proper crisis. . . . In place of fever the balance is often *Critical evacuation:* restored by a *critical evacuation.* If the superfluous matter take to the *Diarrhœa—* intestines, it produces *diarrhœa ;* if to the kidneys, *diabetes ;* if to the *Intestines;* uterus, *menorrhagia ;* if to the skin, *profuse perspiration.* If the re-*Diabetes—* action fail to produce a salutary crisis, the system falls back, collects *kidneys;* new vigor and resumes the conflict, as in intermittent fever, and other *Menorrhagia* periodical diseases. In other instances, such as *hypochondriasis,* it re-*—uterus;* peats the same thing over again, or tries other means of relief, and is *Perspiration* thus said to counterfeit every disease ; that is, it employs many *efforts* *—skin.* to throw *off the incumbrance,* but is generally unequal to the task. Af-*Hypochondriasis—its* ter a longer or shorter struggle, a *confirmed phthisis, diabetes, diarrhœa,* *causes,* *dropsy,* or some other disease, terminates the patient's sufferings (p. 95). *course, and end, if incumbrance are not removed.*

Vagaries of medical practice.   363. In every period of the history of medicine, there has not only been practice opposed to practice and theory to theory, but one fashion has succeeded another with astonishing rapidity. One practitioner treats burns and scalds by heating, another by cooling applications ; one cures the gout by carefully wrapping the feet in flannel, another by plunging them in cold water ; one combats fevers with wine and opium, another by gruel and purgatives. These, though abundantly striking, are but a small sample of the oppositions in medicine. To notice the fashions would be to enumerate the various articles which, from time to time, have entered the materia medica, and almost every possible manner in which these can be prepared and compounded. (Journ, 1810, Vol. VI, p. 287.)

About " specifics."   364. From a belief that there is no disease without a corresponding remedy, medical men have been much in search of antidotes. The task of finding *a specific for each disorder,* reminds me of the labor of the Chinese in inventing a distinct character for every word in their language. However numerous and diversified the hair-splitting systems of nosology may represent diseases, *the means of cure,* like the simple sounds in language, *are few and obvious. Galen* remarked *that bleeding and purging were the two legs of physic, and it is doubtful how* *Purgatives the " legs of physic."* far *the art has been improved by the legs which have since been added* (ibid.)

BRIGGS, H., M. D., *Physician of the Royal Dispensary of Liverpool ;
History of a case of tetanus cured by purgatives.   Liverpool,* 1809.
See EDINB. MED. & SURG. JOURN., 1809, *Vol. V.*

365. *Remarkable case of Luke Gaskell, given in detail.*—The cure
was perfect in four weeks. On the fourth day of the case, *Dr. Briggs*
says :—" I had all along been aware of the awful responsibility I in-
currred by departing so widely from the usual practice in tetanus, and
now my resolution failed me altogether. I was terrified with the apprehension that I had already delayed the free exhibition of opiates too
long, while yet I was loth to relinquish the use of purgatives (p. 154).
On a cool review, I asked myself whether, if the case should prove
fatally, as I then feared it would, I could with justice affirm, *that purgation had been fairly tried and failed*, whether on the contrary the exacerbations that had occurred ought not to be ascribed to the interruption of the plan, rather than to the plan itself? (p. 155). Finally, I concluded to adhere to the plan of purgation, and to discontinue the internal use of opium (ibid).

*Locked-jaw
—remark-
able case ;
cure by pow-
erful pur-
gation.
" Nil despe-
randum."*

366. After the cure, he says :—" If there be any point in medicine,
on which, after having been engaged in dispensatory practice for sixteen
years, I have arrived at any certain conclusion, it is this, that *in gastrodynia*, and many other *spasmodic affections, brisk purgatives* will be
found incomparably *better antispasmodics* than any of that tribe to
which this epithet is usually applied. I believe, too, that their operation
is *strictly antispasmodic*—that *their first effect* is, to supersede the
spasmodic action ; for I have often known complete relief to be obtained
before a stool was procured, in so much, that I have more than once
been asked by patients, ' if I had not given them laudanum ?' " (p. 161).

*Spasms of
the stomach.*

*Purgatives
the best
" antispas-
modics."*

I am inclined to think, that the more drastic purges were laid aside
for no sufficient reason. . . *The more active purgatives* appear *literally*
to have possessed *antispasmodic* virtues (p. 162).

*Drastic
purges.*

The quantity of medicine taken from first to last for twenty-five
days is certainly very large, as follows :—calomel 320 grains, scammony 340 grains, gamboge 126 grains, powdered jalap 6 ounces, infusion
of senna with tincture 10¾ pounds, colocynth-pill nearly 2 ounces, of
which the greater part was taken within the first week.

During forty-eight hours (on the 5th and 6th days) was given scammony 210 grains, gamboge 89 grains, jalap 1½ ounce, infusion of senna
2¼ pounds, calomel 80 grains ; and all this without causing sickness or
griping, but on the contrary with most decided benefit (ibid.)

367. In short, if a remedy be indicated at all, surely *the dose* should be
regulated, *not only by weight and measure*, but *by the effect*. And when
there is such a strong concatenation of morbid actions, as in *tetanus*, it
might perhaps have been expected, a priori, as it has *proved in fact*, that
*nothing but the most active purges, in large doses, and frequently re-
peated*, would *avail to break the train* (p. 163). The whole quantity of
opium taken was 100 drops in two days, and so far from answering any
good end, it seems manifestly to have *prevented sleep*, as well as to have
impeded the operation of the purgatives (p. 164).

*The effect,
not the quan
tity of the
dose to be
considered.*

This is the most important evidence, in respect to purgatives, we have yet published.
Our directions for the use of Brandreth's Pills need no modification. Dose, from 2 to 20, or
any quantity required to purge.

RUSH, BENJAMIN. M. D., *Medical Inquiries*, 4 vols. *Philadelphia*, 1809.

Disease a unit.

368. *There is but one fever.* However different the predisposing, remote, or exciting causes of fever may be, still I repeat, there can be but one fever (vol. III., p. 16).

All forms of disease local, etc., from the sanguifer-ous system.

369. I infer the unity of fever, further, from the *sameness* of the products or effects of all its different forms (ibid., p. 17). All ordinary fever being seated in the blood-vessels, it follows, of course, that all those local affections we call pleurisy, angina, internal dropsy of the brain, pulmonary consumption, and inflammation of the liver, stomach, bowels, and lungs, are *symptoms* only *of an original and primary disease in the sanguiferous system.* The truth of this proposition is obvious, from the above local affections succeeding primary fever, and from their alternating so frequently with each other. *There being but one fever*, of course *I do not admit* of its artificial division into *genera and species* (ibid. p. 33).

Nosological arrange-ments of dis-eases objec-tionable and useless.

370. *Pulmonary consumption* is sometimes *transferred into head-ache, rheumatism, diarrhœa* and *mania.* The *bilious fever* often appears in the same person in the form of colic, dysentery, inflammation of the liver, lungs and brain, in the course of five or six days. Phrenitis, gastritis, enteritis, nephritis, and rheumatism—all appear at the same time in gout and yellow fever. . . . *Much mischief has been done by nosological arrangement of diseases. They erect imaginary boun-daries between things which are of homogeneous nature* (ibid., p. 34).

Consequen-ces of artifi-cial nomen-clature.

371. They gratify indolence in a physician by fixing his attention upon the name of a disease, and thereby leading him to neglect the ranging state of the system. They moreover lay a foundation for disputes among physicians by diverting their attention from the simple, predisposing and proximate to the numerous remote and exciting causes of disease, or to their more numerous and complicated effects (ibid., p. 35).

The mate-ria medica denounced.

372. The whole *materia medica* is infected with the *baneful conse-quences* of the nomenclature of diseases, for *every article in it is pointed only against* their *names*, and hence the origin of the numerous contra-dictions among authors who describe the virtues and doses of the same medicine (ibid).

A good time coming, when the unity of dis-ease will be acknowl-edged and acted upon.

373. By the rejection of the artificial arrangement of diseases, a *revolution must follow in medicine.* Observation and judgment will take the place of reading and memory, and prescriptions will be con-fined to existing circumstances. *The road to knowledge in medicine* by this means will likewise be *shortened*, so that a young man will be able to qualify himself to practice physic at as much less expense than formerly, as a child would have to read and write by the help of the Roman alphabet, instead of Chinese characters (ibid, pp. 34, 35).

374. The efficacy of this remedy (purgation) in the cure of *dropsies*, has been acknowledged by physicians in all ages and countries (vol. II, p. 182). Both *drastic and gentle purgatives* act by diminishing the action of the arterial system, and thereby *promote the absorption and discharge* (ibid. p. 183). *Dropsy:— action of purgatives.*

375. However *varied* morbid actions may be in their *causes, seats and effects*, they are all of the same nature, and the time will probably come when the *whole nomenclature* of morbid actions will be absorbed in the simple name of *" Disease "* (ibid., p. 234). *All diseases one cause. (Apothegm.)*

376. A *mild remittent*, and *yellow fever* are different grades of the same disease (ibid., p. 256). *A mild remittent, but diluted yellow fever.*

377. If we mean by *gout* a primary affection of the joints, we have gained nothing by assuming that name ; but if we mean by it a disease which consists *simply* of *morbid excitement invited by debility*, and disposed to invade every part of the body, we conform our ideas to facts, and thus *simplify theory and practice* in chronic diseases (ibid., p. 272). *Gout;—a local deposit from general derangement : this view simplifies theory and practice in chronic diseases.*

378. The *gout affects* most of *the viscera*. In the *brain* it produces headache, vertigo, coma, apoplexy and palsy ; in the *lungs*, pneumonia, notha, asthma, hemoptysis, consumption ; in the *throat*, inflammatory angina ; in the *uterus*, hemorrhagia uterina ; in the *kidneys*, strangury, diabetes, and calculi ; in the *liver*, inflammation, suppuration, melea, schirrhus, gall-stones and jaundice (ibid., pp. 258, 259). *All* these *diseases have but* ONE CAUSE, and they are *exactly the same*, however *different the stimulus* may be from which they are derived (ibid., p. 261). *Gout, consumption, asthma, etc., all diseases from but one cause.*

379. Thus *rheumatism*, the *gout*, the *measles, small-pox*, the different species of *cynanche*—all furnish examples of the connection of local affections with general diseases ; but the *apoplexy* and the *pneumony* furnish the most striking analogy of *local affections succeeding a general disease* of the system (ibid., p. 86). *Local affections and general disease.*

380. *Pneumony is apoplexy of the lungs*, allowing only for the difference of situation and structure (ibid., p. 87). *Pneumony.*

381. After the production of *predisposing debility* of the system from the action of remote causes, *the fluids are determined to the weakest parts* of the body. Hence the effusion of serum or blood takes place in the lungs. When serum is effused, a pituitous or purulent expectoration takes place ; when blood is discharged a disease is produced which has been called hemoptysis. The pneumony is produced by remote exciting causes which act on the whole system (ibid.) . . The expectoration which terminates the disease in health is always the effect of effusions produced by a general disease (ibid., pp. 87, 88). *Unity of disease further demonstrated.*

382. Who has not seen the *pulmonary symptoms* alternately relieved and reproduced by the appearance or cessation of a diarrhœa or pains in the bowels ? (Ibid., p. 85.) *Consumption—nature tries to cure by spontaneous purgation.*

7

The unity of disease.
383. Science has much to deplore from the multiplicity of diseases. It is as repugnant to truth in medicine as polytheism is to truth in religion. The physician who considers every different affection of the different systems in the body, or every affection of different parts of the same system, as distinct diseases, when they arise from one cause, resem-

The recognition of this doctrine is of the highest importance to humanity.
bles the Indian or African savage who considers water, dew, ice, frost and snow, as distinct essences; while the physician who considers the morbid affections of every part of the body, however diversified they may be in their form or degrees, as derived from one cause, resembles the philosopher who considers dew, ice, frost and snow, as different modifications of water, and as derived simply from the absence of heat (vol. III., pp. 146, 147).

Humanity has likewise much to deplore from this paganism in medicine. The sword will probably be sheathed forever as an instrument of death before *physicians* will cease to add to the mortality of mankind by *prescribing for the names of diseases* (ibid., p. 147. Account of the bilious yellow fever of 1793).

Experience of Dr. Rush.
384. *How Dr. Rush came to believe in the efficacy of purgation.*— Condensed from pp. 222–230, vol. III. :

I gave gentle purges and vomits, bark in all its usual forms, applied blisters to the limbs, neck and head, attempted to rouse the system by wrapping the whole body in blankets dipped in warm vinegar (p. 223), rubbed the right side with mercurial ointment, with a view of exciting the system through the liver ; none of these remedies were of any service. I returned to bark, wine, and the use of cold water (p. 224). . . Had the authority of Dr. Cleghorn for the former, who says : "The bark, by bracing the solids, enables them to throw off the excrementitious fluids by the proper emunctories," &c. No better success, however, attended my efforts (p. 225). . . I ransacked my library, and pored over every book that treated of yellow fever (p. 226). . . I recollected that I had among some old papers a manuscript account of the yellow fever as it prevailed in Virginia in 1741, which had been put into my hands by Dr. Franklin, a short time before his death. I now read it a second time, and paused upon every sentence. I was struck with the following passages (p. 227) :

Franklin on yellow-fever. Purgation indispensable. The abdominal viscera chiefly affected.
385. (*Dr. Franklin, loquitur*): "It must be remarked that this evacuation (meaning the purges) is more necessary in this than in most other fevers. *The abdominal viscera are the parts principally affected* in this disease, but by this timely evacuation their feculent corruptible contents are discharged before they corrupt and produce any ill effects ; and their various emunctories and secerning vessels are set open, so as to allow a free discharge of their contents, and consequently *a security to the parts themselves* during the course of the disease. By this evacuation the very minea of the disease, proceeding from the putrid miasmata fermenting with the bilious and other humors of the body, is sometimes *eradicated by the timely emptying the abdominal viscera*, in which it first fixes, after which a gentle sweat does, as it were, nip it in the bud" (ibid.)

Purgation promotes sweat by re-
386. "When *the primæ viæ*, but *especially the stomach, is loaded with an offensive matter*, or contracted and convulsed with the irritation

of its stimulus, *there is no* procuring a *laudable sweat* till that is re- moving impurities which prevent exudation.
moved; after which a necessary quantity of sweat breaks out of its own
accord, these parts promoting it, when, by an absterging medicine, they
are eased of the burden or stimulus which oppresses them" (p. 228).

387. "All these acute putrid fevers require some evacuation to bring All fevers require purgation.
them to a perfect crisis and solution, and that even by stools, which must
be promoted by art, when nature does not do the business herself"
(ibid.)

388. "On this account, *an ill-timed scrupulousness about the weak-* The weaker the subject, the greater the necessity for full purgation.
ness of the body is of bad consequence in these circumstances; for it is
that which seems chiefly to make evacuations necessary, which nature is
ever attempting, after the humors are fit to be expelled, but is not
able to accomplish for the most part in this disease. And I can affirm
that I have given a purge in this case when the pulse has been so low
that it could hardly be felt, and the debility extreme, yet both one and
the other have been restored by it" (pp. 228, 229).

389. Here I paused. A new train of ideas suddenly broke in upon Weak purges useless.
my mind. I supposed that my want of success, in several of the cases
in which I attempted the cure by purging, was owing to the feebleness of
my purges (ib., p. 230).

390. *By full and continued purgation I cured perfectly four out of* Astonishing effects of full purgation—the seemingly dead restored to life.
the first five patients, notwithstanding some of them were advanced sev-
eral days in the disease. One gentleman had passed *twelve hours with-*
out a pulse, and with a cold sweat on his limbs. His relations had given
him over. *Dr. Mitchell's* account of the effect of purging in raising the
pulse excited a hope that he might be saved, provided his bowels could
be opened. *Purges* were given to him three or four times a day; at
length they *operated and produced two copious fetid stools. His pulse*
rose immediately. A universal moisture on his skin succeeded. In a
few days he was out of danger, and soon afterwards appeared in the
streets in good health (p. 232)... In three days he had taken eighty
grains of calomel, and rather more than that quantity of rhubarb and
jalap (ibid.)

391. This practice could be said to be almost uniformly effectual in Calomel with bark or opium useless.
all those cases which I was able to attend... Many used calomel in
connection with bark, wine, and laudanum, without any good effects...
I can never forget the transport with which *Dr. Pennington* ran across Dr. Pennington and strong purges.
Third Street to inform me "that after he began to give *strong purgatives*
the disease yielded in every case" (ibid., p. 235).

392. Never did I experience such sublime joy as I now felt in con- Dr. Rush rejoices.
templating the success of my remedies. It repaid me for all the toils
and studies of my life. The reader will not wonder at this joyful state
of my mind when I add a short extract from my note-book of the 10th
September: "Thank God! *out of one hundred patients,* whom I have
visited or prescribed for, this day, *I have lost none!*" (Ibid., p. 234.)

All kinds of purges used; the great object being ree stools a day. 393. My practice was, to give *a purge every day while the fever continued.* I used castor-oil, salts, cream of tartar, rhubarb. Calomel and jalap were often ineffectual, then I added gamboge. The purges seldom answered the intention for which they were given unless they produced four or five stools a day (ibid., p. 240). . . *When purges were rejected or slow* in their operation, I always directed *opening clysters every two hours* (ibid., p. 241).

The advantages of purgation stated in seven propositions. 394. *The effects of purging were as follows:*

1. It raised the pulse when low, and reduced it when it was preternaturally tense or full.

2. It revived and strengthened the patient. This was evident in many cases in the facility with which patients who had staggered to a close-stool walked back to their bed after a copious evacuation.

3. It abated the painful symptoms of the fever.

4. It frequently produced sweating, when given on the first or second day of the fever, after the most powerful sudorifics had been given to no purpose.

5. It sometimes checked the vomiting which occurred in the beginning of the disease, and it always assisted in preventing the more alarming occurrence of that symptom about the fourth and fifth day.

6. Removed obstruction from the lymphatic system.

7. Discharged the bile through the bowels as soon and fast as it was secreted, and prevented, in most cases, yellowness of the skin (ibid., p. 243).

Sympathy. 395. One of the laws of sensation is, that certain impressions which excite neither sensation nor motion in the part of the body to which they are applied, excite both in another part. Thus worms, which are not The weakest part suffers. felt in the stomach or bowels, often produce a troublesome sensation in the throat. . . In like manner the irritants which produce fever, in ordinary cases pass through the bloodvessels, and convey their usual morbid effects into a remote part of the body, which has been prepared to receive them by previous debility (ibid., pp. 60, 61).

No amount of purgation injurious. Cures obtained by very large doses. 396. *It is not an easy thing to affect life, or even subsequent health, by copious or frequent purging.* Dr. Kirkland (Treatise on Inflammatory Rheumatism, vol. I., p. 407) mentions a remarkable case of a gentleman who was cured of a *rheumatism* by a purge which gave him *between forty and fifty stools.* This patient "had been previously affected by his disease sixteen or eighteen weeks." Dr. Mosely not only proves the safety, but establishes the efficacy of numerous and copious stools in the yellow fever. *Dr. Say* probably *owes his life to three-and-twenty stools,* procured by a dose of calomel and gamboge, taken by my advice. *Dr. Redman* was purged until he fainted by a dose of the same medicine (ibid., pp. 243, 244).

Diarrhœa never kills, but the disease which is the cause of the diarrhœa. 397. But who can suppose that a dozen or twenty stools in a day could endanger life that has seen a *diarrhœa* continue *for several months,* attended with fifteen or twenty stools a day, without making even a material breach in the constitution?* Hence Dr. Hillary (Diseases of Barbadoes, p. 212) has justly remarked, that "*it rarely or never happens that the purging in this disease, though violent, takes the patient off, but the fever and inflammation of the bowels.*" *Dr. Clark* (Diseases in Voyages to the Hot Climates, vol. II., p. 322) in like manner remarks that *evacuations do not destroy life* in the dysentery, but the fever,with the emaciation and mortification which attend and follow the disease (ibid., p. 245).

398. I have remarked in the history of *this fever* that it was *often cured* on the first or second day *by a copious sweat.* It would be absurd to suppose that the *miasmata* which produced the disease were discharged in this manner from the body. The *sweat seemed to cure* the fever only *by lessening the quantity of the fluids,* and thus *gradually removing the depression* of the system. . . The reason why a few *strong purgatives* cured the disease at its first appearance was, because they *abstracted in a gradual manner* some of the immense portion of stimulus under which the arterial system labored, and thus *gradually relieved* it from its low and weakening degrees of depression. . . *Bleeding* was *fatal in these cases,* probably because it removed this depression in too sudden a manner (ibid., pp. 277–279). *Sweats (crises) and purges.*

Bleeding fatal.

399. *Baron Humboldt* informed me that *Dr. Caristo* had assured him that *bark hastened death in every case* in which it was given in the yellow fever of Vera Cruz. If, in any instance, it was inoffensive or did service in our fever, I suspect it must have acted upon the bowels *as a purgative. Dr. Sydenham* says that *bark cured* intermittents *by this evacuation,* and *Wm. Bruce* says it operated in the same way when it cured the bilious fevers at Massuat (ibid., p. 293). *Bark destructive except when it acts as a purgative.*

400. *The result:*

Whilst *Dr. Rush* was working from eighteen to twenty hours a day, healing and saving by hundreds, *the old-school physicians,* who derided his innovations, persisted in the use of *bark, wine, and laudanum,* and thus succeeded in *killing their patients "secundum artem."* *Bark, wine, and laudanum.*

401. The *Rev. Mr. Fleming,* one of the ministers of the Catholic church, carried the purging powders in his pocket, and gave them to his poor parishioners with great success. He informed me that he had advised four of our physicians, whom he had met a day or two before, " to renounce the pride of science, and to adopt the new mode of practice, *for that he had witnessed its good effects in many cases* " (ibid., p. 314). *Clerical evidence in favor of purgation.*

402. *Reason and humanity awake* from their long repose *in medicine,* and unite in proclaiming that it is time *to take the cure* of pestilential epidemics *out of the hands of physicians,* and *to place it into the hands of the people, . .* The safety of consigning to the people the cure of pestilential fevers, especially the yellow fever and the plague, is established by the *simplicity and uniformity of their causes and of their remedies.* *Reason and humanity are opposed to medical monopoly.*

403. *Dr. Lind* has remarked that a greater proportion of sailors who had no physician recovered from the fever than of those who had the *Popular compared with medical treatment.*

The worst best medical attendance. The fresh air of the deck of a ship, a purge
diseases are
the simplest of salt water, and the use of cold water, probably triumphed over the
to cure. cordial juleps of the physician (ibid., p. 319).

Other medi- 404. For a long while *air, water*, and *even the light of the sun*, were
cal monopo-
lies consid- *dealt out by physicians* to their patients *with a sparing hand.* They
ered and
their *hum* possessed for several centuries the same monopoly of many artificial
bug de-
nounced. remedies. But a new order of things is rising in medicine (ibid., p.
320). It is not more necessary that a patient should be ignorant of the
medicine he takes, to be cured by it, than the business of government
should be conducted with secrecy in order to secure obedience to just
laws. Much less is it necessary that the means of life should be prescribed in a dead language, or dictated with the solemn pomp of a ne-
cromancer. The effects of imposture in anything are like the artificial
health produced by the use of ardent spirits. Its vigor is temporary,
and is always followed by misery and death (ibid., p. 321).

Medical mo- 405. I would as soon believe that ratafia was intended by the author
nopoly fur-
ther consid- of nature to be the only drink of man, instead of water, as believe that
ered. the knowledge of what relates to the health and lives of a whole city or
nation should be confined to one, and that a small and privileged order
of men. But what have physicians, and what have universities and
medical societies done, after the labor and studies of so many centuries,
Medical Ig- towards lessening the mortality of pestilential fevers? They have either
norance and
contradic- copied or contradicted each other in all their publications. Plagues and
tions. malignant fevers are still leagued with war and famine in their ravages
upon human life (ibid., p. 323; cf. Asclepiades, 63).

406. A Mohammedan and a Jew might as well attempt to worship
Why Dr. the Supreme Being in the same temple, and through the medium of the
Rush would
never "con- same ceremonies, as physicians of opposite principles and practice at-
sult" with
the bark- tempt to confer about the life of the same patient. What is done in
wine and lau-
danum men. consequence of such negotiations (for they are not consultations) is the
ineffectual result of neutralized opinions; and, wherever they take place,
should be considered as the effect of a criminal compact between physicians to assess the property of the patients, by a shameful prostitution
of the dictates of their consciences. . .
The extremity of wrong in medicine, as in morals and governments,
is often a less mischief than that mixture of right and wrong which
serves, by palliating, to perpetuate the evil (ibid., p. 349).

Purge until 407. In one very malignant case the *most drastic purgatives* brought
BLACK (FETID)
FÆCES—cri- away, *by fifty evacuations*, nothing but natural stools. The *purges* were
sis—come
away, and *continued*, and finally *black fæces* were *discharged*, which produced *im-*
fear not. *mediate relief* (ibid., p. 375).

408. I observed the same relief from *large evacuations of fetid bile* in
This plan the epidemic of 1797 that I have remarked in the fever of 1793. *Mr.*
always re-
moves debil- *Bryce* has taken notice of the same salutary effects from similar evacua-
ity; tions in yellow fever on board the Busbridge Indiaman in 1799. "It
was observable that *the more dark colored and fetid such discharges were
the more early and certainly did the symptoms disappear.* Their good

effects were so instantaneous that I have often seen a man carried upon deck, perfectly delirious with subsultus tendinum, and in a state of the greatest apparent debility, who, *after one or two copious evacuations of this kind,* has returned of himself, astonished at his newly-acquired strength " (Annals of Medicine, p. 123).

409. *Very different are the effects of tonic remedies* when *given to remove* this apparent *debility.* The clown who supposes the crooked appearance of a stick, when thrust into a pail of water, to be real, does not err more against the laws of light than that physician errs against a law of the animal economy who mistakes the debility which arises from oppression for an exhausted state of the system, and attempts to remove it by stimulating medicines (vol. IV., p. 38). *whilst tonic remedies destroy.*

INTERESTING ARTICLE.

BARLOW, EDWARD, M. D., *Pathological and Practical Observations. Bath,* 1810. *See* EDINB. MED. AND SURG. JOURN., 1814, *Vol. X.*

410. *Purgatives* are *of three sorts : some* evacuating the fecal contents of the intestines ; *others* acting on their exhalent arteries, and producing copious watery stools—and a *third* class stimulating the mucous follicles which so abundantly line the intestines and causing them to expel the mucous matters they so copiously secrete. When the bowels are merely inactive, their secretions healthy, and no constitutional disease present, the *simple aperients* of the *first* class suffice to obviate costiveness and prevent feculent accumulations. The *second* are requisite when, in addition to unloading the intestines, it is desirable to abate internal action or allay fever, by reducing the quantity of the circulating fluid ; and *the third* are required either when the mucous secretions are so morbid as to give rise to diseases, or when they are too copiously generated in consequence of increased action of the vascular system (pp. 431, 432). *Purgatives evacuate fecal matter, produce watery stools, expel mucous matter, first, in inactiveness of the bowels, obviating costiveness; second, in irritated action or fever, reducing the circulating fluid; third, in morbidity or superabundance of mucous secretions.*

Brandreth's Pills in one medicine accomplish the three indications required. In doses of from one to four Pills, they evacuate the fecal contents of the intestines ; from four to six they operate upon the exhalent arteries and produce copious watery stools ; in doses of from six to ten pills they stimulate the mucous follicles which so abundantly line the intestines, causing stools of pure mucous. In headaches, dyspepsia, apoplectic and paralytic symptoms, and in gout and rheumatism, no cure can be obtained without the expulsion of large quantities of this mucous, which Brandreth's Pills effect with entire safety.

411. When it is considered that the *diseases of repletion* are by far the most numerous that the human body is liable to ; that the alimentary canal affords one of the most important outlets for discharging the redundancy of the system ; that it is also a principal one for getting rid of the excrementitious impurities, with which in such diseases *the blood* is speedily *adulterated,* and that the diseased secretions which accumulate within it are oftentimes a means of continuing, of complicating, and even of creating various diseases in different parts of the body, the *value of purgatives* cannot fail to be duly appreciated. *Diseases of repletion;—purgatives cannot be dispensed with to remove the excrementitious matter from the blood.*

It remains for me to show that such *morbid secretions* do exist within the stomach and intestines, and that they do produce therein the effects now attributed to them, being *the direct cause* of some *local complaints,* while they beget also, *by remote sympathies, diseases in distant parts* (p. 432). *Morbid secretions in stomach and intestines. Sympathy.*

412. Of the existence of superabundant mucous in the stomach and intestines during inflammatory complaints, sufficient proof will be afforded merely by *inspecting the discharges* brought off by particular evacuants, or occasionally by the natural efforts. With respect to the stomach this examination may mislead, if only superficial; for the mucous being clear and colorless, is not readily distinguishable from the watery fluid surrounding it; if, however, a rod or wire is passed through the liquor, and elevated, it will raise the mucous existing therein, and sufficiently manifest its dense and viscid nature (p. 433).

Examine the discharges of intestines and stomach.

413. It is this mucous that is produced by increased arterial action, affecting the mucous glands of the stomach in common with all the other parts. To it, and to the action which produces it, superseding the healthy action of these parts, do I attribute the incipient nausea of fever and of constitutional inflammation; and *its expulsion* I deem *important,* both as *removing an injurious accumulation,* and as *enabling the secreting vessels,* thus disencumbered, *to continue those efforts, whose direct tendency is to relieve the general circulation,* however inadequate they may be, when unassisted, to accomplish this purpose. Similar secretions are going forward also at such times throughout the whole course of the intestinal canal, and are evidenced by the quantity of mucous which a dose of calomel or antimony, administered under such circumstances, uniformly expels (ibid).

Superabundant mucous creates disease.

Purgatives assist the action of the secretories in expelling mucous.

414. The want of sufficient attention being given to the peculiar effect produced by different purgatives, may perhaps suffice to account for the uncertainty and indecision which still prevail in their employment. If this mucous matter is recently formed, and in no great abundance, a *common purgative of the drastic kind* will suffice to remove it, together with all such fecal lodgments as may have taken place in the intestines. *A source of injurious irritation is thus removed; the various secreting and excreting vessels are left free to perform their natural functions; and the progress of nature, in her force to restore health, goes forward uninterruptedly.* If the mucous secretions are *of older formation and consequently more viscid, more tenacious and more difficultly expelled,* the *common purgatives fail* to give relief, and a doubt is cast on the propriety of employing them, and on the veracity of previous reports of successful cures. *The error here, however, is in employing a purgative inadequate to producing the effect required. . . .* If *saline purgatives* are given with the expectation of cleansing the intestines when loaded with mucous secretions, they will very imperfectly effect this purpose (pp. 433, 434).

How to select the purgatives;— when the mucous matter is of recent formation, drastics suffice;

when it is of old formation, powerful purgatives.

Salts ineffectual

415. The *quantity* of this mucous secreted *in acute diseases* is very considerable. It lines both the stomach and intestines, and causes many powerful medicines to pass through them without producing their ordinary effects; for, *in consequence of the interposed mucous, the medicines come only imperfectly or not at all in contact with the living fibre, which alone they are capable of stimulating. It passes through, therefore, as if either the living fibre were torpid, or the medicine inert,* when *neither supposition is correct;* and to mistake and accident we are occasionally

Large quantities of mucous from acute diseases hinder the operation of many purgatives.

indebted for illustration of this subject, which perhaps regular prac- *Large doses often have but moder- ate opera- tion.* tice would more slowly and imperfectly afford us. For the errors of dispensers and the stupidity of patients have not unfrequently afforded me instances of *inordinate doses of purgative medicines* being given, *with only moderate and salutary operation* (p. 434).

416. Case of *scarlatina* given.—*Purgatives* were, in consequence, thenceforward more freely employed, and the *effect regarded more than the dose* necessary for producing it ; and although the inflammatory fever ran high, and was not allayed for many days, there did not occur a speck of ulceration on either tonsil. Neither did any of the ordinary sequelæ attend the disease, but the recovery was progressive and complete. *Scarlatina. The effect and not the dose to be considered.*

We may hence infer the difficulty of establishing the precise doses of medicines to be admitted, and must be conscious of the superior advantage of *attending solely to the sensible operation,* when this is capable of being ascertained, *disregarding altogether the quantity of medicine necessary for effecting it.* This is always possible with respect to purgative medicines, and to be accomplished by *regular inspection of the alvine evacuations,* without which the practitioner must remain in much doubt concerning some of the most important operations going forward within the body, and must labor under great disadvantages in accurately applying the remedies it is necessary to employ (p. 435). *Inspection of the evac- uations rec- ommended.*

417. Morbid secretions are very frequently formed in the stomach, which occasion a large proportion of *gastric diseases.* To particularize only one. Conceiving the *pain in gastrodynia* to proceed *from a contractile effort of the stomach to throw off* from its surface the mucous which offends it, I have for many years laid aside the use of *opium and stimulants,* which *merely repress the effect, without at all removing the cause,* and which even tend to add to this by stimulating the glands to increased secretion of the offending mucous, and *have trusted solely to such medicines as act by expelling that matter, to whose presence I attribute the complaint.* . . *Morbid mat- ter in the stomach oc- casions gas- tric dis- eases. Gastro- dynia.* *Opium and stimulants do not re- move the cause—pur- gatives ex- pel the offending matter.*

I own I am averse to relieving the pain by *opium,* or by any means but a removal of the offending matter—*as the relief to pain consequent upon such evacuation may be relied on as announcing the radical cure of the complaint.* In some hundred cases that I have now treated on these principles I have *in no instance given a grain of opium, or failed in giving decided relief.* Almost the only medicine I employ as a purgative compound consists of extract of colocynth, calomel, and antimonial powder (p. 436).

418. The disease of *colic* I believe to be *precisely analogous* with gastrodynia, both *in its pathology and treatment,* and to differ only in being more prone to pass into inflammation. The remote sympathies which different parts of the body evince under disordered condition of the stomach and digestive organs have often engaged the attention of practitioners (p. 437). *Colic—its treatment.*

419. I have mentioned that in all *complaints attended with fever,* or *constitutional inflammation,* the gastric and intestine secretions are *Fever and constitution- al inflam- mation.*

Morbid secretions and increased arterial action.

quickly increased. Accumulations of morbid secretions oftentimes take place in the alimentary canal, of slow and gradual formation, and not referable by any well-marked connection to a state of generally increased arterial action. The former state may even be superinduced upon the latter, and thus an additional complication, both of diseased action and of diseased condition, ensue. A disease, in which this morbid state of the secretions exerts considerable influence, is *rheumatism* (ibid.) Cases follow :

Rheumatism.

Gout. Pathology. Cure by purgatives.

420. Admitting, then, the pathology to be correct which attributes *gout* to the existence of a *state of plethora and inflammation in the blood-vessels*, and the influence of *vitiated secretions within the alimentary canal*—which latter may be regarded in a great degree as the natural product of the former—does it not seem to be fully within our power to bring this hitherto intractable disease under the control of rational practice? And may we not hope to treat it as effectually, and much more safely, by the well-ascertained powers of such a remedy as a combination of colocynth, calomel, and antimony presents us with, as by the less manageable means of white hellebore, or the precarious and uncertain " eau médicinale," *i. e.. " colchicum ?"* (P. 441.)

Colchicum.

Applicable to Brandreth's Pills.

421. The means I would recommend are advocated not for their possessing any secret or unexplained power over disease, but from their being *pointed out by a rational pathology, and fully established, both with respect to their safety and efficacy, by extensive experience* (ibid.)

B. G. B., *Observations on the Treatment of the Sick returned from Corunna.* See EDINB. MED. AND SURG. JOURN., 1810, *Vol. VI.*

Fevers. Calomel—can never supersede purgatives in the cure;—sometimes cures as a purgative.

422. There appears too great a desire of discovering something like a *specific for fever* to the very great neglect of obtaining evacuations. Calomel seems to be regarded in this way, and is abundantly employed with a view of producing some particular irritation of the system that will arrest the progress of or remove the complaint.

Whatever this medicine may do, after evacuations have been promised, I feel certain of one thing, that it will never supersede the necessity of evacuations in fever ; and I question very much if *its good effects in fever*, and in all inflammatory complaints, do not *depend upon its evacuating qualities* (p. 170).

Dr. Freind on fevers—evacuations alone can cure; without them—death.

423. Those, however, who attempt to cure *inflammatory fever*, or *inflammation, by any other means than by evacuation of some sort or other, will lose many an opportunity for doing good ;* and, in confirmation of this opinion, I will quote the authority of the very learned *Dr. Freind :* " Hoc unum libi spondeo te experiundo comprobaturum, quod silicet ex febribus multæ evacuantibus solis, etiam si haud alio fueris remedio usus, cedere consuescant ; vix ullæ antem, quæ paulo vehementius invaluerint, medicina qualicunque, si ab hoc evacuandi instituto decesseris, restingui possint." (Commentaries on 1st and 3d books Hippocrates.) *Dr. Freind* here observes *that many fevers will yield to evacuations alone, when no other remedy is used ; but scarcely any will be removed,*

when the fever is great, by any remedy whatever, if evacuations are NOT employed. I have no hesitation in saying, when this plan is speedily adopted, that the most beneficial effects will generally result, and that a great many cases of *inflammatory fever* which would otherwise have ended fatally, or become putrid, and have been protracted for a fortnight or three weeks, or even longer, *will by this system terminate favorably in a week* (pp. 170, 171).

TUOMEY, MARTIN, M. D., *A Treatise on the Principal Diseases of Dublin. Dublin,* 1810.

424. *Bilious fever.*—Purgatives must be steadily persevered in throughout the complaint, for it is upon them we must chiefly rely for success; and as the *accumulation of foul matters* in the alimentary canal is *constantly and copiously produced*, so there is no disease in which the free and regular use of purgatives causes less distress or gives more uniform relief. It frequently happens that from the operation of a purgative a large quantity of foul excrements come away; and yet in ten or twelve hours after there is another large evacuation, so as often to cause just surprise how so much could be generated in so short a time; and these copious and foul evacuations continue for several successive days without inducing proportionate weakness, but, on the contrary, they procure great mitigation of the symptoms. Even *delicate and young females* are relieved, *without being exhausted*, by these evacuations (p. 8). *Bilious fever. Copious and foul evacuations —impart strength but induce no weakness.*

425. So far from producing weakness, we have often observed with pleasure the *renewal of strength, which these evacuations occasion*, when a languor or depression of the animal powers, even to faintness, had previously existed. But we have likewise remarked that, as soon as the alvine excretions have assumed a natural appearance, a much smaller evacuation has actually produced a considerable reduction of strength (p. 9). *Evacuations strength—remove debility.*

426. It is remarkable that we are disappointed of any substantial improvement in the state of our patient *whilst the dark fæces remain behind*, notwithstanding the quantity of the evacuations procured (ibid). *Dark fæces are critical.*

BUCHAN, A. P., M. D., *Bisnomia. London,* 1811.

427. Is it credible that a human infant should be so imperfectly organized that it cannot pass over the years of childhood, naturally the most healthy period of life, except the biliary system be ever and anon expurgated by calomel? or that the early and habitual use of this mineral poison can be unattended with injurious consequences? Perhaps the time may come, when the *most judicious plan of curing* internal as well as external complaints, will be acknowledged to *consist in removing all impediments to the natural exertions* made by the vital energy to restore health (p. 71). *Childhood and calomel. The good time to come.*

CLARK, JOSEPH, M. D., *On the Bilious Colic and Convulsions of Early Infancy.* Dublin, 1811. *See* TRANSACTIONS OF THE ROYAL IRISH ACADEMY, 1811, *Vol. XI.*

Childhood— Convulsions —the old practice fatal —PURGATION the cure.   428. In the beginning of my practice, as long as I pursued the beaten track of employing mixtures of rhubarb and magnesia, solution of manna in fennel-water, chalk, musk, opium, and blisters, recovery from *convulsions in early infancy* was a rare occurrence. After six years' close attention to the subject I am convinced that *in colic and convulsions* nothing but a *brisk expulsion of the contents of the bowels* is likely to afford permanent relief. A dose or two of castor-oil, or a common purgative enema, may remove slight attacks of this nature. It is in general *after* the failure of such measures that a physician's advice is required (p. 124).

Evacuations—as the quantity so is the relief.   429. The *purgation must be very active and continuous* to be efficient. In the course of recovery the quantity of evacuation seldom fails to astonish the attendants, who cannot well comprehend whence it all can be derived. *The relief obtained is uniformly proportioned to the quantity discharged* (ibid.)

ARMSTRONG, JOHN, M. D. *Observations on the Origin, Nature and Treatment of Typhus Fever*—in MEDICAL INTELLIGENCER, 1812.

Typhus.— Many of its symptoms from wanting 'ecarbonization of the blood.   430. The want of due decarbonization of the blood is the cause of many of the most remarkable symptoms attendant on *typhus. Blood not duly decarbonized,* operates more or less as *a narcotic* on the brain, and tends materially to influence the animal heat and the heart's action ; and *hence* partly arise the *muddled state of the brain,* the *smothered heat* of the surface, and the *soft, compressible pulse,* &c. Why typhus-fever *Intermittent or remittent form— causes of.* assumes *in one person an intermittent, and in another the remittent or continued form, is most probably owing to the dose of the poison,* or the condition of the recipient, or both conjoined (Med. Int., No. 30, May, 1812).*

The Morbid Anatomy of the Bowels. Liver and Stomach. London, 1828.

Small-pox, measles, scarlatina — blood-diseases.   431. The contagions of *small-pox, measles* and *scarlatina* first operate on the blood, and that fluid being thereby changed, the solids are specifically affected, especially the skin and mucous membranes of the air-passages ; and these affections, too, if left to themselves, and even *Nature compared to a tidal flowing river.* often in despite of medical applications, *have a determinate course, the blood apparently,* like the water of the Thames, *requiring a certain time for its purification,* which it effects, perhaps, *by throwing off the effete and superfluous matters.* through the secretions and excretions (Art. I, p. 10).

Letter to Dr. Boot, contained in Dr. Boot's edition of Armstrong's Works.

Much learning often is folly in practical matters.   432. I have never yet met with a *learned physician* who was a good *practitioner.* At the bedside such men are ˙lost in the conflict of authority.

HARTZ, WILLIAM, M. D.   *On the use of Purgatives in Purpura.*
Dublin, 1813.   *See* EDINB. SURG. AND MED. JOURN., *Vol. IX.*

433. *Purpura.*—Convinced by my previous ill success of the inefficacy of mere tonics in bad cases, and favorably impressed by the occurrence of *cholera* previous to the appearance of the petechiæ, I determined
in this case to direct my whole attention to the state of the abdominal
viscera, and accordingly prescribed *brisk purgatives.* From the good
effects of the first, I directed its *repetition* for a few successive nights.
To my surprise the hemorrhage soon ceased, the spots rapidly disappeared, and in less than ten days the patient recovered, under every
possible disadvantage of constitution, of air, and of diet.   Encouraged
by the unexpected result of this unpromising case, I *no longer hesitated
in employing purgatives,* and *trusting to them only* in both species of the
complaint.   It was often necessary, however, to purge to a great extent
(p. 186).

[margin: PURPURA— the regular practice un-successful—successful—purgation cures. Important case.]
[margin: Full and free purgation re-quired.]

434. It appears from the observations of *Burserius,* that *Strack* supposes *petechiæ* to originate *from vitiated bile in the primæ viæ,* and from
a tenacious mucus adhering to the intestines, and that he accordingly
proposed *strong cathartics* as the proper remedy for the disease.   I have
carried this theory farther, and have, not without advantage, allowed it
to influence my practice in *typhus,* when petechiæ are present, and many
very desperate cases have appeared to me to *owe their recovery, almost
from the jaws of death, to the powerful and repeated interposition of
purgatives* (p. 187).

[margin: Typhus. Petechiæ from vitiated bile.]

MEDICUS.   *On Pathology.—See* EDINB. MED. & SURG. JOUR. 1815.
Vol. XI.

435. *Disordered actions* of the human body are, generally speaking,
the means which nature employs for the expulsion or removal of offending agents; thus if the stomach be excited *to vomit,* the cause producing
that disturbance is removed by that action; thus also *diarrhœas* carry
off noxious matters; and the emunctories of the body are generally
cleared out for the same purpose (p. 335).   As a machine, the human
body may be said to "go," at the same time that it includes powers
for repairing all injuries that otherwise would prevent its going, and
these reparatory processes include almost all the symptoms of disease
(p. 336).

[margin: Natural cure by vom-iting, diar-rhœa, etc.]

436. We will suppose, for example, that the stomach, unable to perform healthy digestion, presents to the liver, as it passes to the duodenum,
an ill-concocted chyme or chyle.   Does it not become necessary that the
liver should pour forth a bile suited to the purpose it has to answer?—
a purpose far different from what would be required if a healthful
digestion had taken place in the stomach.   Such a bile cannot be deemed
improper, since it answers the purpose for which it was intended, namely, of carrying through the bowels what was noxious, and of effectually

[margin: The stomach —vicarious function of the liver.]

assisting in assimilating such parts as are healthy and proper. To attack the liver, therefore, because it has done its duty, would be adding to the

Mistakes of practice— checking the vicarious function pro- duces liver- complaint.

evils which already excited its powers, and would be exhausting those means of resistance and reaction which were appointed for the most beneficent of purposes. *To oblige, by medicine, the stomach to retain such substances as, in a state undisturbed by medicine, it would reject, is the readiest conceivable method of calling forth the symptoms of " liver affection," and a general disturbance of the alimentary functions.* And thus it happens that the more extended reactions of the constitution follow these circumstances, and thus, by a very easy process of reasoning, shall we arrive at those causes which produce *gout, asthma, cutaneous diseases,* and in short a long train of grievous maladies (p. 336.)

Purgatives restore healthy di- gestion.

437. During healthful digestion, feelings are excited far different from those which arise when the meal has not been regulated by mode- ration and sobriety ; and how often are means applied to appease the tumult occasioned at such times, and thus so many noxious agents are introduced, which become all the causes of great and extended future mischief (p. 337).

Foulness of the bowels curative.

438. It has been said that foulness of the bowels is a common cause of disease. It appears to me that *when the bowels produce the foulness, so often observed, such foulness proves curative.* It is a reaction of the liver (?) against a constitutional disturbance, which in the end proves curative. Immediately on discovering this foulness, we feel satisfied that *on its removal* the various symptoms of disease will disappear (p. 339).

Reaction tending to reparation of the constitu- ion.

439. There is *a balance in the constitution* consistent with every nat- ural effort ; it may be called the *diathesis,* such as *gout,* and a variety of *other inflammatory affections,* and these states of balance involve their own series of phenomena. Thus the head may be oppressed with a super- abundance of blood, and may be liable to affections under one form or series ; another may involve rheumatism ; another, gout, &c.; and all of them, extended reactions of the system, tending towards a reparation of the constitution.

It may be observed that foulness of the bowels cannot exist to the full extent at which it appears at any one period ; for the quantity that on some occasions is discharged would be more than the canal was capa- ble of containing. It must, therefore, be *the result of successive deposi- tions from some great secreting organs.* For instance, during the exist- ence of disease, wherein there are great determinations of blood, ape- rient medicines bring away evacuations of no particular character; but *after a little time the circumstances of the case alter ; heavy, lumpy, and discolored evacuations begin to appear, and continue to be parted with. As soon as these appearances arise, the symptoms of the original disorder begin to diminish, and, in the course of a short time, disappear altogether.* It must have occurred to every practitioner who has strictly examined these circumstances, that he has found a difficulty in accounting for the quality and extent of this collection of foulness (p. 339).

440. It must also have been frequently observed that *affections of the head, epilepsy, chorea, local diseases* of various kinds, and great and extended *affections of the skin,* have all *given way as soon as the bowels have expelled a quantity of foul and fetid evacuation.* During the progress, however, of these maladies, the bowels have not shown the same character until the disorders have attained *a particular stage, and then the progress towards health is decided.* Could we succeed in bringing about this stage, many very grievous maladies might be cured; that is, we might induce thereby the various organs of the alimentary canal to render the more extended reaction of the system unnecessary. I do not mean to deny that there is occasionally a very *great accumulation in the bowels, so foul a state* of them that *worms* occur, which appear there to have found *a proper nidus ;* and that other great sympathetic affections take place arising from these accumulations (ibid).

Dark and fetid evacuations break the power of disease and produce reactions.

Worms.

441. If we trace these affections, we shall find *many natural efforts made to remove* such accumulations and foulness; and even that many very distant reactions occur tending to relieve the body of the grievance. Thus the *blood* returning through the "*vena portæ,*" is delayed, and as the heart acts uniformly, more blood flows to the head than usually, in consequence of this *remora* in the return of blood from the lower circulation. This fullness of blood in the head occasions many reactions, amongst which we may rank *epilepsy,* which shakes the whole body in convulsions, and *is the means of removing worms and other foulness* from the bowels, as under the influence of that disorder the alvine and urinary excretion are violently expelled (pp. 338, 339).

The natural cure—distant reaction.

The blood—its course.

Epilepsy.

442. *Why disease and cure are units, physiologically accounted for.* —The *tendency of disease* is either to *spontaneous cure* or to the *extinction of life* (p. 340).

Disease and cure—units.

443. *The human stomach* is an organ endowed by nature with the most complex properties of any in the body, and forming *a centre of sympathy* between our corporal and mental parts of more exquisite qualifications than even the brain itself. Yet the knife and eye of the anatomist do not discover the whole importance of the station it holds in the economy. We must look to the living system for those nice connections of cause and effect, and that source of association which gives it a relation to so many organs, both in the healthy and disordered state. ....We find all those viscera which assist in preparing the chyle and the assimilation of food, joined in a circle of nervous communication of which the stomach is the centre. One portion of nerves is distributed over the whole, so that, while they are employed in one purpose, disorder cannot take place in any one of them without the whole being thrown into confusion. These associated organs are regulated in their apparently disturbed state by laws tending to the relief of that perturbation. By these associated powers the causes of perturbation are removed, and the effects of such reaction are eventually rendered harmless. (Condensed from pp. 345 to ult.)

The stomach —its intimate relation with the whole body.

Sympathy explained through which all the organs suffer in order that one may be saved.

444. *The nerves of the stomach are connected,* through the great sympathetic nerve, *with almost every other nerve in the body.* The lungs,

Lungs, heart, etc., have nervous re-

lation with the stomach, and act with it in the "curative process," which is removal of noxious and offending agents. heart, and diaphragm, are also furnished with nerves which communicate with the great sympathetic. This nerve is the grand link or chain which connects the vital, animal, and natural functions with each other. *It is no very difficult matter to trace the curative actions that take place in consequence of this nervous connection*—how the heart may vary its pulsations agreeably to the impulse it receives through this nerve; how the liver and intestines are apprised of the necessity of varied exertions, agreeably to the kind of digestion that is to pass the sphere of their duties, &c.; all, I say, for the beneficent purpose of ultimately removing from the system the noxious influence of offending agents, such influence as, were it not for those wise provisions of nature, would prove destructive to the human frame (ibid).

More of this "curative process." If the stomach is unfit to effect this cure, excite with purgatives. 445. These several reactions of the body seem all calculated to become effectual, when the system is in a state agreeable to the laws of nature. A really *curative process* may be so far *altered* in its ultimate results *by improper habits of life*, that it may not be enabled to answer the purpose intended, or it may run into an excess, and even occasion detriment to the subject (ibid).

The "curative process"—conclusion. 446. We now see why the operations of the stomach, liver, and bowels are so effectual in removing very great and extended disorders of the system; and why, when required, such medicines as call forth these *reactions of the stomach and primæ viæ*, are the true means of cure. So that, whether a disorder originates in the stomach, proceeds to distant organs through the stomach, or is a disease arising primarily in a distant part of the frame—still such reactions are capable of affording relief (ibid., p. 345, sq., cf.).

PRITCHARD, J. C., M. D. *Remarks on the Treatment of Epilepsy and some other Nervous Diseases. See* MED. AND PHYS. JOURN., 1815, Vol. XI.

Nervous diseases— cure by purgatives. 447. I consider the introduction of the free use of *evacuating remedies* into the treatment of *nervous diseases* as one of the greatest improvements of the medical art which has taken place of late years. Imperfect as our knowledge confessedly is with respect to the pathology of nervous diseases, and inadequate as our remedies frequently prove themselves to be, we have yet the satisfaction of perceiving that we are evidently in the right path; and that, when we have not the means of cure in our power, *we can at least often palliate, without* incurring the *Epilepsy.* risk of *making matters worse* than we found them (p. 459).—Cases of cures of *epilepsy* given.

Neurosis. 448. I have tried the use of *evacuant remedies* in several other disorders of the class *neurosis* with *success ;* but *in none with more singular advantage than in mania*, in which distemper I have had extensive opportunities of witnessing their effects, having been for some years one of the physicians to a hospital where a great number of lunatics were admitted. I am firmly persuaded that if medical practitioners would *depend more on physical and less on moral remedies*, they would succeed in a greater proportion of cases, especially recent ones, than generally happens (p. 456).

449. *Indications* to be obtained by the use of *purgatives* are :

1. By *removing sordes* from the intestinal canal. *Indications of purgatives.*
   I am every day surprised at the prodigious accumulation of fecal matters which I find to take place in the intestinal canals of patients of all years.
2. As *depleting* the system.
3. As *determining* the fluids from the head.
4. As setting up a *new action* in the system.
5. Purging is a powerful means of *stimulating* the absorbent system, as we witness its effects on dropsical patients.
6. A course of moderate purgation is one of the most efficient methods of *invigorating* the digestive organs, improving appetite, and removing visceral obstructions (p. 466).

DICKSON, D. J. H., M. D., *Superintending Physician to the Russian Fleet. On the Utility of Depletion in a Fever among the Russian Sailors. See* EDINB. MED. AND. SURG. JOURN., 1816, *Vol. XII.*

450. It is now well understood that the *value of purgatives is not limited* to the *mere removal of the fecal contents* of the bowels, but that they may be so managed as *to obviate or relieve a tendency to topical congestions* elsewhere, and also to produce a considerable *effect upon the general system*, by the increased quantity of fluids they cause the various glands and exhalent arteries to pour into the intestines. Thus they become more *universally useful* in diseases in general, in proportion as they are *more uniformly applicable*. . . . They were here considered not only indispensably requisite in the first instance, and assisted by enemas, when necessary; but they were liberally exhibited throughout the disease; and very often the bowels could not be kept sufficiently active unless they were repeated day after day (p. 175). *Purgatives —their value unlimited. Action on glands and exhalent arteries.*

451. Though not a new, it is a very important observation, that all uncertainty as to their full operation can only be removed by inspection, without which the practitioner is very apt to be led to imagine by the patient from his own report, or that of the nurse, that he has been sufficiently purged, when, at most, he may have had only two or three partial scanty dejections. . . *While we are producing foul, dark, fetid evacuations, we may naturally expect that we are benefiting and relieving the patient.* By those that have not had much acquaintance with fevers it is *hardly possible to calculate the quantity of medicine sometimes required to overcome the torpor of the intestinal canal, the morbid accumulations that have been discharged after repeated purgations, and in some cases the speediness of their reproduction* (p. 175). *Inspect the evacuation in order to exact sufficient purgation.*

452. In *tropical fevers* especially, I have seen very striking examples of the *abatement of fever and delirium after the operation of purgatives,* and it is therefore of great consequence to be aware that the febrile symptoms are often maintained or renewed *by the retention of* *Tropical fevers.*

Purges must be continued until natural stools ensue.

ritiated secretions, or other morbid contents of the intestines, as also of the quantity of dark-colored offensive matter that is often discharged after the patient has been thought sufficiently purged, and its speedy accumulation in some cases, in order to estimate the extent to which it may be necessary to persist in the use of evacuations (p. 176).

NAVAL SURGEON. *Medical Topography of New Orleans, with an account of the principal diseases that affected our Fleet and Army on the last Expedition against that City.* See EDINB. MED. & SURG. JOURN., 1816, Vol. XII.

Dysentery— Its origin from the liver.

Morbid matters the cause which must be removed. They injure the fabric of the passages— cause flux, ulcerations, etc.

453. *Dysentery.*—In short, to give a condensed view of the whole matter, the phenomena of the cases that recovered, as well as the morbid appearances of those that died, impressed upon my mind a conviction that *the diseased condition of the liver was the soil from which dysentery drew its malignant growth, strength, and nurture.* This was the "fons et origo mali," by it the dysentery was excited, *and only by its removal could the disease be removed.* I can readily conceive that from the disease of any gland, the fluid it secretes may acquire acrimonious properties sufficient to injure the fabric of the passages through which it is destined to pass.

We generally observe in dyspeptic complaints, or after a period of constipation, when the bile, from *remora* in the bowels, becomes morbid in quantity or quality, either that spontaneous diarrhœa comes on, or, after a brisk cathartic has been exhibited, that the dislodged bile excites a sensation in the rectum, as if boiling lead were voided. When the state of the liver is still more morbid, may not the bile acquire the property of exciting *flux*, and of *excoriating and ulcerating the villous coat of the colon and rectum?* (Pp. 142, 143.)

Typhus and the bugbear "debility." Calomel and James' powder.

Neglect of evacuation —its consequence in typhus. Bark, wine, opium.

454. The imaginations of professional men in tropical climates were formerly held in subjection by that bugbear, *debility,* and its train of needless horrors. Systems of nosology had been pleased to style the disorder "*typhus icterodes;*" consequently active depletion was carefully shunned. The practitioner stood fidgeting with his calomel and his James' powder. The disease *took its hue* from the species of treatment employed at first. The *neglect of evacuation* allowed the excitement to riot and revel unchecked; hence came *petechiæ, hemorrhages,* &c. .. Then indeed the disease was pronounced "*malignant, pestilent,* and *highly putrescent,*" and the golden opportunity occurred for throwing in—as the phase is—his bark, his wine, and his opium against that debility, about which at a wrong time he was over-solicitous. That cabalistical word "*typhus,*" I verily believe, has slain its thousands and its tens of thousands (pp. 147, 148).

DROPES, RICHARD L., Surg., *Remarks on some Remedies which are Used in Fevers. London,* 1817. See EDINB. MED. AND SURG. JOURN., 1817, *Vol. XIII.*

Fevers.— Emetics, diaphoretics, and pur-

455. FEVERS.—*Emetics,* I am convinced from experience, *have most frequently proved injurious,* and have seldom failed to *aggravate the symptoms* in a very obvious manner. *The great concussion they give*

the *whole system, particularly the brain,* almost invariably increased the violent pain so often felt in the head, and especially over the eyeballs; and this, it is to be presumed, by increasing the morbid action of the vessels of the encephalon. *The only cases* in which *emetics are admissible* are those in which an obstinate vomiting takes place, owing to some crudities in the stomach, which require to be evacuated (p. 59).

natives compared. THE SUPREMACY OF THE LATTER maintained and proved.

456. *Diaphoretics.*—I believe that it is on the principle of the heat of the body being morbidly increased, owing to obstructed perspiration, that sudorifics are prescribed for the purpose of removing this obstruction, and lowering the temperature. However, I conceive this practice is not well founded. *Diaphoretics,* before they can have the desired effect, *almost always increase the morbid action,* and most *obviously have an injurious tendency.* Besides, we have other means of lessening vascular action and reducing morbid heat without being attended with the same inconvenience as sudorifics. Every day we see patients attacked with fever completely recover without there being the smallest tendency to a diaphoresis through its whole course. *When these medicines have been chiefly relied on, I have always observed the disease to be much protracted, and the cure extremely tedious* (p. 60).

Sudorifics rather injurious, and by no means apt to bring forth a cure.

457. *Purgatives.*—The generality of physicians place too little dependence on *these,* and trust too much to other remedies. I know of no general means attended with so much success as the liberal employment of *cathartics.* They should be given *in large doses,* and *often repeated,* till the patient becomes convalescent, which is generally in a few days from their first employment (ibid.)

Purgatives the only reliable remedy, when given in large doses, often repeated.

458. When given merely as *aperients* their effects are only trifling; but *when administered with sufficient freedom,* WITH A DETERMINATION OF REDUCING INFLAMMATION, *their curative powers are often astonishing* (p. 61).

Aperient and full purgative action contrasted.

WILSON, ANDREW, M. D., *Practical Observations on the Action of Morbid Sympathies. Edinburgh,* 1818.

459. Nerves possess muscular fibers and blood-vessels, and are subject to foreign influences; and *the condition of the blood must influence their actions* by influencing their secretion (text condensed from pp. 20, 21, and 82).

Nervous diseases from impure blood.

460. There is no department of the nervous system by which, if certain or peculiar irritating causes are applied, some other department of the same system may not be influenced, so as to draw the organ to which they belong into morbid action by sympathetic affinity (pp. 165, 166).

Sympathy of the nerves.

461. Certain *acrimonious matters applied to* the extremities of the *gastric and alvine nerves give* a variety of *deranged actions of the brain,* although otherwise in a sound state, and the accelerated pulse of the whole arterial system, from inflammation found in a small portion of its capillary branches, is at once perceptible both to the eye and touch. . .

Morbid matters in the stomach and disorders of the brain, strictures, etc.

Gastric irritation gives *spasmodic affections of the bladder and kidneys.* . . . Irritation of the lower extremities will excite nausea and vomiting (pp. 166, 167).

462. Of all the organs of the human body the gastric and alvine department is that which is most extensively and constantly exposed to the action of these causes; a surface which extends from the cardia to the rectum, every part of which is provided with nerves of the greatest sensibility (pp. 167, 168).

463. *Fever* is excited *by acrimonious irritation in the alimentary canal*, or by the increased secretions which take place in the liver and other abdominal glands (p. 19).

464. The natural and healthy action of *the heart* and the whole vascular system is impaired and reduced below its natural standard, as exhibited in *palpitations, languid pulse, torpor of the limbs, syncope*, and even *death* itself, in consequence of the mere application of a peculiar offensive substance to the digestive organs (p. 19).

This paragraph applies to and explains the action of *poisons.*

465. The approach of *typhus* and *yellow fever* is at all times attended by decided symptoms of an existing *diseased state of the stomach and bowels, i. e.*, with those signs which are known to point out their contents to be of a morbid, irritating nature; but whenever *the alimentary canal* happens to be *loaded with irritating matter*, some derangement of the healthy operation, either of the general system or of some particular organ of the body, is the certain result; and when this state happens to be united with any other cause of fever (as infections), its effects are always thereby much aggravated. It is therefore reasonable to use *every exertion in such cases to expel it as quickly as possible* (pp. 107, 108).

466. ☞The method which the most eminent practitioners have adopted from experience as the most advantageous is by *discharging from the primæ viæ, as expeditiously as possible, their irritating and offensive contents*, and in reducing the febrile heat by cold applications (p. 128). It is also worthy of remark, as it further demonstrates the agency of the contents of the stomach and intestines, in producing organic inflammation, that *in these cases which terminate most favorably the stools are all along abundant and bilious*, with some occasional bilious vomiting; and that by these free discharges, the intestinal contents being carried out of the body as they are collected, their agency as a supervening cause of the febrile state is greatly removed, and they are not left to acquire that degree of acrimony which is necessary to the establishment of inflammation (pp. 129, 130).

467. A powerful *morbid sympathy* is called into action (in acute rheumatism), and becomes established betwixt the irritated digestive organs and the ligaments of the joints; the adjoining tendonous expan-

sions, the membrane of the muscles, and occasionally the muscles them- Pains continue until the primary cause is removed.
selves, often forming organic obstructions, and exhibiting all the severe
phenomena of *acute rheumatism* (p. 210). . . The *primary cause in the
digestive organs* is entirely overlooked, and so is left to continue its
action with full vigor; consequently the daily repetition of the spasmodic paroxysm depending upon it, keeps up the local inflammation on
the sympathizing membranes, and often extends it (p. 220).

408. These shiftings of the pains, and change of place from one part *Atonic rheumatism.* Pains shift, as the morbid matters change their location.
of the body to another, depend on the occasional change of place of the
irritating matter contained in the intestines, to one with which some
other distinct part of the body has a more direct sympathetic affinity
than that which the pain has left (p. 249).

469. The character of *atonic rheumatism* consists in a painful affec- *Atonic rheumatism* —its character.
tion of some muscular parts, or of their membranes. The pains are not
so severe as in acute rheumatism; they very frequently wander from
one part of the body to another, although it often happens that they remain fixed in one part for a long time. . . A particular muscle, or a
portion of its fibers, become frequently so affected by the sympathetic
spasm as to be impeded in its free action; the pain being constantly
aggravated by the slightest movement of the part, although quite easy
when the muscle is at rest (p. 247).

470. The *remote cause* of these phenomena is decidedly seated *in the The cause of all rheumatic complaints is in the digestive organs.
digestive organs* in *atonic* as well as in *acute rheumatism.* They are in
their nature spasmodic, only the seat of the morbid sympathy most commonly appears to be one less susceptible of that inflammation which
forms the secondary disease of acute rheumatism (p. 248).

471. In the *treatment of acute rheumatism* much attention is due to To remove the cause the *most free evacuation* is required.
the state and circumstances attending the primary gastric fever. Expe-
rience has supported the opinion that, *in proportion as the primary
cause of disease is removed, the sympathetic effect on the membranes of
the joints begins also to subside* (p. 221). In order to accomplish this
object the *most free evacuations from the stomach and intestines* are required, and the patient generally bears them well (p. 222).

472. But of a much more painful nature than the atonic rheumatism *Lumbago, hip disease,* and *tic-douloureux,* from disease of the alimentary canal.
are the cases of *lumbago, sciatica, tic douloureux,* and *periodical or inter-
mitting rheumatism.* They are with great certainty to be traced from
the same remote cause, and, like the former, are only sometimes attended
with gastric fever, but are *uniformly associated with decided signs of a
diseased state of the alimentary canal* (p. 249).

473. All *local applications*, independent of clearing the alimentary *Local applications* only palliate; the cause must be removed to cure.
canal from its contained acrimony, can go no further than *merely* to *pal-
liate the effect of this cause*, but without curing the disease, which will
not happen while the power of the other remains in action (p. 257).

Erysipelas. Cure by removing the morbid cause.

474. *Erysipelas* is intimately connected with the state of the digestive organs, which is clearly demonstrated by the well-known fact of its appearing in various degrees on the skin, *in consequence of certain kinds of food having been taken into the stomach,* and this not only in too short a space of time after to admit of the chyle impregnated by them to be taken into the circulation, but while they as yet remained in the stomach, *and the inflammation disappearing as soon as those contents were thrown off* (p. 371).

Sore-throat in scarlet-fever from stomach-vapors.

475. From the *great similarity of the general symptoms* exhibited in *scarlet fever to those* exhibited *in typhus fever,* it will be obvious that the treatment here ought to be very similar to that adopted to those under typhus; which is, in the first place, pointed to the *mitigation of the two great supervening causes of fever—irritation in the primæ viæ* and *excess of caloric*—especially to that which is seated within the digestive organs; *the very exhalations* from which, ascending to the fauces, do, beyond a doußt, tend to *keep up the inflammation,* and, consequently, the ulcerated state (pp. 142, 143).

Purgation removes debility, and gives strength.

476. *That free evacuations increase debility is in reality an unfounded apprehension. . ,* Whatever will act upon the morbid cause, so as to evacuate it from the body, so *far from weakening,* will assuredly *tend to restoration of the strength;* and *this is a fact* which unvarying experience has proved in every instance where nature has not been already exhausted by other means (pp. 60, 61).

The advantage of full purgation.

Examination of dejections.

477. The intention is not merely to preserve the bowels soft, but to discharge from the intestines *a lurking cause of disease;* to accomplish which purpose *very full evacuations* are *always necessary,* procured by the help of the *most active purgatives* administered in appropriate doses; remarking the nature of what comes off till it puts on a healthy appearance (p. 62).

Impurities far more weakening than the fullest purgation.

478. To restore health, purgatives must be perseveringly applied (in typhus fever), as it is certain that *the retention of any sort of noxious matter in the primæ viæ,* the tendency of which is in general to lessen the energy of the nervous system, *is infinitely more debilitating* to the human frame *than the temporary fatigue* attendant on the moderate operation either of an emetic or purgative medicine, besides the harm which may ensue from the noxious matters being partially reabsorbed (pp. 110, 111).

Measles.

Sympathy between stomach and lungs;—purge the acrid matters away.

Bleeding and mild purgatives equally useless, and why.

479. That a state of morbid sympathy betwixt the stomach and lungs does actually exist in many cases of *measles* I believe to be certain. My belief is founded on the very *great relief* from pneumonic symptoms received *by a free discharge of acrid matter* from the stomach and intestines—a relief which can be accounted for from no other law of the animal economy. Repeated *bleedings* will, no doubt, tend to lessen the vascular action, but probably in no high degree, while the secondary cause of fever continues to give its irritation to the nerves of the stomach and bowels; and it is obvious that *venesection cannot act as a means of removing this cause, neither,* indeed, are the more *lenient*

cathartics to be depended on for this purpose; for although they will to a certainty open the bowels, yet they very frequently pass along and *leave the offending cause behind.* It is the more active powers of *drastic purgatives alone* which are here *to be confided in* (pp. 136, 137).

HAMILTON, JR., JOHN. *On the Use and Abuse of Mercurial Remedies. Edinburgh*, 1819.

480. In *pleurisy*, from the time that the influence of mercury becomes evident, the general strength rapidly declines (p. 7).

Pleurisy—baneful effects of mercury.

481. If there be *ulcerations* in any part of the body, they must as certainly degenerate into malignant sores, under the influence of mercury, as blistered surfaces or scarifications mortify in cases where the living powers are much exhausted (p. 9).

Ulcers— become malignant by mercury.

JOHNSON, JAMES, M. D. *Critical and Explanatory Remarks in his Periodical,* MEDICO-CHIRURGICAL REVIEW, *established in* 1819.

482. *Purgatives* in *intestinal inflammation* have been objected to on the ground that they are quickly rejected by vomiting; but this objection is not valid. . . If the first purgative be rejected, it is repeated by *Dr. Pring* in an hour or two, and so on, with various forms of purgatives, until the bowels are opened, when in general we find the ball at our own feet (vol. IV., 1823, p. 259).

Intestinal inflammation. Give purgatives until the stomach retains them, and the cure is effected.

483. *Dr. Pring* says, "*typhus* has two origins, one from external affection, and the other from a spontaneous generation of disease in the subject affected by it" (ibid., p. 250).

Typhus— its origin.

484. His favorite practice is purgation of a very active kind (Pr., p. 102); has seen his patients stimulated into fatal apoplexy (ibid., p. 251).

Apoplexy from stimulants.

485. In the treatment of any form of *chronic disease*, whether in the digestive organs or elsewhere, purgatives frequently increase the symptoms *at first*, an effect which is rather desirable than otherwise, and *it proves that the remedy has a relation with the disease*, and is capable of subverting this state, *if continued for a sufficient length of time* (ibid., p. 275).

Chronic diseases. Effect of purgatives showing the remedy to have a relation with the disease.

By the use of Brandreth's Pills the vital forces change chronic affections into acute. Then further purgation with them soon effects a cure.

486. *Dr. Abercrombie* is of opinion that *the only remedies* of real efficacy *in epilepsy* are *purgatives* and a strict vegetable diet, with total abstinence from strong liquors (ibid., pp. 127, 128).

Epilepsy. The cure by purgatives.

487. *Constipation in Pregnancy.—De Lemazurien* was sent for on the 8th of July, 1823, to see a woman in the seventh month of her pregnancy. Abdomen much distended, transverse arch of the colon

Constipation.

Fatal consequences of the neglect of purgation in pregnancy. greatly distended, pulse and appetite feeble, dyspnœa, sleeplessness, faintness, pains in the loins. Lavements were ordered, but it was determined to wait till the accouchment was over before the evacuation of the bowels should be attempted.

After child-birth, clysters being employed, the fecal accumulation appeared to break up, and there was an evacuation of two or three pounds of hard brown fetid matter, but there remained a collection too large for expulsion. The patient was worn down by nausea, fever, colicky and other pains, and died 21st September.

The colon from the cæcum to the rectum was found to be intensely inflamed. It was a foot in circumference throughout its whole length, was filled with gas and with 13½ pounds (French) of solid fæces (1824, vol. I., pp. 233, 234).

This case was simple. Two or three doses of Brandreth's Pills would have certainly relieved, by thoroughly removing all the fecal contents of the bowels. And no danger incurred at any period of gestation to either mother or child by the use of this safe but certain medicine.

Epilepsy. 488. *Epilepsy.*—The views of *Dr. Chapman* coincide with those of *Dr. Pritchard*, in placing the cause of apoplexy very frequently in the bowels. He was led to the use of purgatives by the total failure of the ordinary plans of treating the disease: " *it will not do, however,*" he says, " *merely to evacuate the bowels ; cathartics must be repeated day after day without interruption*, unless absolutely forbid by circumstances " (vol. IV., 1823, p. 73).

The cause, seated in the bowels, to be removed by continued purgation.

Nervous diseases from retained excretions. 489. The *retention of biliary, urinary, intestinal and cutaneous excretions* is often the remote cause of diseases of the nervous system, as well of the *neuralgic* as of the *spasmodic* and *maniacal* groups (New Series, 1852, vol. X., p. 97)

Neuralgia from morbid matter in the blood, which acts on the part predisposed, to induce local disease. 490. Whenever there exists " induced local susceptibility " *morbid elements in the blood* act most obviously in inducing *neuralgia. Malaria* may be present therein, yet remain latent and harmless until this state occurs. So also the *materies morbi of rheumatism or gout* may fly about until it is specially manifested in some locality rendered more susceptible by predisposing causes. It may be observed that poisons in general have a specific elective affinity for certain portions of the nervous system (New Ser., 1852, vol. X. p. 103).

All our knowledge of medicine is from experience. 491. We find that under certain circumstances a drug does good, and we employ it when those conditions present themselves. The *modus operandi* is often *totally unknown*, and though it would be very satisfactory to know it, yet we can dispense with it, and from experience alone prescribe our remedies with very considerable success (New Ser., 1851, vol. VIII., p. 204).

Erysipelas from retained and putrid fæces. 492. The condition of the alimentary canal should be carefully watched in *erysipelas*, for we have long suspected that it arises more frequently from its derangement than the generality of the profession are aware. *Excrementitious matter allowed to putrify* in the fecal tube will not only operate as an irritant upon the whole system, but from the close and constant sympathy which holds between the cutaneous and mucous surfaces, may be expected to exert a deleterious influence more immediately upon the skin. Hence the *erysipelas bilcosum* and *gastricum* of many writers (p. 371, Ser. I., 1828, vol. IX).

493. In the concluding stages of the *putrid fevers*, when the bowels had been long neglected before assistance was procured, we have seen the most tedious and inveterate forms of the disease (ibid). *Putrid fevers inveterate from neglect of bowels.*

BOYLE, JAMES, Surg., *A Treatise on Epidemic Cholera in India.* London, 1821.

494. It sometimes happens, after patients are despaired of, they *have a critical evacuation of viscid bile.* When this circumstance takes place the patient *invariably recovers.* I have known it to occur in cases when the pulse had been almost imperceptible for twenty-four hours. I looked on the obstruction of the biliary ducts as a source of irritation to the nervous system generally, and the nausea and sickness of the stomach as an effort of nature to free herself from an unaccustomed evil. These views and a general want of success in practice induced me to embrace ideas perfectly new on the subject. *Emetics and purgatives* were adopted as the most likely means to answer the various purposes of clearing the stomach, removing obstructions of the biliary ducts, and exciting a new action in the vascular system (pp. 51–61, condens.). Many successful cases given. *Cholera—its cause, and purgation its cure.*

The very course I pursued in London in 1831, and again adopted in New York in 1849, 1853, and 1866.

CHAPMAN, N., M. D., *President of Academy of Medicine in Philadelphia. The Elements of Therapeutics and Materia Medica,* 2 Vols. *Philadelphia,* 1821.

495. *Gout.*—My impression, very concisely stated, is, that this disease, if not *originating in,* has a most intimate connection with, certain state of *the alimentary canal.* It generally commences with those symptoms which denote a *depraved condition of the stomach and bowels* (p. 190). *Gout—its origin.*

496. I have now for many years habitually employed purgatives in the paroxysms of gout, and with unequivocal advantage. Not content with simply opening the bowels, *I completely evacuate by active purging the whole alimentary canal.* This being accomplished, all the distressing sensations of the stomach which I have mentioned are removed, the pain and inflammation of the limb gradually subside, and the paroxysm, thus broken, speedily passes away. *To effect these purposes, however, it is often necessary to recur to the remedy frequently* (ibid.) *Cure: by powerful purgation.*

497. *Palsy.*—Dissatisfied with this course (the usual routine of bleeding, blistering, and stimulating embrocations to which he formerly had recourse) I have for many years abandoned it, and *rely now almost exclusively on evacuating the bowels* by *the drastic purgatives.* Of the propriety of the change I can entertain no doubt, the success having *Palsy. Bleeding rejected. Purgation highly successful.*

exceeded my most sanguine expectations. To do justice to the practice, *it should be steadily persevered in*, and aided by such remedies as the case may from time to time demand (p. 193).

LLOYD, EUSEBIUS, A., M. D., *Treatise on Scrofula. London*, 1821.

Scrofula.   498. The very great influence which *evacuations from the bowels* have over the rest of the body cannot be denied by any impartial ob-
Purgation—its action explained. server ; it is therefore certain that by increasing or diminishing them we are able to produce *a decided effect on the whole*, or, as I have proved before, *on a particular part of the body*. Thus, if there is much general irritation, or local irritation and inflammation, *by increasing the intestinal evacuation*—taking care, however, not to irritate the bowels—*we may very much relieve* both the one and the other (p. 162).

When Brandreth's Pills are the purgative there is no danger of irritating the bowels.

NICKOLL, WILLIAM, M. D., *General Elements of Pathology. London*, 1822.

Unity of the human body.   499. We speak of the body as being composed of distinct sets of structures—the vascular, the nervous, the muscular; or else we treat of it after the manner of geographers, as consisting of the head, the thorax,
Disease not local but general. the abdomen, &c. Whichever mode we adopt, we acquire a habit of considering each portion which we enumerate as a distinct and isolated fact. The consequence is, that when any deviation from health occurs, *our attention is fixed upon the diseased condition of this particular part of the body*, while every other portion is supposed to preserve its former healthy state. It is evident that *each part cannot be considered as a distinct insulated republic, but as a constituent portion of the general commonwealth*, whose health is dependent upon a certain condition of every portion of the body- (X.)

SHAW, JOHN, M. D., *On Partial Paralysis; a Paper read before the Medico-Chirurgical Society of London, in April*, 1822 ; *a Narrative of the* DISCOVERIES *of* SIR CHARLES BELL *in the Nervous System, by Alexander Shaw, Surg. London*, 1839.

Nerves.   500. By experiments upon the *portio dura* he (Sir Ch. Bell) demon-
Those with one root have only one function; those with two roots a double function, namely motion and sensation. This is true of nerves both that originate from the brain and from the spinal marrow. strated that it was a motor nerve exclusively, and had no power of bestowing sensation. When cut across, in the living animal, the motions of a certain set of muscles were immediately arrested, but the sensibility of the surface supplied by the nerve remained undiminished. Upon submitting the fifth pair to experiment, a totally different set of phenomena presented themselves. This nerve, although it arises from the brain by two roots, has one of its origins nearly four times larger than the other. . . It was found that when those branches which proceed simply from the larger root were cut across, only one endowment—sensation—was destroyed; whereas upon cutting across those branches in which the fibrils of the two roots were united together in the same sheath, not only sensation, but the power of motion, were destroyed (pp. 9, 10). An attempt was made to apply the new observations, in a similar manner,

to the pathology of the spinal marrow. Certain affections of the upper or lower extremities, supplied by these spinal nerves, sometimes occur, in which the sensation of the limb is destroyed, while the motion remains entire, and *vice versa* (p. 11).

501. Now, as it has been established experimentally that motor power belonged to the anterior roots, and sensation to the posterior, it was concluded that when motion, in these cases, was lost, it depended on a morbid condition of the anterior or motor column of the spinal marrow; while, if sensation was lost, it depended on disease of the posterior or sensitive column (pp. 11, 12). *The cause of impaired motion and of impaired sensation.*

These butcheries lead to little good in a practical way.

502. I shall make a few remarks upon a question which has particularly excited the attention of physicians of all ages, since the time of Galen, " Why sensation should remain entire in a limb when all voluntary power over the action of its muscles is lost; or why muscular power should remain when feeling is gone ? " . . In answer, *Galen* said : *that two sets of nerves went to every part ; one to endow the skin with sensibility, the other to give the muscles the power of voluntary action.* This opinion was probably founded on a mere theory ; but the facts lately discovered, and the observations which have been noted in attending to the phenomena of disease, though they do not afford absolute proofs of Galen's supposition, still go far to establish the *fact,* " *that every part of the body which is endowed with two or more powers, is provided with a distinct nerve for each function* " (p. 13). *Further explanation of the above.* *Galen's opinion.*

503. The *form of the nerves,* which at the same time endow the skin with sensibility and the muscles with the power of voluntary motion, is such that they appear to be single cords ; but if we examine the *origin* of any of these nerves, we shall find that it is *composed of two packets of fibres,* which *arise from distinct parts of the spinal marrow.* These origins are soon *enveloped in the same sheath, so as to appear to form a single nerve* (p. 13). *The form of nerves originating from a double root.*

504. It is not too much to suppose that either of these origins may be affected, while the other remains entire. To prove this by ocular demonstration will perhaps be impossible. But we have already seen examples of the consequences of injury to a nerve that has a single root, viz., the " portio dura ; " for, if we cut it, there will be only one set of actions paralyzed ; while by dividing a nerve which has a double origin, viz., the fifth, we shall destroy two powers, namely, voluntary motion and sensibility. We know, also, that when we cut through the trunk of a nerve going to the hand, we destroy both sensibility and the power of motion. . . If the view here taken be correct, it may lead to this rule of practice : If only one set of functions of a spinal nerve be deficient, we should apply our remedies to that part of the system from which the nerve arises ; but if both functions are impaired, we must direct our inquiries to the state of the nerve in the whole course, from its origin to *Local applications and general treatment. Nervous affections as proceeding from impure blood, or fetid matters in the bowels, always indicate purgation assisting the local application and perfecting the general treatment.*

its distribution, as the loss of power is probably owing to some affection of a part of the nerve after the two sets of filaments, by which it arises, are united together (pp. 13, 14, 15).

— It may here be observed that Mr. Shaw was a pupil of Sir Charles Bell's, and that his treatise was based upon the latter's opinion, given in a short "Essay on the Anatomy of the Brain," printed and distributed among his friends in 1809 or 1811. (See A. Shaw, p. 14.)

PRING, DANIEL, M. D., *An Exposition of the Principles of the Pathology and of the Treatment of Diseases.* *London,* 1823.

Inflammation, peritoneal and intestinal—purge without fear of increasing the inflammation, and why not.

505. In *enteritis* and *peritonitis* I have trusted more to purgatives than to bleeding, and I have no reason to regret this confidence. The *use of purgatives, it has been objected, must increase inflammation ; the effect,* however, *is otherwise ;* and the testimony of experience must on this as on other occasions, supersede all a priori reasonings. But as a matter of reasoning, the conclusion against purgatives on this ground is not legitimate (p. 219).

Argument original and logically stated.

506. It does not follow, that an agent which is related with a secreting function so as to increase it, should also be so related with *inflammation,* which *frequently suspends secretion,* as to augment its intensity.

The danger is in not purging with sufficient energy.

On the contrary, in the way of reasoning, it would appear that if secretion is suspended by inflammation, that which restores secretion must diminish inflammation.

Setting reasoning for the present aside, I suspect that *in cases in which* PURGATIVES *have been* SUPPOSED *to increase intestinal inflammation, it is because these means were* INADEQUATELY EMPLOYED (ibid.).

Dyspepsia.

507. *Dyspepsia,* whether simple or accompanied by disordered function of the liver, chronic pains in the side, &c. *When the inconvenience attending purgation has passed away, then an improved state* of the digestive organs succeeds (pp. 307–309, condensed).

Chorea. Purge until healthy stools appear.

508. *Chorea.*—In the few cases which have occurred to me of this disease, some of which were severe ones, it has yielded to purgatives in about three weeks. The stools have commonly in about this period assumed a healthy appearance, and the spasmodic action of the muscles has quickly ceased (p. 245).

Chronic rheumatism—cured by free purgation.

509. A gentleman had *chronic rheumatism,* chiefly affecting his knees and shoulders. He went out on a cold damp day ; in the evening he had rigors ; the rheumatic pains left the extremities, and he was taken with *something like syncope,* sense of constriction at the bottom of the throat, and pain in the chest, with a fluttering irregular pulse of 160 a minute. I gave him *a full dose* of calomel, salts, senna and jalap, which produced *eight or ten stools in as many hours.*

The next day he was able to lie flat in his bed. The purgings were continued. In four days his pulse came down to 60, and in a few days he began to recover rapidly (p. 217).

510. *Humoral Pathology* may be said to have been perfected by *Humoral pathology.*
Boerhaave (Preface, p. 1).

511. So unsettled is the state of pathology that those who read are Medical Ignorance. skeptics in all its doctrines; and those who do not read are left to the norance. guidance of a sort of intuition, which is not always productive of happy results, but very frequently suggests, through the course of a long life, only reiteration of the same error (p. 1).

512. It appears to me, then, in the case of the " peccant humors," *The peccant humors.* that their phenomena are not produced by a mechanical agency. It is *Original views of their* more agreeable with the results of analytical inquiry to conclude *that* action. *the animal poisons contain latent properties of a vital kind, which are related with those of the same kind in living bodies ; that the phenomena* of disease or death, which ensue from the operation of the animal poisons in living bodies, are according to the nature of the properties which are engaged in this relation (p. ii.).

513. In my own experience it has been invariably the case, that *Bleeding induces deter-* those who have sustained great losses of blood suffer more or less from *mination of* what is called *determination to the head.* The symptoms most common- blood. ly are *intense pain* and *throbbing* in the forehead or back of the head, with a pulse seldom under 90 (p. 23).

514. It is common in severe and threatening forms of *cerebral dis-* *Bleeding in orders, notwithstanding previous loss of blood, to resort to the lancet,* and *cerebral disorders fatal.* to repeat copiously and frequently, if the symptoms continue. I have observed that this practice has *generally* had *a fatal termination* (p. 86).

515. I have been in the habit of confiding in *purgatives* to the almost *Cerebral* total neglect of the lancet; but these purgatives have not been of a *diseases.* milk-and-water kind. I have given 6 grains of calomel, 6 grains of *Purgatives of the* James' powder, followed by a 2-ounce draught of senna and salts with *strongest kind to be* half a drachm of jalap in it. If this has been rejected, it has been re- *exhibited.* peated in less than an hour, and *repeated* as often as it was rejected, *until it has produced copious evacuations from the bowels* (ibid).

516. One, and perhaps an important *effect* of such *purgatives,* is to *The purga-* make a *great revulsion to the whole intestinal canal,* which is commonly *tive action* followed by almost perfect relief to the head, and perhaps an immediate *explained.* subsidence of the pulse to 100 or 110. The tendency to disorder of the head is afterwards easily kept within safe bounds by small repeated doses of purgatives (ibid).

CRAMPTON, JOHN, M. D., *On Tinea.* See TRANSACTIONS OF THE KING'S AND QUEEN'S COLLEGES OF PHYSICIANS IN IRELAND. *Vol. IV.*, 1824.

Ringworm. Cure—purgation.

517. *Tinea, or Ringworm.*—Having exhausted my patience with trials of all enumerated topical remedies, the treatment which I finally adopted was, first to use simple poultices, aided by *a constant use of purgatives*, and the tepid bath (p. 60).

> In scald head and ringworm the patient should use Vinegar of Bloodroot as an external application twice or thrice a day, and Brandreth's Pills so as to purge freely. Read directions.

HOSACK, DAVID, M. D., *Medical Essays.* New York, 1824.

Fever. Hosack's definition—Its effects if purgation is neglected. If nature does not remove impurities, art must, or death follows.

518. "*Fever* is *a disease of the whole system ;* the absorbing, the circulating, and the excreting systems of vessels are all affected by it. . . Fever cannot long continue without inducing debility in the heart and arteries. It not only wastes the power of the solids, but by the derangement of the functions and excretions, and especially by the retention of those materials which should have been thrown out of the system as noxious, which in health are constantly ejected, the circulating fluids become changed and vitiated, and thereby become additional sources of irritation to the heart and arteries " (vol. II., p. 93).

From this view we infer that, unless by some salutary power inherent in the system itself, or by some means suggested by art, the greater irritability of the whole system be diminished, or the morbid changes induced in the fluids they circulate be counteracted, these causes of fever mutually operating upon each other must increase and fever be continued, until the vital principle be totally expended (pp. 93, 94).

Effects of retained fæces.

519. *Attention* should be *daily given to the bowels for the purpose of evacuating their offensive contents, especially of the lower tract of the alimentary canal ;* for, these malcontents being retained, not only in some instances become the source of irritation to the intestines themselves, producing diarrhœa, but by their absorption into the mass of circulating fluids, which are thereby rendered still more malignant, they necessarily constitute fresh sources of febrile excitement (p. 98).

Typhus fever. Mercury increases its malignity.

520. I believe that the *typhus fever* of our country owes much of its malignity to the indiscriminate use of *mercury* (p. 101—Report to the Governors of New York Hospital, Sept., 1819).

Malignant pleurisy. Bleeding destroys. Tonics useless, even injurious. Purgation saves.

521. The prudent physician will of course carefully abstain from the use of blood-letting and other depleting remedies (in malignant pleurisy). But he will not certainly guard against *debility by the excessive use of brandy and ardent spirits.* So far from promoting the excretions of the system they actually *restrain those very evacuations* which it should be an object to promote, and *by which alone we are enabled to counteract the typhoid state* of the body in this or any other febrile disease (p. 197—Letter of Dr. Hosack's to Dr. T. R. Beck, Feb. 3d, 1813, on the fatal epidemic prevailing at Albany).

> Brandy and all alcoholic stimulants retard the decarbonization of the blood, because the oxygen of the atmosphere has greater affinity for alcohol than it has for carbonic acid.

522. *Gout* is exclusively an inflammatory *disease of the whole sys-* Various dis-
tem as well as of the part affected. *Apoplexy, palsy, angina pectoris,* retention of
asthma, habitual catarrh, eruptions on the skin, obstructed viscera, and Impurities.
dropsy, arise from the same habit of body and from the same causes
—the effects of an overloaded state of the blood-vessels (pp. 234, 235).

GOOD, JOHN MASON, M. D., *The Study of Medicine.* 5 *Vols. London,*
1825.

523. *Toothache* is often produced by a remote cause, as sordes, in the *Toothache*
stomach (vol. I., p. 41), or whatever tends to render the fluids acrimo- from morbid
nious, as long use of mercury. stomach;—
Chronic rheumatism, or acrimony in the stomach, produces *nervous* also nervous
toothache (ibid., p. 57).

524. The grand proximate cause of *cardialgia, gravel, and gout,* is *Cardialgia,*
debility of the stomach, whence, among other evils, a morbid secretion gout, from
of gastric juice. The debility is not confined to the stomach, but ex- disorder of
tends to the intestinal canal and the other viscera. the stomach.
The debility is evident from the *habitual costiveness* which so pecu- Costiveness
liarly characterizes this affection. The imbecility of the liver is equally the habitual
obvious from the small quantity of bile that seems to be secreted, or its symptom.
altered and morbid hue, as evinced by the color of the fæces (ibid., p.
159).

525. *The lungs* are also in many instances apt to associate in the *The lungs*
morbid action of the digestive organs, when it has become chronic, and cated; bad
to produce a peculiar variety of consumption—*dyspeptic phthisis* (ibid., blood is
p. 160). consump-
It must be obvious that, if *the chyle* which originates in the stomach tion fol-
should be *conveyed to the lungs in an unhealthy condition,* its peculiar lows.
stimulus must be changed in its mode or degree of action, and the lungs,
in consequence, suffer (ibid., p. 163).
The medical treatment: WE MUST RESTORE THE DEBILITATED ORGANS
TO THEIR PROPER TONE (ibid., p. 164).

526. *Colica—colic.*—Among the chief causes, acrid, cold, or indi- *Colic* from
gestible esculents, worms, calculous or other balls congested in the in- ters.
testines and obstructing their passage, as scybala and indurated fæces
(ibid., p. 195). Persevere in
Cure.—Warm fomentations—clysters. *Purgatives* should be at- purgatives.
tempted by the mouth, though the vomiting is sometimes so incessant
that we can get little or nothing to stay on the stomach. But the attempt must be made, and *steadily persevered in* (ibid., p. 196).

527. *Constipation.*—As the fæces are forced forward by the peristal- *Constipa-*
tic action of the intestines, it is obvious, whenever this action is weakened, bid matters
there must necessarily be a retardation, and, consequently, an accumu- in the intes-
lation of fæces. In some instances this accumulation is prodigious. . . tines.
In one case which ended in death, the cause being mistaken for preg- Interesting
nancy, the colon measured in circumference twenty inches, and on dis- tended colon.
section was found to contain three gallons of fæces (ibid., pp. 232, 233).

Variety of diseased manifestations from constipation.

528. *Effects of constipation*, when long continued: pains in the head, nausea, febrile irritation, general uneasiness in the abdominal region, congestion in the abdominal organs, and hence an impeded circulation of the blood, piles, varices of the lower limbs, colic (ibid., p. 234).

Powerful purgatives.

529. If *laxatives fail*, the *more powerful purgatives* must be had recourse to, *till the patient can habituate himself to evacuate the bowels at a certain hour every day* (ibid., p. 235).

Diarrhœa from acrid ingesta;—purge.

530. *Diarrhœa.*—Chief causes: "*acrid ingesta*" and *obstructed bile*. Often antecedently to the looseness there is a sense of sickness, and perhaps a few slight torminal pains. But if the disorder do not prove its own remedy, it is easily removed by any common *purgative medicine* (ibid., p. 240).

Astringents —their imminent danger.

531. It requires to be *restrained with caution ;* for a sudden cure, and especially a *sudden* transfer to a *state of costiveness, has often produced some severe complaints*, and, in one or two instances, epilepsy and phthisis (ibid.)

Worms.

Purge—and why.

532. *Worms.*—*Dr. Heberden* says: "Till some more certain remedy shall be discovered, nothing will be more serviceable than to keep the bowels loose. By their irritation they augment the secretion of mucous, in which also they involve themselves."

By *keeping the bowels loose* we prevent the accumulation of this slimy material in which the worm burrows, and, if we have reason to believe that such accumulation has taken place, *the best plan is to give active purgatives* (ibid., p. 329).

Piles— physiology.

533. *Piles* derive their existence perhaps in every instance from a *turgid and varicose state of the anal veins*, covered with a slight thickening of the inner membrane of the rectum (ibid., p. 363).

Retained fæces the cause.

534. *Causes :*—Local irritation produced by *indurated and retained fæces*, congested state of the liver and adjoining viscera, &c. If left to themselves, they swell into tumors, and become so painful as to prevent walking or sitting (ibid).

Jaundice— permanent. symptoms indicate the cure.

535. *Jaundice* is easily reproduced in those who are subject to it, *by flatulence, acrimonious or indigestible food*. The bowels are for the most part *costive* and moved with difficulty (ibid., p. 390).

Yellow-gum —purge.

536. *Yellow-gum—jaundice of infants.*—A dose of *any active purgative* will generally be sufficient to remove the obstruction (ibid., p. 404).

Fever— Hippocratic definition.

537. *Fever.*—It was the opinion of *Hippocrates* that fever is an effort of nature to expel something hurtful from the body, either ingenerated or introduced from without (vol. II., p. 44).

538. There is no writer of the present day, perhaps, who has carried this view of the subject farther, or even so far, as *Professor Frank*, who regards typhus, plague, petechiæ, and all pestilential fevers, and indeed *nervous fevers of any kind*, whether continued or remittent, not only as proceeding *from specific contagions* in the same manner as exanthemas, but *from contagions producing* a like leaven in the system, and matured and thrown off through the various outlets of the body, by the same process of depuration (ibid., pp. 45, 46).

"All fevers are from lin-purities from without meeting with impurities from with-in."
Dr. Frank's opinion.

539. *Typhus.*—The term is derived from Hippocrates, and means to *smoulder, or burn and smoke without vent.* When a typhus has once arisen, the effluvium from the living body during its action is loaded with miasms of the same kind, completely elaborated as it passes off (ibid., p. 224).

Typhus. The body exhales miasms.

540. *Dr. Haygarth* and *Dr. Bancroft* show from numerous cases, that the *miasmatic poison of typhus*, when received into the body, continues in a latent state at least for seven days from the time of exposure to the contagion, before the fever commences. . . .
A *peculiar state of the body gives a peculiar tendency both to gene rate and receive typhus*, whilst some seem to be favored almost with a natural immunity (ibid., pp. 227, 228).

The typhus poison latent for seven days;—free purgation will therefore remove the poison before it is elabora-ted.

541. *Dysentery :*—primary a disorder of the colon, so considered by Sydenham and Dr. Cheyne;—first gripings, then dejections, and the fever follows. Sydenham's chief remedy was *active purgation twice every other day*, with warm diaphoretics on the days when the aperient was not employed (ibid., pp. 552–556, cond.).

Dysentery, from the co-lon;—cure: active pur-gation.

542. *Eruptive fevers.*—Whenever any diseased action is taking place internally, there is a constant effort exhibited in the part, or in the system generally, to lead it to the surface, where it can do but little mischief. . . It is by means of the fever that the disease works its own cure, for it is hereby that a general determination is made to the surface, and the morbid poison is thrown off from the system ; but the fever may be too violent, and from accidental causes of the wrong kind (vol. III., p. 5).

Eruptive fe-vers—a nat-ural effort to rid the sys-tem of mor-bid matter. The benefit of purga-tion pal-pable.

543. The *grand principle* in the treatment of *small-pox*, as of all the other exanthemas, is *to moderate and keep under the fever ;* and how ever the plans that may have been most celebrated for their success may have varied in particular points, they have uniformly made this principle their polar star, and have consisted in different modifications of cold water, acid liquors, and *purgative medicines*—heat, cordials, and other stimulants having been abundantly proved to be the most effectual means of exasperating the disease and endangering life (ibid., p. 109).
Dr. Mead seems to have been almost *indifferent as to the kind of purgatives employed*, and certainly gave no preference to mercurial pre-parations. His idea was, that all were equally beneficial that would tend to lower the system ; and in this manner he accounts for the *mild-ness of the disease after any great evacuation*, natural or artificial (ibid., p. 110).

Small-pox.
The fever kept under by purga-tives.
Strong evacuation the principle of cure.
Stimulants increase the power of disease.

Hypochon-dria;—the causes indi-cate the cure. 544. *Hypochondria.*—" *The digestive organs are almost always tor-pid.*" Some kind of acrimony is also almost found in the stomach, and particularly that of acidity. The pain in the epigastrium may be re-lieved by the pressure of a belt broad enough to support the whole of the lower belly. Congestions in one or more of the abdominal viscera are a frequent result, and not unfrequently a primary cause. . .
Hence we see why the *bleeding piles* are often so serviceable as to have obtained the name of " medicina hypochondriacorum " (vol. IV., pp. 158, 159).

Paris, J. A., M. D., *Pharmacology, 6th Ed., London,* 1825.

Purgatives. Hamilton en-dorsed. 545. *Purgatives.*—The extent of their importance and value were, however, never justly appreciated until the valuable publication of *Dr. Hamilton* on this subject. . . . His practice has clearly proved that a state of bowels may exist in many diseases, giving rise to a retention of feculent matter, which will not be obviated by the occasional adminis-tration of a purgative, but which *requires a continuation of the alvine stimulant, until the healthy action of the bowels is re-established.* Since this view of the object has been adopted, numerous diseases have re-ceived alleviation from the use of purgatives that were *formerly treated with a different class of remedies, and which were not supposed to have any connection with the state of alvine evacuations* (p. 167, vol. I.).

Fever. The peristal-tic motion is diminished. 546. Thus *in fever the peristaltic motion* of the intestines *is dimin-ished,* and *their feculent contents are unduly retained,* and, perhaps, in part absorbed, becoming of course a source of morbid irritation. This fact has been long understood, and the practice of administering cathar-tic medicines under such circumstances has been very generally adopted.

Emptying only of the intestines not suffi-cient. 547. But *until the publication of Dr. Hamilton, physicians were not aware of the necessity of carrying the plan to an extent beyond that of merely emptying the primæ viæ, and they did not continue the free use of these remedies through the whole progress of the disease* (ibid).

Purgatives are good in neurosis; 548. *Cathartics are essentially serviceable,* also, in several diseases of the class *neurosis,* which are generally intimately connected with a mor-bid condition of the alimentary passages (p. 168, ibid).

In chorea, hysteria, chlorosis; ("Emmena-gogues.") 549. *Chorea and hysteria* have been very successfully treated in this manner. The *diseases incident to puberty* in both sexes are also *best re-lieved by a course of purgative medicines,* and their effects in *chlorosis* have conferred upon many of them the specific title of *Emmenagogues* (ibid).

Also good as "antiphlo-gistics." 550. But *the therapeutical utility of cathartics extends beyond the mere feculent evacuations* which they may occasion. In consequence of the *stimulating action* which some of them exert *upon the exhalent ves-sels, they abstract a considerable portion of fluid from the general current* of the circulation, and are, on that account, beneficial as *antiphlogistics* (ibid).

Dr. Paris is sciolistic as to the history of purgatives; their use was better understood in the time of Parey (1620) than when Hamilton wrote (1794).

551. For the same reason they may act as powerful promoters of absorption, for there exists an established relation between the powers of exhalation and absorption, so that when the action of one is increased, that of the other is augmented. Certain purgatives, as I have just stated, exert their influence upon the neighboring organs, and are calculated not only to remove *alvine sordes*, but to detach and *eliminate foul congestions from the biliary ducts and pores* (ibid., p. 169).

They promote absorption.

Why not say the truth, and also remove congestions and relieve pain in the most distant organs.

552. There is no principle in physiology better established than that which considers *vitality* as *a power engaged in a continual conflict with the physical, chemical and mechanical laws* to which every species of inanimate matter is invariably subject (ibid., p. 209).

Chemical remedies in conflict with vitality.

— And *yet* CHEMICAL REMEDIES *are* CONSTANTLY PRESCRIBED *by the "* SCIENTIFIC*" physician!*

AÏNSIE, WHITELAW, M. D., *Materia Indica. London*, 1826.

553. *Hepatitis.*—A viscid and badly prepared bile, producing obstruction and irritation, is the most immediate source of evil, and so constantly does neglected *constipation precede* an attack of hepatitis, that we cannot for a moment deny but that it must powerfully contribute towards hurrying on the organic derangement by *binding up what should daily be carried off* (p. 549).

Inflammation of the liver, from constipation, and in hot climates and seasons.

MONAT *and* HENDERSON, *Surgs., Narrative of the March of the 13th Regiment of Foot, from Nuddeah to Berhampoor, in* 1826. *See* MADRAS JOURNAL, *Vol. II.*

554. Two individuals who were largely bled became convulsed and died, and after death it was found that, though the *heart was empty*, the *vessels of the head were loaded with blood*. It was thus clearly indicated that, whatever it was that excited *the heart's inordinate action, bloodletting would not subdue it ;* for, as long as a drop of blood remained, it was sent to the head (Journ., p. 327).

Bloodletting kills rather than it cures.

ANDRAL, JR., G., M. D., *Clinique Médicale. Paris*, 1827.

555. In *indigestion* (embarras gastrique), consisting of loss of appetite, bad taste in the mouth, loaded tongue, irregularity of the bowels, sensation of constriction or weight at the epigastrium, and occasional nausea. This train of symptoms we have often seen to *resist* the application of leeches to the epigastrium, low diet, diluents, etc., and *rapidly give way to the exhibition of a brisk purgative*. Do purgatives, by exciting the stomach and bowels together with the auxiliary neighboring organs, *re-establish the power of digestion ?* Do these remedies change, in some unknown way, the mode of secretion in the liver and pancreas? We know not. But this we know, that the treatment above mentioned is very efficacious, and that the *antiphlogistic treatment* is *useless, if not injurious* (chap. IV. †).

Indigestion. Symptoms.

Leeches do not lessen the irritation; purgation cures it.

Antiphlogistics injurious.

Illustrative case. 556. —— Andral, in illustration, gives many cases; No. VI. is selected. A young man entered the hospital with high fever, violent pulsating pain in the head, obstinate costiveness, and other symptoms. Leeches, the pendiluvium, lavements, and tisans were employed to no purpose. On the tenth day the patient was seized with spontaneous vomiting of a large quantity of green bile, which was followed by a smart purging of yellow liquid matter. Next day every symptom of *Nature shows the way to cure.* his malady was gone. The patient was discharged, "cured by Dame Nature."—*Andral asks, " Would not a brisk purgative or two in the beginning have cured the disorder ? "*

Why of course they would. Six Brandreth's Pills given on the first or second day would have done it.

Purgatives moderate the current of fluids and modify the composition of the blood. 557. *Purgatives,* by revulsion, *diminish the activity* with which the fluids tend to the part originally irritated and congested. . . But another influence which has been less noticed, is that which they may have upon the *composition of the blood,* which they must modify by means of the materials which they extract from it. It may be asked, what is the nature of their influence upon the blood, according to whether they chiefly excite the flow of perspiration, of mucous, or of bile, and what changes of composition they may occasion in the blood? This is undoubtedly an interesting subject for investigation (Quoted in Copland's Dict., p. 250, vol. I, Art. Blood, § 160).

CHAMBERS, WILLIAM, M. D., *Physician to St. George's Hospital. On Continued Fever. See* BRIT. AND FOR. MED. REV., 1827, *Vol. VI.*

Fever. Early and steady purgation. 558. *Continued Fever.*—Those who have been in the habit of treating this disease must have observed that in most instances, when purgatives have been *early and steadily administered,* all the symptoms have in a short time yielded to them (Rev., p. 161).

SCUDAMORE, CHARLES, M. D. *A Treatise on the Nature and Cure of Rheumatism. London,* 1827. *See* BRITISH AND FOR. MED. REV. 1839, *Vol. VII.*

Rheumatism. Bleeding changes acute into chronic rheumatism. 559. In no way is a degeneracy into *chronic symptoms* so certainly introduced as *by* that injudicious employment of *general bleeding* which enfeebles the constitution and still leaves the rheumatic disposition in great force (p. 70—Brit. and For. Med. Rev., p. 343).

Purgatives replace bleeding. 560. In proportion as we employ purgatives with judgment, so do we diminish the necessity of using the lancet (ibid).

Continue purgation until evacuations are healthy. Examine stools and urine. 561. In regard to the freedom and continuance of this treatment, we shall inform ourselves in great measure by the nature of the excretions, alvine and urinary; for, *while the fæces are unnaturally dark,* and the *urine is dense,* of a deep color, &c., it is incumbent upon us to *make daily employment* of purgative medicines (p. 96—Rev., p. 344).

Also continue purgation with Brandreth's Pills while severe pain continues, even if the stools are healthy.

562. A course of *sarsaparilla* often proves useful in that kind of *chronic rheumatism* which is accompanied by general derangement of the constitution, without particular affection of any internal organ.

We see that, as the health of the system improves, morbid irritability lessens, the flesh of the patient increases, his looks and strength improve, and the rheumatic pains pass away (p. 370—Rev. 353).

ABERCROMBIE, JOHN, M. D., *Pathological and Practical Researches on Diseases of the Stomach, &c. Edinburgh*, 1828.

563. It has become *a kind of fashion to refer symptoms to morbid conditions of the liver*, without any good ground for considering them as being really connected with that organ. But as a practical man, anxious to be guided by observation alone, there are three classes of facts which have appeared to me worthy of much attention in reference to this subject, namely:

Dyspepsia and SUPPOSED chronic inflammation of the liver cured by PURGATION.

1. That I have frequently seen such complaints get well under very mild treatment, as *regulation of the bowels*, and a little attention to diet;
2. That I have seen such *patients put through long and ruinous courses of mercury without any benefit*, and afterwards found the *complaint removed by a course of mild laxatives;* and

Mercury useless.

3. That I have known patients die of other diseases while these alleged affections of the liver were going on, without being able to discover in the liver, upon dissection, the smallest deviation from healthy structure (p. 320).

564. In *chronic inflammation of the liver* free and continued purging is expressly recommended (p. 361).

REAL chronic inflammation of the liver— PURGE FREELY AND CONTINUALLY.

ANNESLY, JAMES, M. D., *Researches into the Causes, Nature, and Treatment of Prevalent Diseases in India. Edinburgh*, 1828. *See* MED. CHIR. REV., 1828, *Vol. VIII., Ser. I.*

565. Thus, in recruits and other strangers to the climate, on their arrival in India, when the biliary secretion is much increased, the temporary obstruction produced by exposure, wet, &c., often occasion the most formidable symptoms of disease, and when the obstruction is overcome, an immense quantity of vitiated bile is passed. It is reasonable to suppose, if the gall-bladder and ducts be over-distended with their contents, then vital contractility may be weakened, and thus the evil will be increased, until some internal or external cause supervenes, which shall enable the organ to throw off the load which oppresses it, and discharge its morbid secretion (Rev., p. 419).

Fevers in the East Indies.

Natural or artificial purgation alone can cure.

566. The *accumulation of mucous* on the internal surfaces of the duodenum may also obstruct the mouth of the common duct, and prevent the flow of bile into the alimentary canal, until the obstruction be overcome or removed (p. 307).

Mucous obstruction a cause of fever; remove it by purgation.

BAYLE, M., M. D., *On the Influence of Gastric Affections in the Production of Mental Maladies. See* REVUE MÉDICALE. *Paris*, 1828.

567. *Mr. Bayle* proves by numerous cases that *chronic inflammation of the mucous membrane* of the stomach and bowels produced various forms of *insanity*, and that the form of the mental hallucination was often determined by the physical malady in the stomach.

Insanity from disordered stomach.

BROWN, JOHN, M. D., *Medical Essays on Fever, &c.* *London*, 1828.

Malaria produces
mines dis-
cases, ac-
cording to
dilution.

568. *Malaria* produces *intermittent and remittent fevers, cholera, dyspepsia, bilious diarrhœa, liver disease, jaundice;* and *Dr. McCullock* adds, *rheumatism* and *neuralgia* (p. 46).

COOKE, WILLIAM, Surg., *A Practical and Pathological Inquiry into the Sources and Effects of Derangement of the Digestive Organs. London*, 1828.

Fatal accu-
mulations—
do not rely
upon reports
of evacua-
tion, but ex-
amine.

569. In disease there will sometimes be *fatal accumulation of fæces* in the intestines, when both *the patient and attendants report that the bowels are freely relieved* (p. 129).

Constipa-
tion.

570. *Various diseases arising from constipation cured by full purgation.*

Loose stools
not sufficient
—examina-
tion re-
quired;—no
"HALF MEAS-
URES."

In cases of *constipation* we must be careful that the discharge of loose motion does not deceive us, for this may happen without the bowels being sufficiently acted upon. *We ought never to be satisfied*, in any serious case, *without careful examination with the hand;* for it will frequently happen, even *after fluid dejections*, that *a large accumulation of fæces* shall exist.

Case.

On the 12th of December, 1818, I was consulted respecting a little boy four years of age, who for several days had been unwell. I prescribed a dose of calomel, which, in the course of the day, affected his bowels three times, *the motions being loose and yellow.* His diet consisted chiefly of fluid aliment, and of this he took but little. On the

Fever.

morning of the 13th he had considerable *fever* remaining. *A powerful purgation* (calomel and jalap) was given. Early next morning *he voided an excessive quantity of formed and hardened fæces*, some parts of which were *of a black color. After this evacuation* the febrile symptoms speedily subsided (p. 129).

Impaired
digestion
cured by
FULL PUR-
GATION.

571. I was consulted by an elderly gentleman who had been suffering under *chronic and protracted derangement of the digestive organs,* and *who believed* that he had kept his bowels freely open by ordinary domestic aperients. A *more efficient purgative* was, however, prescribed, and to his surprise and comfort *he voided* as *much solid excrement of a brown color* as would more than half fill a large pot-de-chambre (p. 130).

Active pur-
gation—its
usefulness.

572. *Active purgatives* are not only merely required in cases of accumulated fæces, but are sometimes useful by instituting morbid action, by setting up a temporary disease through the alimentary canal. *Something may be attributed to the increased secretion,* but the maintenance of morbid action has sometimes considerable influence in controlling functional affections which did *not originate* from gastric disease (pp. 131, 132).

Palpitation
of the heart.

573. In evidence of this view is given a case of *palpitation of the heart* cured by purgation (p. 132).

574. A case is given of *peritoneal inflammation* cured by full purgation, when "both the practitioner and the nurse informed me that the bowels were *quite open*" (p. 130).

Peritoneal inflammation.

575. In the summer of 1824, I was called upon by a maiden lady aged 34. She informed me that for some months she had been in such a state of distress, from *mental depression*, that life had become completely burdensome. She had neither inclination for food nor exercise. She slept but little and passed restless nights. I prescribed *laxatives and sea air* for a few weeks. She grew worse. On her return to the city, *powerful purgatives* were employed *three times a day*, and in a week she felt quite a different creature (pp. 192, 193).

Mental depression cured by purgation.

Case.

576. In 1816, I attended a lady who had "not been well" for two years, during which period she had been under the care of a respectable medical gentleman without deriving advantage. She was also subject to *pains in her right side, appetite impaired, countenance yellow, rest disturbed*. Employed active purgation (calomel and jalap). The first day she had *twelve dejections*, the others six or seven each. The pain soon ceased, appetite was good, countenance cheerful, and she was again feeling comfortable.

She was now desired to take half the former dose of opening medicine every third night.

In this case the constipation had existed so long that it seemed *prudent to act freely on the bowels at first, and gradually lessen the strength of the purgative* (pp. 232, 233).

Amenorrhœa cured by full purgation.

Case.

Continuation of the purgative treatment.

577. A lady in the *seventh month of pregnancy* had been affected for some time with what was considered a *quotidian ague*. Every day, at nearly the same time, she was attacked with rigor and violent shiverings which continued for half or three-quarters of an hour, and was succeeded by hot and sweating stages. On being consulted I deemed it expedient to administer some *opening medicine before other steps* were taken. *The bowels being freely acted upon in the course of the next twenty-four hours, the fever did not return* (pp. 285, 286).

Quotidian ague during pregnancy cured by purgation.

Case.

578. A gentleman informed me that he was recently consulted respecting a family with *ague*. *Bark* had been frequently given *without success*. Finding that their *bowels* were much *disordered* he prescribed some *opening remedies, intending* to give quinine afterwards, but the ague had ceased (p. 286).

Another case of ague. Bark useless.

MONRO, ALEXANDER, M. D., *Morbid Anatomy of the Brain.* London, 1828. *See* MED. CHIR. REV., Ser. I., Vol. *VIII.*, 1828.

579. *Hydrocephalus.*—*Brisk cathartics* are to be administered *regularly*, especially at the outset and during the first period of the disease; for the quantity of feculent matter contained within the intestines in many cases is really surprising. One instance now occurs to us. The patient was a young lady who, after an attack of fever, during which

Hydrocephalus caused by retained fæces; always purge fully and freely.

head symptoms predominated, and had not been opportunely nor sufficiently overcome, was seized with all the signs of water in the head;
and as her bowels had been rather disposed to astringency throughout
the fever, they became exceedingly torpid, indeed almost unmanage-
able, on the establishment of hydrocephalus.

Five or six common doses of drastic purgatives were required *before
the bowels would answer*, and *fetid and bulky stools were daily passed
for three weeks* under this stimulation, *without any solid food* having
been taken during that time (p. 38—Rev. p. 385).

Case.

Fetid stools.

580. And instituting a new and healthy action in the secretory appa-
ratus by a degree of *warmth and local remedies* adapted to the sensibility
of the part affected (ibid).

McKENZIE, WILLIAM, M. D., *A Sketch of the Natural Cure of Diseases; in* GLASGOW MEDICAL JOURNAL, *February*, 1829. *See* BRIT.
& FOR. MED. REV., 1847, *Vol. XXIII.*

581. The body is almost altogether fluid; nine-tenths of it are so,
and only one-tenth solid. *The fluid parts are in a perpetual state of
change*, being decomposed by one set of functions and recomposed by
another. . . . Our fluids, by means of digestion, absorption, circulation, respiration, and secretion, are in a constant revolution. By these
processes there is effected an *uninterrupted decay and restoration of the
body;* and one can not doubt that the natural cure of diseases depends
very much on the existence and on the perfection of this revolution.
Nay, it is extremely probable, that *one of the principal intentions served
in this mode of carrying on life is the prevention and removal of disease* (Rev. p. 587).

*The blood,
ever chang-
ing and ever
new, and
disease.*

By purgation with Brandreth's Pills we can change the entire body in from a third to
half the time it is changed in the ordinary course of nature, and with entire safety. Case
of

STEPHENS, HENRY, *Surg. Treatise on Inflamed and Obstructed Hernia.
London*, 1829. *See* MED. CHIR. REV. *Ser. I.*, 1829, *Vol. XI.*

582. *Mr. Lawrence* has, under the head of "slow strangulation,"
described a state of obstructed hernia *from fecal accumulation*, and
without doubt *such a state often exists* (p. 62—Rev. p. 112).

*Strangu-
lated hernia
from re-
tained fæces.*

Brandreth's Pills to this poor patient would have been the complete doctor, producing
certain relief, and, in all probability, would have cured the rupture.

STOKER, WILLIAM, M. D. *Treatise on Continued Fevers, &c. Dublin,*
1829.

583. *Typhus fever* is connected with *morbid changes that previously
take place in the fluids*, and produce *morbid actions*, and sometimes
permanent change of structure in the solid parts. These changes are

*Typhus
fever.*

distinguishable from those which occur *in inflammation,* and the *morbid action* excited relatively by these changes in the *blood* are also distinct. In inflammatory fever, *increased action;* in typhus fever, *debility* is almost the immediate consequence (p. 74). *Dr. Stoker's* definition and modus procedendi,

The remedies employed by me in mixed and typhoid fevers, and arranged according to their relative importance, are:

Mixed fevers—cleanliness, ventilation, cool regimen, plentiful diluents, *and purgatives.* with purgative medicines.

Typhoid fevers—yeast, wine, *and aperients* (p. 113).

584. In both *ague and intermittent neuralgia,* I believe the *disordered function of digestion,* and the consequent morbid condition of the chyle and of the other contents of the stomach, whether ultimately absorbed or carried into the sanguiferous system, or carried *downward by the primæ viæ,* become in their transit a chief cause of all the succeeding symptoms (p. 357). Ague and neuralgia from retained impurities.

585. When these *periodic diseases* become, however, *more established,* it is probable that not only the fluids are further affected, but that consequent changes are excited, and hence *the morbid condition of the fluids* may be *the primary source of organic disease* (ibid). These impurities the cause of organic disease.

The following quotations establish the absolute necessity of having by us a purgative to which we may always apply with safety for relief; and we have it in Brandreth's Pills.

COPLAND, JAMES, M. D. *Dictionary of Practical Medicine.* London, 1830. *New York Ed. by Dr. Ch. A. Lee,* 1846–1852.

586. A belief is too generally entertained *that fecal matters and sordes will not accumulate in the colon* unless the patient has been constipated. *But they may collect in its cells,* the more central part of *the canal allowing daily evacuation;* and they may even *remain there for* a *considerable* period, producing much irritation, and even a relaxed state of the bowels, thereby misleading the judgment of the practitioner as to the pathological state constituting the disorder. . . . In many cases, when the morbid collections have become acrimonious, an irritative *diarrhœa continues for some time,* or recurs at intervals, *before the morbid matters are fully thrown off,* owing to spasmodic constrictions of parts of the bowels. . . On these occasions the evacuation is often preceded by *gripes, tenesmus,* or a *scalding sensation in the anus* (vol. I., p. 450, Art. Colon, § 6). Fecal matter may accumulate where there is no constipation— watch and purge.

Effects.

587. *Purgations* are used in order to *occasion a local determination of blood, and thus derive it from the seat of disease,* to evacuate the viscera, increase the discharge from the mucous surface, and augment the secretions in adjoining organs (ibid., p. 218). Purgatives —their action and aims.

588. The *fetor, &c., of the breath,* and of the perspiration, &c., consequent upon *interruption of the abdominal secretions,* indicate that *impurities have accumulated* in the circulation, and that they are *being eliminated* by the *lungs* and the *skin.* So long as the vital energy is Interrupted secretion— vicarious action of the secretory organs.

sufficient for the due performance and harmony of the functions, injurious matters are seldom allowed to accumulate in the blood to the extent of *vitiating its constitution, without being discharged from it by means of one or more organs.* But as soon as this energy languishes, or is depressed by external influences and agents, and the blood is thereby either imperfectly formed or insufficiently animalized and depurated, some one of its ultimate elements or proximate constituents become excessive, and the chief cause of disorder, *which terminates either in the removal of the morbid accumulation, or in a train of morbid actions and lesions* (vol. I., p. 23 8, Art. Blood, § 116).

Causes of disease.

589. Thus it will appear that changes in the secretions and in the blood itself are most influential in the production, perpetuation, and aggravation of disease. . . Thus, also, it will appear not only that hurtful matters carried into the circulation, and ultimate elements or proximate constituents allowed to accumulate in it, owing to the imperfect performance of some alimentary function, will be removed from it when the vital influence is sufficient for the task, but that both kinds of injurious agents will, *according to their nature,* become productive of a vitiated state of the blood, of the secretions formed from it, and even of the various tissues themselves, when the state of vital manifestation is insufficient to remove them from the frame (ibid., p. 239, § 117, ibid.)

Defective secretion causes absorption of morbid matter vitiating the blood and producing disease.

590. I consider the grand pathological inference to be fully established: that *the interruption or obstruction of any important secreting or eliminating function,* if not compensated by the increased or modified action of some other organs, *vitiates the blood* more or less; and if such vitiation be not soon removed, by the restoration of the function primarily affected, or by the increased exercise of an analogous function, that still more important changes are produced in the blood, and ultimately in the soft solids, if the energies of life are insufficient to expel the cause of disturbance, to oppose the progress of change, and to excite actions of salutary tendency (ibid., p. 240, § 124, ibid.)

Defective secretion counteracted by vicarious action, produces vitiated blood.

591. *Miasmata* produce a morbid impression on the nerves of organic life, followed by depression of the vital influence; *the functions of digestion and secretion languish,* and, owing to the imperfect performance of secretion and assimilation, the necessary changes are not fully effected *in the blood,* and thus the irritating and otherwise *injurious matters accumulate* in it. . . The vascular system becomes excited by the quantity and quality of its contents; and when the vital energies are not too far depressed for its production, the excitement becomes general. The accelerated circulation has the effect of exciting the organic functions, of restoring the secretions which were impeded or interrupted, and thereby of removing the morbid state of the circulating fluid, after which the return of health is rapid. *When,* however, *salutary reaction is not brought about,* owing to the morbid depression of the vital energies and to changes which had taken place in the blood, *the vitiation of the blood proceeds;* the secretions are also vitiated, the solids affected, one or more vital organs suffer in an especial manner, the energies of life are exhausted, and various organic lesions are induced, having reference to

Miasma—action on organic life, impairing the maturation of the blood. Reaction if there is sufficient energy—course of disease, if not.

the previous state of the system, the kind of changes produced in the blood, and the agencies in operation during the progress of the disease (ibid., p. 240, § 125, ibid.)

592. *M. Andral* states that " he has often found *in the blood-vessels a curdy, friable matter, of a dirty-gray color,* and resembling either the semi-concrete pus of chronic abscesses, or the sanies of malignant ulcers, or cephaloid matter, broken down and mixed with blood." And similar instances are recorded by *Bichat, Beclard, and Velpeau.* In all these cases, abscesses, tubercles, or other morbid formations, also existed in some part of the body (ibid., p. 246, § 144, ibid.) *Morbid formations in the body implpart morbid matters to the blood.*

593. *Morbid secretions* should be *frequently evacuated,* in order that vital power may not be further reduced by their *morbid impression* on the *nerves and mucous digestive surface,* and that *the possibility of the absorption* of any part of them *into the circulation* may be thereby avoided (ibid, p. 249, § 158, ibid.) *Evacuate morbid secretions to prevent absorption of impurities.*

594. In all the alterations of the blood resulting from the introduction or absorption of morbid matters from parts previously diseased, *whatever tends to lower nervous and vital power, or to promote absorption —more particularly blood-letting, which operates in both these ways—* ought to be guarded against, and a diametrically opposite plan of cure adopted, not neglecting the promotion of the *depurative and excreting functions* (ibid., § 159, ibid.) *Bloodletting CAUSES ABSORPTION of morbid matters.*

595. *Fecal matters* collected in the *cæcum* often induce *inflammation,* or the paroxysms of pain are very acute, sometimes attended by *vomiting* and all the symptoms of the most severe *colic,* or even those of *ileus* (§ 10). The *symptomatic disorders,* when the viscus is much distended either by fecal or by other matters, or by flatus, are numbness of the right thigh, œdema of the right foot and ankle, sometimes retraction of the testicle, or frequent calls to empty the bladder, and sometimes hemorrhoides, uneasiness and pain in the right iliac region, often extending to the hypochondrium, various dyspeptic symptoms, costive or irregular state of the bowels, occasionally diarrhœa, with scanty, offensive, and mucous stools (§ 11). The efforts made to evacuate the bowels are often attended by severe tormina and even retching. I have seen several cases of *varicose veins* of the leg, or *indolent ulcers,* and a case of *disease of the bones* of the foot, the occurrence of which was evidently connected with great disturbance and accumulations in the *cæcum.* . . The complexion is deficient in clearness, and with the surface often covered with an oily or dirty moisture ; the perspiration becomes fetid and the breath offensive ; the soft solids lose their elasticity, and are slightly emaciated ; . . . and at an advanced stage the symptoms more clearly manifest that the blood is imperfectly depurated, or that it is affected by the absorption of a portion of the excrementitious matter retained in the cæcum. In addition to these symptoms, *general debility and disinclination to any* physical or mental *exertion* are often complained of (§§ 10, 11, 12 ; Art. Colon, p. 330, ibid.) *Fecal matter in the cæcum. Various and direful consequences of such accumulations.*

Cholera—from acrid secretions:—remove these by purgation. 596. Even in *cholera*, in which the eruption of an increased quantity of morbid secretions into the duodenum occasions copious discharges from the stomach and bowels, with cramps, &c., we are not justified in concluding that any organic change is present beyond *simple irritation* of a temporary kind, *excited in the villous surface by the acrid state of the secretions passing along it* (ibid., p. 624; Art. Digestive Canal, § 17, B).

Chorea—Its causes. 597. Among the chief predisposing causes of *chorea* is a *neglected state of the bowels*, leading to accumulations of deranged secretions in the primæ viæ, torpid functions of the liver, and other secreting and assimilating organs. The most exciting causes are the irritations of *worms*, of *morbid matters accumulated* in the bowels (*Stoll, Baldinger, and Wendt*), and *fright*, improper employment of *lead, mercury*, &c. (*De Haen*), *suppressed eruptions and discharges* (*Thilenius, Darwin, and Wendt.*) (Ibid., p. 389; Art. Chorea, § 12, III. 13 B.)

Cure:—remove the cause by purgatives. 598. *Purgatives* have been recommended in *chorea* by *Sydenham, Whytt, Hamilton, Cheyne*, and others (ibid., p. 392, § 23, VI., ibid.) The first indication is to remove *morbid secretions* and *fecal accumulations*, the usual *cause* of the irritation of the organic nerves (ibid., p. 394, § 29, B, ibid.)

Diarrhœa. The retained morbid matter must be purged away. 599. *Idiopathic diarrhœa*, when recent, requires demulcents or diluents merely, in order to facilitate the discharge of acrid or accumulated matter. This having been accomplished, disorder soon ceases. But the *irritating substances may be partly retained and keep up a prolonged or remittent state of the disease*, with *griping pains* and *scanty stools*, which may be partly *feculent, mucous, or serous*—the latter predominating, when the irritation is considerable. In this case much discrimination is requisite in selecting the aperient which is obviously required; for, if it be insufficient, the disorder will be prolonged (ibid., p. 609; Art. Diarrhœa, § 25, VII.)

BRANDRETH's PILLS are all that is needed, and discrimination is *not* required.

Crisis—Illustration of. 600. *Illustration of Crises.*—A person exposed to the causes of *autumnal fever* of a bilious and remittent form, experiences during the earlier stages the usual symptoms of *impeded or interrupted secretion*, and general vascular excitement. *In consequence of interrupted action of the emunctories the blood contains an increasing proportion of effete materials*, particularly of the elements out of which bile is formed. These for a while increase and modify the vascular excitement, or, when excessive in quantity, or especially noxious in quality, even tend to exhaust or depress it. But they at the same time being appropriate stimuli to the biliary and depuratory viscera, serve to restore their impeded functions, to turn the balance of excitement in favor of them, *thereby to reduce the morbid vascular action, to cleanse the circulating fluid from its impurities, and to change in other respects its condition*, and thus *the disease terminates with an apparent collapse, followed by a copious discharge from the bowels, consisting of morbid bile and of the excretions from the intestinal mucous surface—the products of the noxious matters which had accumulated in the blood, but which is now being eliminated from it, by a renovated as well as an increased secreting and excreting function.* Now, this procession of morbid phenomena shows, that the ancients were *not so far* wrong as many of the moderns suppose, *when they believed that critical evacuations were beneficial, chiefly because they conveyed a morbid matter out of the system* (ibid., p. 516, Art. Crises, § 15).

601. As the office of the *excreting organs* is to expel those *elements which are effete, and would be injurious to the frame if retained in the blood,* it must necessarily follow, that any interruption to their function must be highly injurious. The dropsical effusions in various cavities following interruption to the action of the kidneys, fully illustrate this. As a large quantity of ingested matters is carried into the blood, either directly from the stomach or along with the chyle, and discharged from it by the emunctories, it is evident not only that the kind of ingesta will affect very remarkably the properties of the excretions, but that obstruction or interruption of any one of them will be followed by serious effects, *unless some other organ perform an additional office vicarious of that which is suppressed, and even in this case disease will generally ultimately arise* (ibid., p. 668, Art. Diseases, § 99). *(In disease impurities must be removed by the proper emunctories or vicariously; if not fully removed, disease quietly follows.)*

602. What are most *diseases,* but *either suppression or excess in the secretions or excretions?* (ibid.) *(What disease)*

603. *Dropsy from Disease of the Kidneys.*—In a very great majority of instances, where effusion proceeds from this cause, the *irritating nature of the fluid* poured out, superinduces *inflammation of the membranes and cellular tissues* containing it, and thereby aggravates the disease, and *accelerates a fatal issue;* for if it be considered that when the functions of the kidneys are interrupted, *excrementitious or serous plethora* will be the result; and that the watery parts of the blood which are effused from this cause *must necessarily contain a considerable quantity of the injurious matters usually eliminated by these organs,* the *irritating quality* of the accumulating fluid here contended for will be admitted (ibid., p. 705, Art. Dropsy on the Chest. § 52). *(Dropsy—an excrementitious fluid of irritating quality the essence of the disease.)*

604. *Purgatives are very applicable in dropsies generally,* on account of their deobstruent operation when uninterruptedly continued, or of their influence in *deriving from the seat of effusion,* in draining the fluid parts of the blood from that circulating *in the intestinal tubes,* in thereby lessening excrementitious or serous plethora, and favoring the absorption of the effused fluid. They constitute a most important part of the treatment of every form and state of the disease (ibid., p. 710, § 66, ibid.). *(Purgatives, because removing the cause, "applicable in every form and state of the disease.)*

In *hydrothorax, cathartics and purgatives,* especially the *hydragogues,* often afford speedy relief (ibid., p. 739. § 172, ibid.).

605. Frequently *affection of the brain* is induced by irritation of the gastro-enteric surface. In children this is remarkably common, and even in adults a slight degree of disorder of the stomach is often followed by *headache, somnolency* and *incapability of mental exertion.* The occasional dependence of *epilepsy* in adults, and of *convulsions* in *(Stomach-disorder causes numerous diseases of a nervous character.)*

children, upon morbid action in the digestive canal is well known. *Inflammation of the membranes* or *of the substance of the brain*, and *acute hydrocephalus* sometimes also supervene upon gastro-intestine irritation, and in the course of their development render obscure, or entirely mask, the previous ailment. For, as *Lallemand* has remarked, as soon as the cerebral affection even partially obscures sensibility the existence of disorder in the digestive canal is ascertained with great difficulty. In my opinion, the majority of cases denominated "*spinal irritation*" are caused by gastro-enteric disorder (vol. II., p. 30, Art. Gastro-enteric Disease, § 3).

Purgatives—their judicious use removes the cause of disease, and how.   606. *A judicious exhibition of purgatives* will frequently *remove* irritation of the digestive canal, especially if it be caused by unwholesome ingesta or morbid secretions, or fecal accumulations; and even when it cannot be referred to either of these, but rather to the state of vascular action in the digestive surface, the augmented secretion procured by refrigerent or mild purgatives may promote its resolution or diminish its intensity (ibid., § 4. ibid.).

Pneumonia and diseases of the skin from the same source.   607. Even the occurrence of *pneumonia* may be favored by disorder of the digestive canal (ibid., p. 31, § 7, ibid.).

Arsenic injurious in cutaneous disease.   Its connection with *diseases of the skin*, is much more general than practitioners suppose. It is chiefly owing to the irritation of the digestive mucous surface, that the cutaneous affections resist so long the treatment prescribed for their removal. I have repeatedly seen *arsenical* and other irritating medicines exhibited in no small quantities; and although they were evidently exasperating both the internal and external affections they were continued with a perfect belief in their applicability (ibid., p. 33, § 15, IV., ibid.).

Impure blood causes diseases of the liver, kidneys, and skin.   608. When the *disorder* of the gastro-intestinal surface is *attended with a craving or morbidly excited appetite*, food is taken in larger quantity than it can be digested, and much *imperfectly formed chyle is carried into the blood* where it excites *disorder of the liver, of the kidneys*, and often *of the skin*, in the course of the excretion of the unassimilated matters by these organs (ibid., p. 34, § 16, ibid.).

Many diseases from impurities of the blood produced byimperfect excreting function of the skin.   609. The suppression of the *excreting functions of the skin* may be followed—especially if the kidneys do not perform a vicariously increased function—by *catarrh*, or by *rheumatism*, or by *inflammation of the lungs* or *pleura*, or by *diarrhœa*, or by *dysentery*, or by *enteritis*, according as *the predisposition of parts may determine* the morbid action. The cause or causes, whether exposure to cold or to influences depressing vital power, occasion, first, interruption of the depurating functions of the skin, and next, more or less congestion of, or vascular determination to, internal viscera or parts; and, in addition to this latter effect, and as a consequence of the suppression of the cutaneous function, the *blood is loaded with these excrementitious elements* which the healthy action of the skin eliminates. The resulting conditions of the blood and of the circulation are such, in many cases, as kindle diseases, either those above mentioned or others of a slighter or severer nature (vol. III., p. 1137, Art. Therapeutics, § 44).

610. What has been said respecting the functions of the skin, applies likewise to the other excreting and secreting functions. Of all excreting or depurating functions, those performed by the kidneys are the most rapidly fatal when impaired (ibid., p. 1138, § 47, ibid.). *The same is true of the other secreteries and excretories.*

611. *The cure.—It is believed* by many *that the regular and daily evacuation of the bowels is quite sufficient; but this may not always be the case, as to* either the *fecal discharge* or the *biliary secretion*, or even as to *both*. . . Hence the *importance of observing* accurately the appearance of the intestinal excretion, both in health and in disease, and of *having recourse* to such means as those appearances, the frequency of the evacuation, and the associated state of the disease will suggest. The several substances employed as purgatives and cathartics should be suited to the peculiarities of each case, and be conjoined with others of the same class, or with such as may either correct or promote their operation (ibid., § 48, ibid.). *Constant observation of evacuations necessary, and why. This applies to BRANDRETH'S PILLS.*

With Brandreth's Pills you can obtain any desired effect upon the bowels or general system.

612. *The promotion of the several secreting and excreting functions, whenever they are torpid or impaired*, is requisite to *the prevention* of many contingent evils during states of vital depression, by whatever cause produced; but it has a still more general application, for, in all circumstances, in states of excitement and increased vascular action, as well as in those of depression, these functions are very often either torpid, or impaired, or even interrupted, and require restoration; otherwise additional or *more severe and dangerous changes result, and the blood, loaded with excrementitious materials, occasions the most deleterious effects in vital organs* (ibid., p. 1137, § 42, ibid). *Changes in the blood from retained impurities resulting from a deficiency of the secreting and excreting functions, and vice versa.*

613. Next to the sedative or depressing effects produced by the causes of disease, the *impairment of depurating functions* closely follows, the latter being very frequently the cause of the former. These functions are often *restored by the same means as are employed to remove the primary morbid impression* (ibid., § 43, ibid). *Cure:—by removing the impurities.*

614. In *chronic, malignant, and structural maladies*, the constitutional or *vital power is impaired*, and *the blood is altered* more or less as these maladies advance, especially *cancer, tubercle, rickets, &c.*, the alteration of the blood becomes more or less evident, this fluid being thinner, poorer, or deficient in red globules. Hence the necessity of supporting the powers of life by means which will neither excite nor irritate them, and of preserving the healthy state of the blood by conjoining with *those means* such *as will correct or prevent alterations of this fluid*, and will, at the same time, promote the conversion of the colorless or chyle globules of the blood into red globules—will *promote the processes of sanguification and nutrition* (ibid., p. 1142, § 63, ibid). *Chronic diseases from impoverished blood. The cure by promotion of sanguification and nutrition; otherwise using Brandreth's Pills.*

615. A person is exposed to causes, as infections, which depress organic nervous energy, and thereby impair or suppress the more important depurating and secreting functions. The consequences as respects the blood are obvious. This fluid soon abounds in effete and injurious elements, increasing both the amount of the vascular contents, and *Effects of impurities in the blood.*

Brandreth's Pills at these times will surely bring the system into a healthy condition. oppressing and irritating the whole vascular system, although certain organs may manifest these effects in a more prominent manner than others, *until a salutary crisis is observed, and the morbid state of the blood is removed, or until the soft solids are changed, their vital cohesion is loosened, and disorganization ensues* (ibid., p. 1046, Art. Sympathy, § 102).

The mutual action of the excreting organs;—retained excretions pro- duce, among other effects, organic dis- ease—i. e. structural changes. 616. There is very *intimate connection* existing *between the state of the blood and the depurating offices of the mucous surface of the intestines,* especially of the large intestines. This surface, and more particularly the follicular glands, may be considered as eliminating from the blood redundant or decomposed blood globules, and much effete materials, and as thereby contributing, with the other emunctories, to the purity and healthy condition of this fluid. The connection subsisting between *the functions of excreting viscera,* not only as *altering the condition of the blood,* but also as *affecting each other individually;* the influence which the state of one depurating function exerts upon the others through the medium of the blood, as well as through that of the organic nervous system, and the mutual and conjoint operation of all these functions, not merely in changing the physical appearance and constitution of the blood and the states of vital influence, but also in occasioning *structural alterations,* are among the most important topics comprised by a rational system of pathology (ibid., p. 1045, § 96, ibid).

Worms from tenacious mucous and pituitous sordes. 617. *Predisposing causes of worms should,* as much as possible, *be removed or counteracted.* In furtherance of this indication, the diet and the treatment should be adopted that are most efficacious in promoting the organic nervous force and the tone of the digestive organs, and in removing *tenacious mucous* and *pituitous sordes,* which often adhere to the digestive mucous surface, and which often forms the *nidus* in which the *ova of parasites* are lodged and hatched. It will generally be noticed that the *secretions and excretions* which in all persons form the principal part of the *fecal discharge are seldom thrown off from the secreting surfaces so quickly and entirely in the delicate and debilitated as in the robust and healthy,* but remain or are retained in *the former class of subjects, and become the soil in which these animals are reared* (ibid., p. 1547, Art. Worms, § 158, B).

Spasms.

Cure by pur- gatives. 618. *Spasms of the voluntary or involuntary muscles.—Purgatives* are generally beneficial, more especially when the liver or brain is congested, and when the spasm is connected with acidity and flatulence of the digestive canal, or with accumulation of morbid secretions, excretions and fecal matters, as when spasms occur in *colic,* or in the course of *gout, rheumatism, hysteria, hypochondria,* &c. In these, as well as in some cases of other diseases, not only are *morbid excretions thus liable to accumulate, but the blood becomes more or less contaminated by effete materials,* which the impaired functions of the emunctories fail of removing.

Simply evacuating the bowels not suffi- cient. 619. In these circumstances purgatives should be selected with this view, not merely of evacuating the contents of the bowels, but also of promoting the functions of the excretory organs. When *cerebral con-*

gestion is connected with the spasms, then *active derivative purgatives* ought to be exhibited *by the mouth and in enema* (ibid., p. 931, Art. Spasms, § 31, C).

620. But the most remarkable *cause of the slow progress of the therapeutical science* is to be found in the highest and most legitimate ranks of the medical profession—*in the physicians themselves* (§ 9) ; in wrong estimates of the efficacy of particular medicines and agents (§ 7, D) ; in erroneous, limited, or one-sided views of the causes, seats, nature and procession of diseases ; of medical doctrine (§ 4, I.); medical jealousies and contentions ; opposing systems ; plans on means of cure ; jarring views as to the efficacy or operation of certain medicines ; opposite opinions in courts of justice, or otherwise appearing in public ; the publicity given to medical discussions have an unfavorable influence on the public, and prevent many from trusting to medical treatment (ibid., pp. 1130, 1131, Art. Therapeutics, § 12, I). *{Causes of the slow progress of the knowledge of remedies, and of the unbelief therein.}*

621. The blood is found altered in disease :
1. By a change in the proportion of its constituent elements ;
2. By the addition of foreign matters (+) (cf. G. Harvey). *{How the blood becomes impure.}*

AN HONEST PROFESSOR.

MARX, K. Z., M. D. *Professor in the University of Gœttingen. General Pathology. Gœttingen*, 1833.

622. The *conscientious* practitioner can resort but to few remedies ; for whenever the choice lies between what is *harmless* and what " heroic," he must unconditionally employ the former (Preface). *{Materia medica.}*

CHOMEL, M., M. D., *Clinical Lectures on Typhoid Fever. Paris*, 1834. *See* BRIT. AND FOR. MED. REV., 1836, *Vol. II.*

623. *In the stools of patients, at the commencement of recovery from typhoid fever,* there are *always scybalæ ;* on which
Dr. *John Conolly* observes : If *medicine* had produced the same effect *earlier,* which nature did eventually, the symptoms would have been milder, although the course of the disease would not have been cut short (Rev., p. 40). *{Typhoid fever;—the stools of convalescents always contain scybala.}*

" The course of the disease would not have been cut short " may admit of a " perhaps."

LAENNEC, R. T. H., M. D., *A Treatise on Disease of the Chest. Translated by John Forbes, M. D. London*, 1834.

624. I would therefore lay it down as a valuable practical rule in chronic affections of the heart, that previously to having recourse to any remedies intended to act directly on it, we ought to be assured that the digestive organs are in a healthy state, *that their mucous surfaces are* *{Chronic heart-diseases. The first step to be taken; purgation.}*

10

free from irritation, their vascular system not morbidly distended, and that the liver is performing its secreting function freely and regularly (p. 687).

Let Brandreth's Pills be used in accordance with the printed directions, and there will be no medicines required to "*act directly on the heart.*" The mucous coats will be freed from all irritating substances, when the liver and the heart will, as a rule, perform their functions freely and regularly.

CLARK, JAMES, M. D., *A Treatise on Pulmonary Consumption, and Inquiry into Causes, Nature, Prevention, and Treatment of Tuberculous and Scrofulous Diseases in General. London,* 1835. *See* BRIT. AND FOR. MED. REV., 1835.

Cachexia— from dyspepsia and deranged secretion and excretion. 625. *Dyspepsia* is the most fertile source of *cachexia* in every form; it also generates in derangement of the various secretory and excretory functions, particularly that condition of them in which the effete matter is imperfectly carried off (p. 223).

Consumption. Keep the system free from impurities, and you keep off the causes of the disease. 626. So long as the constitution remains unimpaired, the ordinary exciting causes (catarrhs, inflammations) may come into active play again and again, during a whole lifetime, without producing consumption ; but the moment *the tone of the system is seriously lowered by sedentary habits, insufficiency of food, impaired digestion, depression of mind, excessive study, vitiated atmosphere,* a very slight external cause will then suffice to induce the deposit of tuberculous matter (Rev., pp. 71, 72, vol. II.)

CONOLLY, JOHN, M. D., *Editor of the* BRITISH AND FOREIGN MEDICAL REVIEW, *On Clark's Treatise on Consumption.* 1835, *Vol. XXI.*

Consumption always from impurities in the system. 627. *Consumption* is invariably *the consequence of a pre-existing unhealthy state of the constitution,* without which the accidental causes which call it into being would have been entirely incapable of producing it (Rev. p. 71).

CURE OF CONSUMPTION AND DYSPEPSIA.

'' HAMMONTON, N. J., May 7, 1866.

"DR. BRANDRETH—*Dear Sir:* I have long wanted to write to you and express my gratitude for the beneficial effects that have been experienced in my own family, and in hundreds, aye, thousands of others, by the use of Brandreth's Pills. The first year my lamented friend Brockway sold your pills in Boston (1838) I called at his office. I was then in a declining state of health, and my friends, as well as myself, supposed my earthly voyage would soon terminate. Mr. Brockway urged me to take the Brandreth Pills, but having used so much medicine, with no good effect, I was more inclined to let nature take its course, and calmly submit to my fate. Mr. B. offered to give me one dozen boxes if I would try them as prescribed. By this I saw he had great faith in them, and I finally consented to take them, but not as a gift. I went home and went at it, almost hopelessly. After taking one box I began to feel better. Well, sir, when I had used up my twelve boxes, I was apparently a well, healthy man, my weight having gone from 131 pounds up to 152 pounds. I then ordered a supply, and between that time and the present I have retailed three thousand dollars worth of these invaluable pills, and am quite sure that I have thereby been instrumental in saving, not hundreds, but thousands of lives. I have given them to my oxen, horses, pigs, fowls, cats, dogs, and always with the desired effect. I have a wife and nine children, most of them born since I have used the pills. A more healthy family cannot be found

We are frequently asked how it is our children look so healthy. My wife replies that 'We raise them on Brandreth's Pills.' Now, my children overload their stomachs, get cold and out of order, like others, but they have been taught the remedy, and go and take the pills of their own accord. This I consider an important branch of their education, and feel assured, as they shove off upon the voyage of life, that they know how to take care of themselves. I was in trade at my last residence, North Lincoln, Me., for 29 years. I have been here about seven years; I am, therefore, well known, and my statements can be verified by hundreds.   "Yours,

"C. J. FAY."

CONTAGION EVEN HARMLESS TO THOSE WHO USE BRANDRETH'S PILLS.

Each one of us, even the most diseased, has within him a germ or root of that original pure blood of our common mother Eve.

This germ of pure blood supports his life, and constantly struggles to throw out from the circulation corrupt humors into the bowels. Brandreth's Pills assist this regenerating process.

By their powerful aid we constantly make blood of a better quality, until the whole is renewed and purified.

Those who desire to pass untouched by contagious maladies, who wish for soundness of body and mind, or to have healthful children, should use Brandreth's Pills, which cleanse the bowels and the blood of all unhealthy accumulations.

COMBE, ANDREW, M. D. *Principles of Physiology applied to Preservation of Health, &c. Edinburgh, 1835. Letter on the Observation of Nature in the Treatment of Disease. See* BRIT. & FOR. MED. REV., 1855, *Vol. XXI.*

628. Experience shows that *the physician and the remedy are useful only when they act in accordance with the laws of the constitution and the intentions of nature.* . . If this be done systematically, every effort of nature will be towards the restoration of health; and all that she demands from us in addition, is to remove impediments and facilitate her acts (Rev. p. 509, sq.)

Assist nature to remove impediments

629. Instead, therefore, of medicine being superseded, as many suppose, by taking nature for our guide, it will, on the contrary, only begin to take just rank as a science when our allegiance to nature shall become practical, enlightened, and complete. . . *Nature is truly the agent in the cure of disease;* and as she acts in accordance with *fixed and invariable laws,* the aim of the physician ought always to be to facilitate her efforts, by acting *in harmony with, and not in opposition to, those laws* (ibid.).

Medicine and the " vis medicatrix naturæ."

Dr. Combe in 1840 was in New Haven, Conn. We had a conversation with him on the great importance of purgation as a universal remedy. But the doctor could not understand how purgation could be useful after the bowels were emptied of their contents. How long a principle is uncomprehended! and yet this great man might have lived thirty years longer, had he but have only investigated this one of purgation, and been governed by the lights of experience which he would have found to flow from it.

FORBES, JOHN, M. D., *Editor of the* BRITISH AND FOREIGN MEDICAL REVIEW, *commencing* 1835.

630. *Purgation* appears to be banished (in continental treatment of *fevers*), from a fear that it may increase the irritation of the follicles of

Fever.

Purgation does not increase intestinal inflammation. the intestines—a fear which has sprung from too excessive devotion to morbid anatomy. That active purgatives, particularly in the early stages of fever, will increase the follicular irritation, is a *completely theo-* *Practice vs. Theory.* *retical objection.* The reasoning on which it is founded will not bear examination, *and our experience* in this country experimentally *contra-* *dicts it* (Rev. 1836, Vol. III., p. 63).

The Doctor is a friend of Brandreth's Pills.

Leeches, gum-water, and costive-ness. 631. In the treatment of *fevers* we have witnessed more misery and waste of life from *leeches, gum water, and costive bowels* than from any degree of purgation (Rev. 1836, Vol. IV., p. 167).

Poisons destroy the nervous fac-ulty through injury done to the blood. 632. Physiological researches during the last thirty years have satisfactorily proved that most if not all of the agents which exert such destructive energy on the nervous system (as poisons) do it through the medium of the circulation, as shown by the experiments of *Christison* and *Coindet*, of *Brodie*, *Viborg*, and others. And we are much mistaken if future researches do not prove this equally of what we term the *true puerperal fever.* . . The entire absence of coagulum, the perfect fluidity of the blood, apparently both in color and consistence to thin watery claret, tends to confirm these views (Rev. 1836, Vol. II., p. 484).

The materia medica—why so large and full of useless drugs—leads to dangerous results in practice. 633. How many medicinal agents have been indebted for their reputation to fortuitous circumstances. It would be easy to show from the former history of diseases that the medicine employed in the treatment had no influence whatever in effecting the cure, but that the result was entirely owing to the efforts of nature. A physician, for example, employs a certain medicine in a few cases and finds his patients recover; hence he concludes that the treatment and the cure stand to one another in the relation of cause and effect. Misapprehensions of this sort produce a very false and injurious impression upon the minds of students, leading them in their future practice to bleeding, blistering, and treating " heroically " all affections that appear to be violent and intractable (Rev. 1842, Vol. XIII., p. 55).

In tumors, &c., BRANDRETH's PILLS affect FIRSTLY and CHIEFLY the MORBID GROWTH.

Tumors. Another rea-son why BRANDRETH's PILLS remove only impu-rities. 634. " *Nature gives up in the first instance that which is extraneous and parasitical, in preference to what is normal both in structure and in degree of development.*" This is an important law, observable in a thousand cases, without the auspicious operation of which indeed one-half of our labors would be in vain (ibid., pp. 330, 331).

Acute rheu-matism. 635. These recommendations (*continued purging in acute rheuma-tism*) are *in the HIGHEST DEGREE IMPORTANT for the speedy removal of the disease, whether mild or severe:* and the custom of some practitioners who avoid purging from fear of giving occasion to injurious exposure of the person, cannot be too strongly reprobated (ibid., p. 450). *The only remedy purgation.*

636. It is evident then : *The resumé on medical art, nature, etc.*
1. That in a large proportion of the cases treated by allopathic physicians, the disease is cured by nature and not by them.
2. That in a lesser, but still not a small portion, the disease is cured by nature, in spite of them ; in other words, their interference opposing instead of assisting the cure.
3. That consequently, in a considerable proportion of diseases, it would fare as well or better with patients, in the actual condition of the medical art, *as more generally practised*, if all remedies, at least all active remedies, especially drugs, were abandoned (p. 257, vol. XXI., 1846). *These remarks apply to the "regular practice" of the "healing art."*

637. This lamentable condition of medicine, regarded as a practical art, is in truth a fact of such magnitude—one so palpably evident—that it was impossible for any careful reader of the history of medicine, or any long observer of the process of disease, not to be aware of it. What indeed is the history of medicine but a history of perpetual changes in the opinions and practice of its professors, respecting the very same subjects—the nature and treatment of diseases ? And amid all these changes, often extreme and directly opposed to one another, do we not find these very diseases, the subject of them, remaining, with some exceptions, still the same in their progress and general event ? (pp. 257, 258.) *History of medicine— and what it teaches.*

638. To be satisfied on this point we need only refer to the history of any one or two of our principal diseases or principal remedies, as *fever, pneumonia, syphilis—antimony, blood-letting, mercury.* Each of these remedies has been, at different times, regarded as almost specific in the cure of the first two diseases, while at other times they have been rejected as useless or injurious. What seemed once so unquestionably, so demonstrably true, as that venesection was indispensable for the cure of pneumonia ? And what is the conclusion now deduced from the clinical researches of Louis and others ? Is it not that patients recover as well, or nearly as well, without it ? The experiments prove, far better without it (pp. 258, 259). *Bleeding, antimony, mercury— their efficacy doubtful; their effects rather injurious.*

639. If the medical god *Mercury* has lost the domain of *syphilis*, he has gained that of *inflammation ;* and many of our best practitioners might possibly be startled and shocked at the supposition that their successors should renounce allegiance to him in the latter domain, as they themselves had done in the former. And yet such a result is more than probable, seeing that there exists not a shadow of more positive proof, if so much, of the efficiency of the medicine in the latter than in the former case (p. 259). *Mercury— its reign for the future questionable.*

640. *Truth is good.* If the art of medicine, as we profess and practice it, cannot bear investigation, and shrinks before the light of truth, from whatsoever quarter it may come, it is high time that it *Truth above all.*

should cease to be sanctioned and upheld by philosophers and honest men (ibid).

DR. FORBES DESERVES WELL OF ALL MANKIND.

LOUIS, CH. A., M. D., *Physician to the Hôpital de la Pitié. Recherches sur les effêts de la saignée dans quelques maladies inflammatoires, &c. On the Effects of Bleeding in Inflammatory Diseases. Paris,* 1835.

Bleeding proved to be worse than useless in inflammation of the lungs.
641. A volume consisting of numerous cases to test the efficacy of blood-letting in pneumony at the Hospital de la Pitié, in Paris. Some patients were bled on the first, some on the second, some on the third day of the attack, and so on; some seldom, others repeatedly, with the periods from attack to convalescence duly noted. And from these cases he comes to the *inevitable conclusion that bleeding is a noxious, not a beneficial agent, in the disease—that it does not remove pain, and if it at all modifies it, in twenty-four hours it is generally as severe as ever;* that bleeding seems to produce an effect only when used at a period sufficiently remote from the origin of the malady to be perhaps coincident with improvement.

Blisters equally use less.
642. *Mr. Louis* applied to the effects of *blisters* the same experimental analysis, and came to the conclusion that *in pneumonia* they are also *devoid of utility.*

Brandreth's Pills are of absolutely certain benefit in every case of pleurisy; and in all inflammations whatsoever they should be used at once. Then they have never been known to fail.

LOUIS, E. H., M. D., *Pathological Researches in Phthisin. London,* 1835.

Cases the only true evidence of the virtue of a medicine.
643. The *numerical method* is, in fact, the only method in our power to pursue; it *is the only control* we can possess over assertion, the only test for opinion. Its application to a sufficient number of facts, must inevitably give us the most exact and best possible knowledge of those facts, and we .would ask the individual who believes that science is founded on facts, what more he would require? (p. 28.)

By the numerical method we would be judged. Let this method be applied to effects Brandreth's Pills produce upon disease; and what an amount of suffering and sorrow would soon terminate! No inflammation, no cholera, no fever, no pleurisy, no rheumatism, or any pain would cause alarm, because it would be known that a few Brandreth's Pills would soon restore any and every organ to health.

MOORE, G., Surg., *An Inquiry into the Pathology, Causes and Treatment of Puerperal Fever; which obtained the* FOTHERGILLIAN GOLD MEDAL, *March,* 1835. *London,* 1836.

Puerperal fever—early purgation.
644. *Puerperal Fever.—*That *early purgation is* indeed *an essential auxiliary* in the treatment, is amply testified by those who have been most successful (p. 223).

In every case of puerperal fever I have seen, where purgation was used at once when the violent pain in the womb admonished that inflammation had commenced, was cured. The purgative was Brandreth's Pills. Every other case where other remedies than purgative were applied was lost. In fact, forty years ago it was generally understood that puerperal fever meant—death. In 1840 a friend of mine, a physician, lost seventeen cases of this fever one after another. I recommended purgation, i. e. Brandreth's Pills. He followed my plan and gave the pills, and never after lost a case.

PARISÉ, M. R., M. D.   *Pathology of Rheumatism.* See BULLETIN GÉNÉRAL DE THÉRAPEUTIQUE, *July,* 1835, *and* BRIT. AND FOR. MED. REV., 1836, *Vol. I.*

645. *Rheumatism.*—Its change of situation does not change its nature, although it goes by different names. Thus it is *the same disease* which in the head is called *gravedo*, in the neck *torticollis* (*wry-neck*), in the side *pleurodynia*, in the loins *lumbago*, and along the sciatic nerve *sciatica* (Rev., p. 255).

[margin note: Rheumatism. The same disease under various names according to location.]

CURE OF INFLAMMATORY RHEUMATISM.

DR. BRANDRETH :   SING SING, Jan. 25, 1867.

For some years I have been subject to attacks of inflammatory rheumatism, which usually come on every three or four months. My physicians were of the highest reputation. By their advice I took colchicum, citric acid, and other celebrated remedies, but none relieved me or shortened the attacks, which lasted for weeks at a time. In my last attack I concluded to try your famous pills. I was lying upon my bed at the time, suffering the severest pains in my feet and ankles, which no pen can describe.

The first dose of six pills was so effective that in a few hours the pain and swelling sensibly abated, and in forty-eight hours were all gone, and I was cured and have had no return.

I send you this testimonial for the benefit of others who, suffering in a similar manner, may know how they can find certain relief.

I am respectfully yours,   J. D. DUDLEY.

_____

FURTHER PROOF.

To DR. BRANDRETH :   BROOKLYN, Oct. 5, 1866.

It gives me pleasure to state the good I have experienced from your pills. Since I commenced their use I have felt in all respects like a new man, and the rheumatism I took them to relieve has entirely disappeared. At first I was prejudiced against them, because their operation was attended with severe griping; but on a further experience I am convinced such pains were only caused by the medicine struggling with and removing certain obstructions in the bowels. I commenced with taking five pills every night on going to bed, and by an increase of one pill every evening ran the quantity up to twelve pills, which number I continued to take for ten days, and then gradually reduced to five pills at a dose. With the exception of the first three doses I have experienced no pain or griping, but the operation was both easy and pleasant. I took the pills for twenty-four days, and noticed that I passed a great quantity of black, bilious-looking, offensive matter, which I am glad to have got clear of. The Brandreth Pills take right hold of all that is deleterious in the bowels; and, as I said before, I now feel like a new man, and deem it my duty to express my gratitude to you.   Sincerely your friend,

FRANKLIN L. HAWLEY, 238 Classon Avenue.

MCILWAIN, GEORGE, Surg., *Remarks on the Unity of the Body, &c. London,* 1836. *See* BRIT. AND FOR. MED. REV., 1836, *Vol. II.*

646. *The whole of the body sympathizes with all its parts* (Rev., p. 180).

[margin note: Axiom.]

WILLIAMS, ROBERT, M. D., *Physician to St. Thomas Hospital. Elements of Medicine. London*, 1836.

647. Certain diseases—as *typhus, scarlatina, varioli, erysipelas,* &c., are produced *by morbid poisons.* These have definite specific actions—*latent periodicity*—the phenomena varying according to the dose and predisposition of the individual. Generally these poisons act with an intensity proportioned to the feebleness of the patient (Preface).

As the impurity, so the disease. The danger of the malady depends upon the degree of impurity of the blood.

648. *Bleeding.*—From a careful comparison of such evidence as exists, *Dr. Williams* concludes, that since the evidence against bleeding in fever so greatly outweighs that in its favor, it seems demonstrated, and by the most practical experience as yet before the public on any disposed medical question, that *bleeding in the cure of fever* is the exception, *not the rule ; . . that the cause of the disease being a poison, it is necessary to remove the poison from the body* in order to stop the disease (p. 171).

Bleeding does not remove the cause of disease in fever, scarlet-fever, etc.

649. The most effective treatment was found to be as follows :

Ten grains of rhubarb, or a scruple, at whatever stage the patient was admitted, and barley-water enemas, night and morning, with half an ounce of syrup of poppies added. Success is the only criterion in medicine, and certainly this practice has effected the cure of a much larger proportion of cases than any other mode I have witnessed (p. 93).

The benefit of laxatives and injections.

How infinitely superior Brandreth's Pills are to this treatment, as all who know them will admit.

650. The results obtained by the practice of bleeding in *scarlet fever,* as well as by abstracting from it, are given in the following table:

Of 121 *persons,* treated in the Foundling Hospital, in 1786, *by bleeding,* 19 *died,* being about *one in six.*

Of 60 *persons,* treated at the London Fever Hospital in 1829, *by bleeding,* 10 *died,* being the same average ; whilst

Of 125 *persons,* treated *by purgatives and emetics,* only 10 *died.*

Bleeding in scarlet-fever proved to be pernicious by 436 cases.

And if Brandreth's Pills had been the purgative, not five out of a hundred would have died.

LAWRENCE, WILLIAM, Surg., *Treatise on Hernia. London*, 1838.

651. *Strangulated Hernia.*—The notions that purgatives are capable of exciting the mucous membrane of the alimentary passages, and thus producing an aggravating inflammation of the stomach and bowels, is groundless ; and the practical precepts founded on this theoretical and imaginary foundation, have always appeared to me a signal triumph of doctrine over the most unequivocal results of experience and the plainest dictates of common sense (p. 323).

Strangulated hernia. Purgatives are indicated and never injure.

If the bowels should not be relieved three or four hours after the operation, a pill of calomel, or of calomel and extract of colocynth, may be given, followed by a drachm or two of sulphate of magnesia in mint or plain water, and this *repeated every three or four hours until the bowels are freely relieved.* If this do not succeed, a large common injection, with four or six ounces of infusion of senna, or an ounce of castor-oil, should be administered (ibid.)

Give six or eight Brandreth's Pills; they will certainly relieve the bowels, and if given early will probably save the pain and danger of the operation.

KENNEDY, HENRY, Surg., *Editor Dublin Medical Press. Sept.* 23, 1840.

652. *As soon as a quantity of blood is abstracted, that moment the system commences to supply the deficiency.* So impatient is nature at the loss, that if the food taken is insufficient for her purpose, she takes back whatever may have previously been poured out—such as serum, lymph, or possibly even pus. (Cases in proof are given from Drs. *McDowell, Stoker,* and by the author.) *Nature abhors blood-letting;—instead of removing impurities, it restores them to the circulation.*

Never bleed. "Thou shalt not kill."

MORGAN, G. F., M. A. *First Principles of Surgery. London,* 1840.

653. The influence of the blood on the vital functions is proved by the fact that the vigor and activity of animal life depend principally on the condition of the circulating fluid; and according to the qualities of the mass, *when inflammation sets in after severe injuries,* are the subsequent constitutional phenomena in a great measure regulated (p. 179 +). *Good blood greatly assists the recovery from accidents.*

654. There are *two principal morbid varieties* of constitution in which local injuries produce peculiar and extraordinary effects. The one is that of *general plethora,* attributable to over-repletion of the vascular system; the other arises from an *impoverished state of the blood,* coupled, in the worst cases, with a disturbed condition of the nervous system (p. 144). *Morbid state of the blood from two causes.*

655. *Nothing* at the commencement (of inflammation) *will suffice but free and general depletion with purgatives;* and we have by these means known consciousness restored after an unfavorable prognosis had been passed (p. 147). *Inflammation. Free and general purgation required.*

656. If we regard the *morbid alterations in the composition of the blood* as the primary source of fevers, we can easily explain the subsequent derangement in the functions of the organs, and the vitiation of the different secretions during their continuance. In all cases the increased discharge has the effect of relieving the congested state of the mucous membrane (p. 179 +). *Fevers and vitiated secretions from impure blood.*

The believer in the efficacy of purgatives will thank Dr. Morgan for this testimony.

CANSTADT, CHARLES, M. D., *Professor in the University of Erlangen. Special Pathology and Therapeutics founded on Clinical Observations. Erlangen*, 1841. See BRIT. & FOR. MED. REV., 1842, *Vol. XIII.*

Iodine—Its action. 657. The modus operandi of *iodine* consists in *undermining* the universal process of *nutrition* (vol. I., p. 11—Rev., p. 331).

As the blood, so the nervous system. 658. An *asthenic condition of the nervous system* is an affection always coincident with *anemia;* since, on the one hand, a normal condition of that system is indispensable to a right formation of the blood, as on the other normal blood is essential to a healthy state of the nervous system (ibid., p. 33—Rev., p. 332).

Blood and pus. 659. Severe *suppuration* produces precisely the same effects as excessive *venesection;* while precisely the same means which improve the condition of the *blood* produce a similar effect on that of the *pus* (ibid., p. 87—Rev., p. 336).

Inflammation. Nature's attempt to cure —she may overdo it. 660. The phenomena of *inflammation* are *not morbid movements*, but consist chiefly of *energetic endeavors of nature to oppose or rid herself of an injurious agent or influence*. Death may in this way incidentally occur from salutary efforts of nature herself, as when hemorrhagic apoplexy of the brain or lungs ensues from the reaction instituted to repel or extrude some morbific agent or influence operating on these organs or elsewhere (ibid., p. 96—Rev., p. 337).

Mercury— producing salivation— no medicine but a poison aggravating the inflammation. 661. *Dr. Alison* of Edinburgh (Library of Medicine) denies "that *mercury* administered so as to affect the gums possesses any power of controlling inflammation and its consequences." And on this point the present writer, after considerable experience, reiterates an opinion he formerly expressed, that he has more frequently seen *inflammatory symptoms aggravated or transferred to other parts, on that event (salivation) taking place*, than relieved by it (ibid., p. 3—Rev., 338).

Crisis—another view. 662. *The discharges (sweats)* which occasionally signalize the crisis *do not contain the materia peccans.* The crisis itself is the recovery, the discharges being nothing but the effects and proof of the regeneration of the unhealthy functions (ibid., p. 260—Rev., p. 342).

Hypertrophy. Bleeding injurious. 663. *Hypertrophy.—Blood-letting*, if practised *in moderation*, is apt to prove *fruitless; if energetically* employed, it is more likely to *promote anemia, dropsy, and debility* than to cure hypertrophy (ibid., p. 10—Rev., p. 331).

Chlorosis of all forms from imper- 664. The multifarious symptoms of *chlorosis* do not require separate attention; since, depending on a common lesion, to wit, the *deficient* *crasis** *of blood,* they simultaneously disappear when that fluid is brought to its normal state (ibid., p. 40 ; Rev. p. 333). fectly elaborated blood.

HURNEFELDT, F. L., M. D., *Chemistry and Medicine in Close Co-operation.* *Berlin,* 1841.

665. In the *cæcum* there is carried on to a certain extent a repetition of what takes place in the stomach and small intestines. In the *colon* are found the insoluble matters of the food, the bronze coloring matter of the bile, mucous, fat, soluble and insoluble salts, various azotized matters, etc.. besides fetid volatile productions (p. 110). Digestion continued in the cæcum.

These matters being retained and reabsorbed through constipation, what an amount of evil is produced ! Let those who are costive beware. The bowels must be evacuated once at least in the day, or there can be no health and no safety.

MUNNELEY, THOMAS, Surg. *A Treatise on the Nature, Cause and Treatment of Erysipelas.* *London,* 1841.

666. It is an easy thing for the purpose of producing an immediate effect, or " knocking the disease on the head," as it is often termed, to take from a man two, three or four pounds of blood ; but should he survive, the probability is that *he will not for several years, if forever, be the sound man* he was before the shock his system has had inflicted upon it by such heroic proceedings (p. 220).

667. *Purgatives,* in by far the majority of cases, if properly used, *completely obviate the necessity of venesection,* especially if they have been preceded by an emetic (p. 230). *Erysipelas.* Bloodletting and purgation compared.

This is sound doctrine.

CRICHTON, SIR ALEXANDER, M. D., *Commentaries on some Doctrines of a Dangerous Tendency in Medicine, and on the General Principles of safe Practice.* *London,* 1842. *See* BRIT. AND FOR. MED. REV., 1843, *Vol. XV.*

668. *In typhus, bleeding is useless and reprehensible.* Nature's principle of curing this disease is the same as that by which the paroxysm of an intermittent is terminated ; she reduces the quantity of circulating fluids until she brings about an equilibrium between them and the enfeebled moving powers *by excrementitious evacuations* (Rev., p. 465). *Typhus.* Bleeding useless. Nature's cure— another view.

669. The *Liebig theory* of the action of contagious and other animal poisons is, that if the exciting agent be a compound body, *it will reproduce itself ad infinitum,* provided the compound body on which it acts contains elements fitted for such an end. This theory accounts for numerous cures of *syphilis without mercury* by *Dr. Fricke* in the hospital of Hamburg. From *low diet and continued purgation* the parts of the *Syphilis.* Cure without any mercury —merely by purgation.
(*The Liebig theory.*)

* Blood globules. Brandreth's Pills not only take away impurities, but they make the blood richer in Crassamentum or blood globules.

blood are not supplied which are susceptible of the metamorphosis. Thus *the poison becomes starved and purged out ;* the same result being produced as is effected in fever, by the annihilation of the desire for food and consequent suspension of the process of chymification (condensed from pp. 210 to ult. of Crichton).

GULLY, JAMES M., M. D., *On the Simple Treatment of Diseases.* London, 1842.

Nature's mode of cure—another view.

670. *The constant tendency of the diseased body is towards cure,* and this for the most part by the erection of certain modes of vital action in other parts of the frame than that which is morbid, and by the elimination of certain matters from the emunctories. . . Thus a fever usually declines just as the kidneys, the lower bowels, or the skin pour out their respective excretions copiously (p. 32).

These " certain matters " have been obtained from morbid parts invariably.

JONES, HENRY BEALE, M. D., *On Gravel, Calculus, and Gout, chiefly an Application of Professor Liebig's Philosophy to the Prevention and Cure of Diseases.* London, 1842.

Gout— cure by purgation.

671. We may diminish the proportion of the *gouty material in the blood :*

1. *By stopping the supply*—that is, by change of diet; and
2. *By causing an increase of secretion* from the liver and intestinal glands through the action of purgatives.

These medicines will have the further effect of causing the secreted products to be discharged from the intestinal canal, instead of remaining to undergo partial reabsorption (pp. 70 to 74).

LANZA, V., M. D., *Professor of Physic in the University of Naples. Positive Nosology. Naples,* 1842. *See* BRITISH AND FOR. MED. REV., 1846, *Vol. XXIII.*

What retards the true knowledge in medicine.

672. The *chief obstacles* which impede the advance of experimental medicine are the following :

1. The extreme *variety* which prevails in different countries *in plans of cure, popular remedies, medical usages,* &c., whereby *all common grounds of comparison are wanting.*
2. The monster-abuse of *polypharmacy*—the injury it has caused, alike to humanity and to " the art," being notorious.
3. The number of *compound remedies* still in vogue, a clear *relic of barbarism,* which should long ago have been banished by the profession.
Leaving all these behind, medicine must *commence anew* to determine the true power and value of remedies (Rev., p. 63).

The BRAN-DRETHIAN PRACTICE justified.

673. We first find that therapeutics must be *founded on experience.* . . The method of treatment to be adopted in any particular case must be

that which has most *frequently been found effectual* in some previous and analogous case (Rev., p. 15).

MacLeod, Radcliffe, M. D., *Physician to St. George's Hospital. On Rheumatism in its Various Forms. London,* 1842.

674. *Acute Rheumatism.—Purgatives.*—This discipline ought gen- *Acute rheumatism.* erally to be *repeated on several successive days;* indeed, throughout the whole course of a case of acute rheumatism, the due evacuation of the *Purgation* bowels ought to be an indication never lost sight of; and in many cases, *the only depletion re-* where the attack is comparatively mild, *this is the only form of deple- quired. tion required* (p. 34).

Richter, C. A. W., M. D., *Contributions to Scientific Medicine. Leipzig,* 1842.

Important Article.

675. *The* Vis Medicatrix Naturæ.—This power both *organizes* un- Vis medica- organized matter, and *disorganizes* vitalized matters, *separating vitalized* trix. *matter from the system after it has fulfilled its uses in the organism, and* The theory *has become, if detained, a hurtful agent* (sect. 1). of disease;— effete matter retained in the system.

676. If the recomposing and decomposing processes are in *equi-* Nature's way *librium,* there *is health;* but if *the effete matter be not cast off,* or a removing im- *hurtful agent enters* the system from without, the *equilibrium is de- purities from* the system. *stroyed,* and the innate *vital force sets up an action to restore it—the re- sulting phenomena being the phenomena of disease.* So that *morbid action* consists in *an interruption of the renewing or reformative pro- cess, concurrently with* ALTERATIONS IN THE QUALITY OF THE BLOOD, and a reaction of the innate vital force to *restore the normal* state (ibid.)

677. The *hurtful agent is eliminated* from the system through the Localization secreting and excreting organs, or not *being fully eliminated, is localized* of effete mat- ters causes in some one or more special structures, thus giving rise to various con- local dis- stitutional and chronic local diseases (ibid.) eases.

678. *Fever is a healthy process.* The innate vital force, feeling the *Fevers—na- presence of a *hurtful agent* in the system, *attempts its removal after the* ture's effort at a cure;— *same manner as it removes effete matter. If the hurtful agent is not elim-* why she *inated, it is localized in an organ,* and *the innate vital force attempts its* often fails. *removal* by colliquation of that organ, giving rise to various changes of structure, and to *the general symptoms of local diseases.*

Hectic fever is in reality a healing process, *set up to expel the hurtful* Hectic fever. *power from the organ to which it has retreated;* and it is injurious only because the hurtful power is of such a nature, or so situated, as to re- quire for its expulsion a greater effort than the vital machinery will bear; so that the recomposing process is never re-established, and the colliqua- tion goes on until the dissolution of the organism, or death, takes place (sect. ii).

158   THE DOCTRINE OF PURGATION.

How medicines ought to act. 679. *Medicines only assisting the healthy action of nature in throwing off the hurtful power* (ibid.)

And this is what Brandreth's Pills produce. No more: no less.

SCHULTZ, C. H., M. D., *Professor in the University of Berlin. On the Renewal of Human Life. Berlin,* 1842. *See* BRIT. AND FOR. MED. REV., 1845, *Vol. XVIII.*

The blood— Its development. 680. It is necessary that the organic constituents of the blood pass through their embryo state, just as the embryo itself, before they can be perfectly developed; and as the lymphatic glands are the gills and placentæ of the system, if these perform their functions imperfectly, as in **Chlorosis and phthisis.** scrofulous constitutions, a deposit from the unripe blood takes place. Hence the development of chlorosis and phthisis (p. 142; Rev., p. 392).

Elements of General Pathology. Berlin, 1844–45. *See* BRIT. AND FOR. MED. REV., *ibid.*

Blood—Impurities and varieties of diseases. 681. The state of the blood circulating through the secreting organs influences their diseases. (Predispositions in the glandular and secreting systems.) (Rev., p. 345.)

By a stoppage of the depurative process in the liver the whole mass of *the blood* gets *charged with impurities.* The dead vesicles show a tendency even to chemical decomposition, as in stinking secretions, nauseous cutaneous affections, &c. . . The blood acts injuriously on the nervous and muscular system; it is deficient in the stimulating property of healthy blood. Thus the brain, nerves of the senses, and muscles, are imperfectly acted on, are weakened, and at last paralyzed. Apoplexy, intermittent fever, spectral illusions, and even paralysis of the senses, are the result of this state. (Predispositions of the blood.) (Rev., p. 343.)

WILLIAMS, CHARLES J. B., M. D., *Principles of Medicine. London,* 1843. *See* BRIT. AND. FOR. MED. REV., 1844, *Vol. XVII.*

Defective excretion;— a fruitful source of disease. 682. The *excretions are defective in* many idiopathic and symptomatic *fevers,* and there can be little doubt that many of the constitutional effects of these fevers are, in a great measure, due to this important element. *The positively noxious properties which excrementitious matters* **Morbid matters, etc., retained.** *retained in the blood are known to possess, must be taken into account,* when we attempt to explain the state of constitutional irritation and depression, with perversion of functions, which fevers so generally present. *The changes in the blood may also be in part referred to defective elimination of effete matter; and it is when the secreting organs recover their power, and a diarrhœa occurs, or a copious discharge of highly-colored urine, that* THESE APPEARANCES CEASE (p. 81; Rev., p. 479).

Disease from change in the blood. 683. The causes of disease are *changes in the due proportions of the blood,* and otherwise, by respiration, secretion, nutrition, and by foreign matters (ibid.)

684. In the treatment of this element of disease—*foreign morbid matters in the blood*—the two indications which present themselves are, *first, to counteract the injurious operation of these matters ; and second, to expel them from the system.* WE DO NOT POSSESS CHEMICAL ANTIDOTES WHICH CAN ACT ON THE FOREIGN MATTER IN THE BLOOD WITHOUT INJURING THE BLOOD ITSELF. The *other* indication is more *generally* pursued, although *little recognized by practitioners, to expel the offending matter from the system. The excretory organs, especially the kidneys and the alimentary canal, are the natural emunctories through which foreign and offending matters are expelled from the blood.* Let us bear in mind *how often fevers and other serious ailments seem to be carried off by spontaneous diarrhœa, diuresis, or perspiration* (ibid., p. 122 ; Rev., p. 485).

All chemical antidotes INJURE THE BLOOD, although they may expel morbid matters from it. Expel these as nature does.

Cozzi, L., *Professor of Chymistry. Analysis of the Blood in a Case of Lead Colic, in* JOURNAL DE PHARMACIE. *Paris, February,* 1844. *See* EDINBURGH MEDICAL AND SURGICAL JOURNAL, 1844, *Vol. LXII*

685. *Professor Cozzi,* in analyzing the blood of a person severely affected with lead colic, discovered that the lead existed in the state of a salt, or of an oxyde of the metal, in the albumen of the blood (Ed. Journ., p. 553).

Painters' colic. Poison of lead in the blood.

HOUSTON, JOHN, M. D., *Introductory Lecture in Surgery. Dublin,* 1844.

686. The great mind of *John Hunter* saw and believed that the blood possessed in itself an independent life even while circulating loosely in the blood-vessels, but he knew not the nature and the seat of that vitality. The discovery was reserved for the physiologists of our days. There are particles, called globules, floating in this liquid, about the 3000th part of an inch in diameter, or so small that myriads of them are contained in a single drop. It has been ascertained respecting these globules that they are, each and all, endowed with a definite and uniform shape, and with a development, in virtue of which they pass by successive transitions from a condition of origin to one of final evolution—a veritable organization, in other words—properties which give them a claim to the title life, as much as those which justify the application of that term to the ovum, from which proud man himself dates his being. The atomic particles of which the blood is composed being thus individually alive, collectively they form a mass of which it may literally, as well as allegorically be said : *" For it is the life of all flesh ; the blood of it is for the life thereof ; for the life of the flesh is in the blood."*

The blood. Physiology.

Red corpuscles. Description of their individual vitality ; proved by microscopical observation.

The globules are themselves, each and all, possessed of an independent life. I have repeatedly watched them, and have shown them to others, when burst from their cell-membrane, performing sundry independent and apparently voluntary evolutions in the field of the microscope, until to the eye the whole looked like a moving mass of creeping things. In this view, then, the blood is doubly alive as exhibited—first in its forming and taking part in the repairs of the animal machine, and

The globules possessed of independent motion.

secondly, in the independent movements possessed by the ultimate particles of its matter (Lancet, Amer. Edit. 1845, vol. I., p. 214, +).

PIDDUCK, JOHN, M. D., *On the Treatment of Indolent and Irritable Ulcers. London,* 1844. *See* LANCET, 1844, *Vol. II.*

Ulcers—natural outlets. Purge till the discharge is healthy, when they will naturally heal. 687. I regard *the ulcer* as *a natural outlet or issue for the escape of certain morbid principles from the blood,* the retention or suppression of which would have occasioned diseases of a more dangerous tendency. . . If the ulcer or the issue emit a disgusting odor and discharge freely, the necessity for such a drain is unequivocal; it cannot be closed without risk of a worse disorder. But when the odor of the ulcer, or the issue, ceases to be disagreeable, and the discharge is moderate in quantity, and of a healthy quality, it admits of cure with perfect safety (Lanc., p. 405).

BARTLETT, ELISHA, M. D., *Professor of Medicine in the University of Maryland ; Philosophy of Medicine, Philadelphia,* 1845. *On the recent Progress and future Prospects of Practical Medicine. See* BRIT. AND FOR. MED. REV., 1846, *Vol. XXII.*

The materia medica. 688. *The Articles of the Materia Medica.*—There is probably no man more entirely sceptical in regard to their alleged properties and virtues than I am. There is no man who has been in the habit of *using a smaller number of them.* My own opinion is, that the number of substances endowed with active and peculiar or characteristic remedial properties is small. . . In many cases of disease all medicines, using the word in its *common* signification, are evils, and that they may be dispensed with, not merely with negative safety, but to the actual benefit of the subjects. . . The golden axiom of Chomel—that it is only the *second* law of therapeutics *to do good,* its *first law being* this, *to do no harm*—is gradually finding its way into the medical mind, preventing an incalculable amount of positive ill (Rev. p. 237).

Assist nature or let the disease alone. 689. It is coming every day to be more clearly seen that perhaps the most universal and beneficial function of medical art consists *in the removal and avoidance of those agents the action of which is to occasion or to aggravate disease, thus giving the recuperative energies of the system their full scope and action, and trusting to them when thus unembarrassed and free for the cure of disease* (ibid).

BUDD, GEORGE, M. D., *Professor of Medicine, King's College, London. On Diseases of the Liver. London,* 1845.

Liver-disease—and mercury. 690. In this country *mercury* has generally been resorted to, when the local symptoms have led to the suspicion that the *liver* was diseased; but I fear with no benefit to the patients. It has been well observed by Abercrombie : " On the liver-diseases of this country, mercury is often used in an indiscriminate manner, and with very undefined *Ambiguous* notions as to certain specific influence which it is supposed to exert *the action of* over all the morbid conditions of this organ. If the liver be supposed *mercury.* to be *in a state of torpor, mercury* is given to *excite* it ; if *in a state of acute inflammation, mercury* is given to *moderate* the inflammation and *reduce* its action " (p. 99).

COPEMAN, EDWARD, Surg., *A Collection of Cases of Apoplexy, with an Explanatory Introduction. London,* 1845. *See* LANCET, 1845, *Vol. I.*

691. The following collection of cases is published with the view of *Apoplexy.* furnishing sufficient data for determining the comparative merits of different modes of treating apoplexy, and for judging of the expediency *Bleeding fatal.* of resorting to bleeding for the cure of that disease (Introduction). Here follow 250 cases.
The conclusion is, that bleeding, generally speaking, is so ineffectual *The more* a means of preventing the fatal termination of apoplexy, that it scarcely *blood is abstracted, the* deserves the name of a remedy for this disease ; that the treatment *fewer are the chances* without loss of blood was attended with the most success, and that *of recovery.* *the mortality of the disease increased in proportion to the extent to which the bleeding was carried;* the more copious the loss of blood the more fatal the disease (pp. 198, 199 ; Lanc., p. 533).

MACKIN, CHARLES T., M. D., *On the Acute form of Gout, with Remarks on its similarity to Acute Rheumatism. In Lancet, American Edition, Vol. I.,* 1845.

692. In a well-defined attack of *gout,* the pre-existing and gradually *Gout; — a* progressing *derangement of all the organs* which subserve the purposes *local disease from* of *digestion and nutrition, coupled with* the very remarkable increase *derangement of the digest-* of *nervous irritability* observable (as far as my experience goes) inva- *ive organs.* riably antecedent to a paroxysm, are sufficient, in a great measure, to warrant the conclusion that it is one of the most prominent examples of a local disease, depending solely for its origin on constitutional disturbance (p. 312).

693. It is, in the established rules of modern practice, to be taken *Modern* by storm, to be driven from the system " vi et armis," and all the means *practice.* which an already *overgrown materia medica* places within our reach, have been and are brought to bear against it. Patients are cured ; " they get well." . . . From the first recipe traced on sand by the staff of *Anaximander* or *Therecydes* (the inventors of writing) up to the last *A physician's opin-* " fiat mistura," have we one which we can positively say will produce a *ion of his art.* certain and definite effect? No, not one. Medicine is then, as yet, nothing save a nice balance of contingencies (pp. 312, 313).

A knowledge of Brandreth's Pills would have changed this opinion.

694. The premonitory signs of its approach are generally to be found *The precur-* of a well-marked and definite character, so much so that in many in- *sory symp-* *toms as indi-* stances he who has undergone a previous attack, can foretell with uner- *cating the seat of evil*
11

to be the stomach and intes-tines, and removal of the morbid matter in them to con-stitute the cure. ring certainty the coming of a "*fit*," as it is termed, some time anterior to the appearance of the unwelcome visitor. The *first symptom* which excites observation, is a considerable *increase of nervous irritability*, and a general *peevishness* and *hastiness of manner*. The *sleep is restless* and unrefreshing, disturbed with *frightful dreams*, tossing of the limbs, etc. The *appetite* (though not invariably) *falls off*. There is *gastro-in-testinal derangement*, with a *sense of fullness and oppression* subsequent to meals; *dyspepsia* and *heartburn* are pretty constantly present. As the symptoms become aggravated, the patient is annoyed with *flatulence*, accompanied with *sour eructations*. . . .

There is a bitter, or at all events, a vitiated taste in the mouth, espe-cially on first rising in the morning; headache in those of plethoric habit; the bowels are costive or relaxed—in either case the secretions are dark and offensive. The urine is of a saffron tinge, often scanty in quantity, and charged with lithic acid. These form the more remarka-ble prodromata, and, curiously enough, are observed to possess a distinctly intermittent character (p. 313).

— These are, as the author expresses himself in another place, " not the ' *hints*,' but the ' *positive directions*,' laid down for the man-agement of the disease, for our guidance and instruction, by *Dame Na-ture* " (Lancet, A. E., Vol. I., p. 672).

The last warning.   695. Of the near approach of the " fit " the patient is warned by being seized at intervals with *flying or transitory pains* in different parts of the body, mostly affecting those portions of the frame already weakened by previous illness (ibid.).

The parox-ysm a salu-tary process of natural cure.   696. A most remarkable fact connected with the disappearance of the paroxysm is that the patient, with the exception of being more or less crippled for a time, experiences a sort of general renovation of the system, and his state of health is better and more vigorous subsequently than prior to the fit. It seems as if the localization of this disease were a salutary process instituted by the " vis vitæ " for the more effectual and complete removal of the cumulative disturbance of the general economy (ibid).

The disease is general; its appear-ances local.   697. I have also observed that very slight causes will bring about the development of *the elements* of gouty inflammation, *with which the sys-tem appears to be charged*. I have known so trivial an accident as striking the great toe against a stone in walking produce a paroxysm. This peculiarity is often witnessed in those who are of confirmed gouty diathesis. Indeed, a man constitutionally subject to the disorder ap-pears " to wear his heart upon his sleeve," slight accidents, otherwise of no moment, being sufficient to induce an attack of this extraordinary disease (p. 314).

SARA, ROBERTS, *Professor of Medicine in the University of Milan. Sui Pregi é Doveri del Medico. Milan*, 1845.

SIMPLE REME-DIES the best.   698. A physician of no great reputation would positively compromise his interests, if he limited himself to the prescription of *simple remedies*.

The general ignorance obliges him to be a proselyte of the *polyphar-* Humbug es-
macia; and indeed it is very easy to unite to any medicine a greater or sential to the
"profession."
less number of substances which are quite incapable of modifying its
properties. And it is also useful frequently to vary the medicines,
because the public readily disbelieves in the knowledge of a physician
who always prescribes the same remedies (p. 115).

699. The principal means of obtaining success in practice is to limit Success in
one's self to a *reasonable system of expectation,* and to prescribe in cases practice—
how to
in which *no active medicine is clearly indicated,* substances incapable of obtain.
exciting remarkable changes in the animal economy (p. 120).

TAYLOR, J., M. D., *Clinical Remarks on Cancer. See Report of the
University College Hospital in* LANCET, *1845, Vol. II.*

700. The commonest way in which *cancer* is propagated is *by the circu-* Cancer—
lation of the cancer-cells in the blood, and *the arrest of them in the capil-* cells in the
blood.
laries, when they multiply and form tumors. In this case (the reported Purge and
one) there was no ulceration. The organs that are secondarily affected in removing
prevent their
by cancer have always some connection with the seat of the primary accumulation
in the arte-
disease. We can easily see the connection between cancer in the breast ries.
and lungs. In passing through the pulmonary capillaries the cancer-
cells are arrested, and thus the cancer is formed (p. 602).

VOGEL, JULIUS, M. D., *The Pathological Anatomy of the Human Body.
Leipzig,* 1845. *See* BRIT. AND FOR. MED. REV., *1846, Vol. XXII.*

701. *Gases* may be developed in the human body from two distinct Foul gases
sources—from *food in the intestinal canal in the act of decomposition* from decom-
position.
and from *decomposition of the tissues* of the body itself. The gases
produced in the intestinal canal occasionally permeate through its walls
into the peritoneal cavity (Rev., p. 324).

WADDY, J. M., M. D., *On Puerperal Fever. See* LANCET, *1845, Vol. I.*

702. When the *intestines are burdened with fecal accumulations* the Effects of re-
constitution becomes affected in various ways; thus *cerebral and vis-* tained fæces.
ceral congestions, phlebitis, &c., may be the result of pressure on the
larger vessels. The intestines are distended beyond their tone, and give
rise to *flatulency, anorexia, indigestion,* and there is probably *absorption
of putrid matters,* which may all tend to promote a highly unfavorable
state of the general system (p. 674).

703. The phenomena of the *typhoid and ataxic (nervous) fevers,* Fever—the
whether common or puerperal, will be best explained as the *consequences* effort of na-
ture to elimi-
of poison—either generated within or introduced from without—*the* nate poison.
fever being strictly an effort of nature to throw off injurious matter
from the living body (pp. 698, 699).

Remittents. 704. *Remittent and intermittent fevers*—the consequence of *nature's endeavors to eliminate a poison* from the system by the biliary organs (ibid.)

IMPORTANT QUESTIONS.

Rapidity of the pulse. 705. Does the rapidity of pulse (in fever) depend upon a law of nature to make up, by *rapidity of distribution and change*, for a deficiency of vital principle in the blood, or is the heart directly *stimulated into increased action by morbid matter in the blood?* (Ibid.)

. CLENDINNING, DR., *Report to the Royal Medical and Chirurgical Society, January* 13, 1846. *See* LANCET, 1846, *Vol. I.*

Hydrocephalus from SUPPRESSED DIARRHŒA. 706. T. S. *Allen*, Surgeon to St. Marylebone Infirmary, has seen in more than 500 cases of *diarrhœa in children*, whose ages varied from 3 months to 3 years, that in at least 6 to 1 the diarrhœa was symptomatic —*a salutary effort of nature to relieve the system*—to suppress which, by *opiates and absorbents*, was to *invite head-symptoms, hydrocephalus, convulsions, and death* (p. 101).

HALL, MARSHALL, M. D., *Practical Observations ·and Suggestions. London*, 1846. (+)

Bleeding a refuge of ignorance. 707. That invariable refuge of the timid and ignorant—the lancet!

Milk-fever— cure by depletion with nature's mode and by purgation. 708. I am of opinion that what is designated "*milk-fever*" is frequently symptomatic of the condition of the mammæ. The remedy for this febrile state is therefore *depletion of the milk-ducts.* As a prevention of milk-abscess and milk-fever, and with other hygienic objects, the infant should be put to the breast at the moment it is born. If, in spite of this, the breasts become in the slightest degree tumid, or febrile action is set up, another and a stronger infant should be applied without delay. *This is nature's mode of relief, and infinitely more efficacious than the application of leeches.* . . The patient must take barley-water as her sole nourishment, and the bowels must be freely purged.

HARRISON, J. B., Surg., *Essays on General Pathology. London*, 1846- 47. (+)

The blood may become impure in three different modes. 709. In the first place, it is manifest that the presence of *foreign matter in the blood* must induce a state of derangement. In the next place, it is equally clear that if the *blood do not undergo those changes*, which it is destined to receive during its transmission through the lungs, it can no longer preserve its healthy constitution. In the third place, the *blood itself may be imperfectly elaborated* (No. V.)

Medical men have small faith in their own remedies. 710. It is well known that *the faculty do not themselves take medicines in the same manner that they prescribe* them to be taken. They have not, it must be owned, that large credence which they require from others. There is not with them the regular taking of spoonfuls at stated intervals, and the expectancy and confidence of the forthcoming result, which they ask of others.

LEESON, JOHN, M. R. C. S. E. *Liebig's Philosophy applied in the Treatment of Functional Derangement and Organic Disease. London*, 1846.

711. There are about *four hundred and ten preparations* in the pharmacopœia of the Royal College of Physicians. Now, any practical man of ten or twenty years' standing must have found that *four hundred* of these preparations *are of little or no value whatever* in the treatment of any form of disease, and that about the *remaining ten* might have assisted him in reducing, at one time or other, cases occurring in every department of his practice. Nearly all the waters, confections, decoctions, extracts, infusions, liquids, mixtures, essential oils, spirits, tinctures, have little or no influence over any form of disease, when used as internal or external remedies. Many of the *mineral preparations are absolutely injurious* in their effects under every circumstance, while the retention of other remedies is burlesque and nonsense (pp. 10, 11). *The pharmacopœia.*

712. Fancy *aluminum, antimony, silver, arsenic, barium, bismuth, calcium, copper, iron, mercury, magnesia, lead, potassium, sodium, zinc* (all of which are to be found in the London pharmacopœia of one hundred years' standing, with the exception of barium and bismuth), as medical agents which are yet authoritatively retained, and which have been at one time or other plied as sovereign remedies for many inveterate forms of disease, although most of them, if not all, are abandoned by every practitioner of standing and experience as the most dangerous applications for any kind of medical purposes (pp. 12, 13). *Metallic remedies.*

MAGENDIE, M., M. D. *Introductory Lecture in the Collège de France*, 1846. *See* LANCET, 1846, *Vol. I.*

713. When disease requires assistance, we may still by well-judged intervention *assist nature in overcoming the functional derangements* which gave rise to the disease (p. 238). *Assist nature by art.*

714. *Tartar emetic*, when brought into contact with the blood, has the power of *dissolving the globules* (p. 363, citation in the paper of Butler Lane, Surgeon). *Tartar-emetic.*

WILSON, J. A., M. D., *On the True Character of Acute Rheumatism; in* LANCET. 1846. (+)

715. *Inflammation* is but an *expression of the nutritive function endered difficult* for the time in particular structures. Inflammation originates no movement, creates no function, brings no new elements into operation; it is *not an acquired principle, but an innate faculty* held in trust by every living structure from the beginning, for the means of self-protection, and as a security under injury for redress. Thus considered the *arthritis of acute rheumatism* is respected by the physicians as salutary under circumstances, and as working with the fever to a cure. *Inflammation—not a disease, but nature's warning.* *Rheumatism.*

Acute rheu-
matism.

716. *Opium in acute rheumatism.*—The healthy relations of this drug with the blood (and it is prescribed on no other indication) are not such as to authorize its employment in a disease whose principle of cure is one of unrestrained spontaneous action.

Opium and lancet:— poison and bloodshed denounced.

717. These *approved principles of* cure by *poison and bloodshed* rest professedly on more than conjectural science for their authority; they are not set forth diffidently, as the experimental misgivings, by small induction, of a theory yet to be realized, but are proclaimed as the dicta of a bold and successful experience; they are blazoned as heroic mottoes above the vulgar host, that seeing them we may know our leaders and be prepared to follow them.

Localization of fevers according to the poisonous matter in the general circulation.

718. As *the scarlet-fever* localizes itself especially *in the throat, the measles in the* mucous lining membrane of the *lungs,* the *epidemic typhus* in the *cæcum and lower ilium,* and the *erysipelas fever in the* integuments of *the head and face,* so is the *rheumatic fever determined* by special effects of inflammation *to the larger joints of the body* and the surrounding articular structures; but the heat, swelling, and redness thus induced are no more the cause of the constitutional disturbance in acute rheumatism than the scarlet-rash, or the small-pox pustule of the fevers that bear their respective names. They are but the partial expression, by impaired nutrition, of a disorder that is general to the system.

Disease from change in the proportion of the natural elements of the blood.

719. Assuming the evil was in the blood, not so much from impurities as a change in the relative proportions of its necessary elements, we might rationally expect the composition of some structures or products to be more influenced than others by an excess or deficiency of principles important to their very existence, since the greater frequency with which particular parts are affected only indicates that the tissues of which they are composed, and the fluids which permeate to them, are such as to be especially affected by a morbific cause which prevails to a greater or less degree throughout the system.

The blood feels and lives.

720. There is *in the blood* an *independent faculty of sensation* which by physiologists is not as yet acknowledged. In disease, as in health, it is sentient of its own states, as it is inceptive of its own actions, and through it we feel much of what, in idle phrase, is made exclusive to the nerve.

Acute rheumatism can cure itself.

Bleeding, opium, and calomel, if they do not kill, complicate the disorder.

721. The *fever of acute rheumatism* is competent to the task of its own cure. Yet the patient is made to *pay by the lancet for its acuteness,* and swallows every specific for gout and neuralgia in right of his rheumatism. . . From this practice, there is reason to believe that many of the *dangerous complications* so frequent of late years in the pathology of acute rheumatism do in truth proceed. In the well known combination of *opium and calomel,* this mischievous diligence of treatment receives its most frequent illustration. The objects proposed in this heroic formula are the immediate and complete extinction of fever, pain, and inflammation.

It is a rude and empirical practice which seldom succeeds, and failing of success is most injurious to the patient; it has destroyed very many who, under less popular and energetic methods of treatment, would have recovered. . . Failure of cure injurious to the patient.

There is more wisdom, for there is less cruelty, in *homœopathy*, *hydropathy*, or *animal magnetism*. Yet the courage is with those who refuse to prescribe.

LET YOUNG MEDICAL MEN PONDER.

722. *Purgation.*—Its simplicity ill accords with the impatient violence and affected combinations of modern therapeutics; yet of constitutional methods of cure, no one, by long practical experience, has been more thoroughly approved. *Purgation* —its simplicity.

723. To *secure effects* by perspiration, *opium, antimony, ipecacuanha, ammonia*, have been *unsparingly added to the system, already tasked* by an active disturbing principle, to its utmost means of resistance. Hence, from undue haste, violence, and inconsistency of action, a great loss of the credit which would otherwise have attached to the sweating practice in rheumatic fever. Forced sweat.

Imperfect sweating causes offensive matters to remain in the ducts and pores.

Sweating to be beneficial must come on spontaneously, with no aid from drugs,.

DICK, ROBERT, M. D., *The Treatment of Dyspepsia.* *See* LANCET, 1847. *Vol. I.*

724. *Cæcum.*—In all cases of constipation or torpor of the bowels, attention to the cæcum is important. It is here that fecal accumulations are, on several accounts, apt to take place. The circumstance of *the large bowel* here *forming a cul-de-sac*, out of which, moreover, the fecal matter, during 14 or 16 out of the 24 hours, can only escape by a course counter to gravity, disposes not a little to the collection there of excrement. And indeed, in most cases of constipation, in cases of chlorosis, &c., we shall generally both see and feel *a fullness of this part*, sometimes of remarkable and even *alarming extent and hardness*. . . . And I have no doubt that in not a few cases a state of chronic irritation of (sub-) inflammation and even of ulceration of the mucous membrane of the cæcum, is induced from the long contact with hardened fæces which, moreover, have become preternaturally fetid and undergone certain irritating chemical decompositions. In such circumstances either round or irregular masses of a fatty looking substance may often be detected in the evacuations. This consists of inspissated mucus, secreted by a *surface highly irritated or (sub-) inflamed*. A slight prolongation or increase of such irritation will convert this inspissated discharge into a purulent one (Lanc., p. 32). Constipation;—its cause in the cæcum; supervening inflammation from hardened fæces.

725. In impure states of the fluids we prescribe purgatives on the following assumption, namely, that *if we, by artificial means, afford nature the opportunity, she will, by emunctories whose action we excite, discharge herself of morbid principles,* retaining those that are healthy. This, indeed, is the *grand general law, in faith of which we venture, in any case, artificially to meddle with nature* (ibid. p. 88). The BRANDRETH'S PILLS.

SHERWOOD, JOHN BURDETT, M. D., *On Dyspepsia. London*, 1847.

Unity of disease. 726. I am of opinion that the proximate cause of all diseases consists in *some alteration in the force, quantity, or quality of the circulating fluid ;* and that, of those affecting the general system, *vitiation of the blood* is an *invariable accompaniment* (Preface).

JOHNSON, EDWARD, M. D., *On Life, Health, and Disease. American Edition. New York*, 1850.

Purgation accelerates the change of matter. 727. *Purgation*, like exercise, accelerates what *Liebig* calls *the change of matter*—that is, the daily disorganization and reorganization of the elements of the blood and vital organs, by *more rapidly expelling* the old and worn out material *and supplying* its place with new (p. 96).

Old age the only legitimate cause of death. 728. There is but one legitimate cause of death, and that is old age. *If any man die while any of his organs is unimpaired, he dies prematurely*, and before he has fulfilled the final cause of his existence (p. 98).

Health and disease. All the legitimate effects of medicine attained by purgatives. 729. *The health* of the body depends upon the healthy performance of the nutritive actions, and *disease* consists in the unhealthy performance of these actions, or of one or more of them. *Medicines*, therefore, *have no real value nor power* over disease, *excepting as they have the power of increasing or diminishing the activity of the nutritive actions, absorption, secretion, circulation, &c.* (p. 88).

If from indigestion or overfeeding our food does not become blood, the system is filled with gases, etc. 730. We cannot derive any benefit from what we eat except from that portion of it which in due course becomes blood. *All* that we eat, therefore, *beyond what can be converted into blood*, is either changed into fat, or *is left in the stomach* and bowels *to run into fermentation*, serving no other purpose than to *distend these organs with* all sorts of *pernicious and offensive gases* (pp. 81, 82).

Imperfect digestion—(constipation)—how it impoverishes and poisons the blood. 731. The *result of improper digestion* is that the necessary change which should be wrought upon the food in order that it may nourish our bodies, is very imperfectly effected—*the chyme is of unsound quality.* The next result is this: the chyme, by admixture with certain other juices which it meets with in the bowels, is destined to become chyle. But the chyme being of vicious quality, *the chyle* which is formed from it *must also be vicious.* At all events it must be deficient in quantity; certainly *it is impossible* to suppose *that as much perfect chyle can be elaborated out of bad chyme as of good.* You might as well hope to *Good illustration.* make *as much good butter out of bad cream, or out of cream and water, as out of pure cream.* The chyle, therefore, is deficient in quantity; but this chyle is destined to become blood. The chyle, therefore, being deficient, the blood resulting from it must also be deficient (p. 125).

The blood the nutriment of the body. 732. *But the blood is in fact the real food on which the body feeds,* and this food being scantily supplied, the strength of course is ill-supported. But there is another mischievous result of this condition of the stomach and bowels, beyond that of unhealthy and deficient gastric juice. In that condition of the health which I am endeavoring to describe, the stomach and bowels actually secrete *air*. It is a thoroughly established fact that *air-wind—flatus*—is actually formed from the blood, and poured into the stomach and bowels by those arteries which ought to form only gastric juice. Now, *this wind* not only does no good in the stomach and bowels, but it does a vast deal of harm. For, besides the evil effects which it produces by its pernicious qualities, it *violently distends these organs*, stretching and separating, and thus greatly *weakening and destroying the firmness* and compactness *of their ultimate tissue* (pp. 125, 126).

Wind secreted, and its effects.

WEGG, WILLIAM, M. D., *Observations Relating to the Science and Art of Medicine. London*, 1851.

733. A highly important *action of medicines* upon the intestinal surface remains to be noticed, as affecting its excretory function. I do not mean the process which eliminates from the villous surface a fluid largely composed of water, containing the remains of the epithelium, &c., and which almost any irritating cause may excite, but the *excretory function of the glands which thickly stud the surfaces of the bowels, and especially those of the large intestines*. Although the lungs, liver, kidneys, and skin contribute largely to the depuration of the body, there is little doubt that these glands *contribute greatly to the same result*, very probably by expelling matter different from that which those other depurating organs eliminate (p. 213).

Purgative medicines—their action on the colon.

HASPEL, A., M. D., *Medical Staff of the Algerian Army. Maladies de l'Algérie. Paris*, 1852. *See* MED. CHIR. REV., *New Ser.*, 1852, *Vol. X*.

734. In this season of the year (*autumn in Algiers*) every individual seems to be endowed with an especial susceptibility to the development of typhoid symptoms, when he becomes the subject of *dysentery, intermittent or remittent fever*. But these *accessory phenomena*, the stupefied countenance, the restlessness, heat of the belly, &c., *quickly disappear, at the same time with the principal disease, under the influence of an evacuating plan of treatment*. We must *distrust* the fulness of pulse, the false plethora, which manifest themselves during the prevalence of the great heats, and which *seem to call for bleeding*. If we yield to this *perfidious indication*, we find our patients fall into a state of *adynamia*, without the dysentery undergoing any amendment; or, *if the abstraction of blood produce any relief, it is but temporary, to be speedily followed by a sensible aggravation of all the symptoms* (p. 58).

Malignant fevers abound.

Purgation the cure.

Bleeding kills.

735. Mr. Haspel refers to the advantages derivable from purgatives, recorded by the old writers, and considers that their disuse in recent times has arisen rather from the *prevalence of theoretical views* of the inflammatory nature of diseases than as a result of experience.

He speaks highly of *emetics at the very outset* of these diseases (pp. 9, 11, 39 ; Rev., pp. 106 sq.)

Theory and practice.

CARPENTER, C. WILLIAM B., M. D., *Principles of Human Physiology.*
London, 1853.

Pure blood resists all contagions. 736. I firmly believe that *if the blood of a person of sound constitution be kept in a state of perfect purity by* the moderate use of *wholesome food and drink*, by the respiration of *pure air*, by *adequate exercise* not pushed to over-fatigue, and by personal *cleanliness, he is as completely protected against* the invasion of *cholera* as he who has been effectually and recently vaccinated is proof against small-pox. . . *The same is true of all contagions and diseases*, and hence the *universal value of purgatives*, which quickly restore the above conditions, if any aberration has taken place (chap. IV.)

DICKSON, SAMUEL H., M. D., *Professor Med. College of South Carolina. Elements of Medicine. Philadelphia*, 1855.

The blood— how it becomes impure (passively diseased). 737. *The blood is often indirectly poisoned* by the influence of contingencies which *prevent* the *elimination* of such *effete matters* as must be got rid of to keep it in a normal condition. We have reason to infer the existence within it of injurious ingredients, whose presence we cannot demonstrate by the ultimate results. The blood may thus become, so to speak, passively diseased (p. 111).

Influenza and purgatives. 738. In the cure of *influenza, purgatives* aid in reducing to its proper level the vascular excitement; while we " derive" from the head and throat *by determining* to the gastric intestinal surface (p. 313).

The blood— in what way it becomes impure. 739. The blood is found altered in disease:
1. By a change in the proportion of its constituent elements;
2. By the addition of foreign matters (p. 111).

Demands careful attention.

What foreign matters chymists have found in the blood. 740. A great variety of *foreign matters* may be absorbed into, mixed with, and detected in the blood. *Kramer* found in it *silver*, after the nitrate and chlorate had been taken. *Œsterlein* discerned globules of *mercury* in it, as well as in the saliva and urine of persons who had been taking mercurials. *Heller* found *iodine* and *bromine* in the blood of patients to whom these remedies had been administered. *Nitrate, hydriodate, and carbonate of potass, antimony*, and *carbonate and sulphate of iron* have been found in similar circumstances. *Quinine* may be discovered in the *urine*, which it must reach *through the vessels;* and *lead* is shown in the *gums* and in the *brain* of those poisoned by that metal (p. 111).

CONSEQUENCES.

Other impurities. 741. The *foreign matters which*, as causes of diseases, *enter the blood*, are not always, however, to be thus exhibited by chemical tests and reagents; but their *presence can be inferred as indisputably* though less palpably. . . *Blood thus poisoned becomes in its turn poisonous.* The glands are irritated by it, and the secretions and excretions become morbid (p. 112).

742. The *sugar excites the kidney into diabetes*, the carbon and *urea* oppress the brain with *coma*. Its chemico-vital relation to the tissues undergoes essential changes, and *infiltration and exudation, congestion, dropsy*, and *hemorrhage* follow. It ceases to be nutritious, and *atrophy* and *marasmus* follow, or its nutrition is perverted and morbid, and we have *hypertrophy*, or *deposition of scrofulous, tubercular, typhus or cancerous matter* (ibid.)

Various forms of disease induced by impurities.

BENNETT, JOHN HENRY, M. D., *Editor of* EDINBURGH MEDICAL AND SURGICAL JOURNAL.

743. The *mortality from pneumonia* has *diminished* since large *bleedings* have been *abandoned*. (Present state of theory and practice of medicine. Journ., Vol. I., 1856, p. 19.)

Bleeding in pneumonia.

744. *Pericarditis.*—Some few years gone by, the practice was to meet the violence of the inflammation by the extremest antiphlogistic measures ; the lancet was plied with a most unsparing hand, and with the most unhesitating faith in the propriety of its use. But where are the believers in, or imitators of, such a practice now ? This " heroic and certain method," as it was called, of arresting the destructive agent—*of exterminating the disease*—has been convicted of error, and condemned by a late authority as "*uncertain and very dangerous.*" Again : "*after blood-letting*, rapid induction of the *mercurial influence* is of the greatest consequence," wrote an authority in a most unhesitating style some fifteen years ago. But now we find one of the most observing and practical physicians* among us admitting, that the firm faith which he himself once reposed in the efficacy of the remedy had been undermined by the truth-telling effects of further experience. In short, " the errors and absurdities," says Dr. Markham, " into which men have been led through this hastening to be wise—the fallacious and extraordinary proceedings in practice it has involved them in—he who is desirous of learning will find recorded on every page of the history of medicine. By thus casting dust in the eyes of others, and perverting our own wisdom, we raise up positive barriers to the advance of true knowledge ; for now the mist of delusion which our faulty haste has generated must be swept away before the honest face of the simple fact can be made available to light our slow steps along the difficult passes of new knowledge (Journ., vol. I., 1856, pp. 1038, 1039).

Pericarditis.

Bloodletting and mercury condemned.

745. The very discordant opinions which equally honest and equally skilled observers maintain—observers not living in separate ages, or in different countries, or in separate cities, but exercising their art upon the same disease, under the same roof, in the same public hospitals— must have a meaning. Is it not one which is oftener than we care for to confess, responded to by our consciences at the bedside of the patient ? (ibid., p. 1039).

Medical ignorance or prejudicial stubbornness.

* *W. O. Markham*, M. D., in his " Diseases of the Heart, their Pathology, Diagnosis, and Treatment." London, 1856.

Inflamma-tion :—nei-ther bleed-ing nor mer-cury cures. 746. None but men ignorant of pathology now talk of "knocking down" *inflammation with blood letting, or with mercury.* Indeed, why these remedies are employed at all, *has,* to use the word of *Dr. Mark-ham,* "*yet to be shown*" (ibid., p. 1042).

BENNETT, J. HUGHES, M. D., *Professor of Medicine in the University of Edinburgh. Observations on the Results of an Advanced Diag-nosis and Pathology, etc. Edinburgh,* 1856. *See* EDINB. MED. AND SURG. JOURN., *Vol. I.,* 1856.

Past expe-rience and theories—of no use in medical treatment by the faculty—begin "de novo." 747. *Medicine is not a scientific art,* which is *dependent* for its principles on the study of and commentary *on the older writers.* . . . On the contrary, *it is the book of nature, which is open to all,* that we ought to peruse and study; and why should we read it through the eyes of the sages of former times, when the light of science was comparatively feeble and imperfect? . . . *The lesson which a careful study of the history of medicine has forced upon me, is the necessity of reinvestigating,* with all our improved modern appliances, the correctness or incorrect-ness of *existing dogmas,* in order *to establish an improved practice for the future* (Propos. I.; Journ., p. 773).

Small-pox. The pustules —the matter of disease se-creted from the blood. Bloodletting is injurious. 748. *Dr. Wm. Addison* (Cell-therapeutics, 1856) correctly points out that in the distinctive *eruptive fevers,* such as *small-pox,* the numerous small *abscesses in the skin eliminate the morbid poison,* which formerly existed in the blood, and are in this way essential to the cure. This provident action he denominates "*Cell-therapeutics.*" In all such cases *experience has shown* that time and a natural sequence of changes is necessary for a restoration to health, and that the idea of cutting short such changes by *bleeding is alike erroneous in theory and injurious in practice* (Propos. III.; Journ., p. 777).

Bloodletting —the theory far more ap-plicable to purgation. 749. Large and early bleedings have been practiced under the idea that by diminishing the amount of the circulating fluid—
1. The *materies morbi in the blood* would be *diminished,*
2. *Less blood* would flow *into* the inflamed parts;
3. That the increased quantity of *blood in* the parts would be *les-sened;* and
4. That the character of *the pulse* was *the index* as to the amount of fluid that ought to be drawn (ibid.; Journ., p. 776).

Bleeding re-moves the good and allows the bad to re-main. 750. The careful investigations of chemists, and especially those of *Andral* and *Gavarret, Simon, Becqueril* and *Rodier,* and others, have further shown us, that whilst *venesections greatly deteriorate the blood, rendering it poorer in corpuscles and richer in water, they have no effect in eliminating morbid products,* and that in the vast majority of cases ELIMINATION IS IMPEDED BY BLOOD-LETTING (ibid.; Journ., p. 778).

Inflamma-tion;—the natural and the purga-tive cure the same. 751. *Inflammation* having occurred, the great work now to be accom-plished is to break up the exudation that has poured out, to *remove the pressure* it exerts *on the nerves and blood-vessels,* and *render the whole capable of being eliminated from the economy,* either directly, by dis-charge externally, or *indirectly, first, by passage into the blood, and secondly, by excretion through the emunctories* (ibid.; Journ., p. 779).

752. Now, it requires to be shown that draining the body of blood cannot in the slightest degree influence the congestion in the inflamed part. *There* the vessels are enlarged, the current of blood is arrested, the blood-corpuscles are closely aggregated together and distend the vascular tube, and are *in no way affected by the arterial current*, even when increased in its neighborhood. That opening a vein can alter *this* state of matters is scarcely to be conceived; and if it could, how would this assist in removing the exudation which has coagulated outside the vessels? (ibid.; Journ., p. 780.) *Inflammatory action described — bloodletting useless — Indication for purgatives.*

753. So far from getting rid of inflammation by weakening the pulse, we not only fail to do so, but *prolong* the time for the transformation of the exudation. This, indeed, is acknowledged by *Louis, Chomel and Grisolle,* who distinctly show that *the progress of a pneumonia is never shortened by bleeding* (ibid.; Journ., p. 781). *Bleeding prolongs disease.*

754. It is injurious to *diminish by bleeding the nutritive processes* themselves, when they are busily engaged in operating on the exudation, and eliminating the morbid products (ibid.; Journ., p. 781). *Bleeding retards recovery.*

755. The phenomena of *fever and excitability following inflammation,* have been wrongly interpreted. *In themselves they are sanative,* and indicate the struggle which the economy is engaged in, when attempting to get rid of the diseased processes; and we only *diminish the chances* of that struggle terminating favorably, by *lessening the vital powers* at such a critical juncture (ibid.; Journ., p. 782). *The crisis must not be interrupted by bleeding.*

756. Assuming it as granted that in some cases the pain is *for a time* relieving by bleeding, and that in *pneumonia* the respiration *temporarily* becomes more free—at what cost are these advantages obtained, should the patient be so weakened as to be unable to rally? Even if he does rally, a large *bleeding* almost *always prolongs the disease* (ibid.). *Bleeding a dangerous palliative which prolongs the disease.*

757. *Clinical Lectures on the Principles and Practice of Medicine. New York Ed.,* 1860. *Hepatization of the lungs.*

In all *hepatization,* the object of nature is *to reconvert the solid exudation* once again into fluid, whereby it can be *partly evacuated* from the bronchi, but principally *absorbed into the blood,* and *excreted from the economy.* Gradually the solid amorphous mass is converted into a fluid crowded with cells. This is *pus.* The cells, after passing through their natural life, die and break down, whereby the exudation is again reduced to a condition susceptible of absorption through the vascular walls, and once again mingles with the blood, but in an altered chemical condition. *After undergoing various changes in the blood, the exudation is finally removed from the economy* (pp. 265, 266). *The natural and the purgative cure the same.*

PICKFORD, J. H., M. D. *Hygiene. London,* 1858.

758. *Malaria* is modified by altitude. If the elevation be considerable, the temperature will necessarily restrict the fever to the intermit- *Dilute the impurity and*

you dilute the disease.

tent form; whilst *in the plain* beneath, the same noxious emanations would produce, *in tropical climates, remittent or yellow fever, plague or pestilential cholera* (§ 966, p. 172. Cf. Brown).

576,000 reations for purgation during epidemics, contagions, malarious influences, etc.

759. A healthy adult respires twenty times in a minute, and takes into his lungs, at each respiration, twenty cubic inches of air, or 576,000 cubic inches in twenty-four hours. This respired air comes into contact, at each inspiration, with 201,600 square inches of mucous surface of air-passages and cells. Is it, therefore, matter of surprise that *atmospheric air, contaminated* by infectious or contagious matter, or poisoned by malarious, miasmatic or paludal emanations, should exert its baneful *influence on the blood and on the organic nervous system*, through the nerves distributed to the enormous superficies with which it comes in contact at each inspiration? The wonder is, that any of us escape! (§ 932, p. 165.)

Insensible perspiration—its amount;—analogy with urine.

760. The sum of the *cutaneous and pulmonary secretions* amounts, according to the best authorities, to two pounds, eleven ounces, three drachms, and twelve grains in twenty-four hours. *The cutaneous exhalation is a true secretion from the blood*, somewhat analogous to that of the *urine*, of those matters which, at the temperature of the body, are capable of assuming the gaseous form, as carbonic acid and water (§§ 1101, 1102, p. 206).

HAZARD, THOMAS R., of Vaucluse, R. I. *Purgatives.*

761. Doctors' and undertakers' fees are so high that it is very inconvenient for persons of small means to be sick or die in these times. That most of the maladies that prevail in our climate may be prevented by proper care I have no doubt; and that most of the sicknesses that do occur may be cured at a trifling expense and loss of time, I am, after half a century's observation and experience, equally certain. I think men and women would now survive to the average age of seventy, instead of half that term of years, if they would live and practice in harmony with the laws of their being; which, like all Nature's works, are ever found to be as simple as they are grand, when understood.

762. Moses was inspired to utter a great truth when he declared that " *The life of the flesh is in the blood.*" Action is life; and the blood is the organ by which it is communicated to every member of the body. It follows that if the organ be out of tune, the music or harmony of life cannot be complete, however cunningly it may be piped upon. If there is discordancy in the instrument, it is not the fault of the law—which is ever perfect in itself—but it is the fault of man's animal propensities that transgress the law.

763. The blood that imparts life and nourishment to the system feeds upon the food we eat, the fluids we drink, and the air we breathe. To preserve its purity we should eat to live, rather than live to eat. Eat slowly, chew the food well, drink sparingly, even of water, and be temperate in all things, and one half of the primary causes of disease

will be removed. Hilarity and cheerful conversation whilst at the table greatly assists digestion. A hearty, prolonged, explosive laugh will well nigh split a pine-knot on its passage to the stomach.

See to it, as far as is practicable, that you breathe uncontaminated air; for every breath we draw comes in contact with the blood, and imparts to it its own quality, whether it be the savour of life to life or of death to death. Look especially to your sleeping-rooms that they are daily (and if small nightly) ventilated. Avoid beds, and particularly pillows, that are filled with blood-shotten feathers. Keep the pores of the body open and clean by frequent bathing, for each of these are pipes that gives tone to life's *organ*. Above all things look to it that there is no decaying vegetable matter of any kind near or under your sleeping apartments, for probably more sickness occurs from this cause than any one other. If at any time you begin to feel dull and heavy and *good for nothing*—if you lose animation, and your flesh feels numb and sore; if your mouth grows *clammy*, and your tongue *furs;* if your eyes feel as if they had *sticks* in them, or your head, or side, or back begins to ache, or old sores and weak points of the system *grumble;* if you snuffle, or your voice grows husky, accompanied with a hacking as if to clear the throat—lose no time in ascertaining and removing the local cause, if possible, before you are stricken down by disease. Proceed first to your cellar, especially if you sleep on the ground-floor. Examine it well in every nook and corner. You may, in your researches through its dark labyrinths, perchance stumble upon a dead cat, and perhaps some festering rats ; but heed them not. Their aroma is not pleasant, but it is not deadly poisonous; but, if you should fall in with a rotten turnip or potato, or cabbage, or any other decomposing vegetable, eject it at once a stone's-throw from your house, with every vestige of its remains, even to the earth it has impregnated ; for the miasma that arises from a peck of decomposing vegetables of any kind, if inhaled into the lungs, and consequently blood, especially during sleep, is sufficient, with the aid of the lancet or of a little morphine, to kill a regiment of hardy men, and the stronger and more robust they are the more certain will be their doom. I have myself known, many years since when the lancet was in vogue, scores of hardy young men and women perish under such circumstances in a single country town of this State, whose lives might have been easily saved, I am entirely confident, under a different mode of treatment. I have now in my recollection a certain Doctor Sangrado, who then practiced in that town, of whom it might with truth be said "Death followed after him." He seldom entered a family at the season of year when these morbid attacks were most rife, without sending one, two, or three, and even five in one instance, to their graves. Weakly patients, whose strength of constitution was not competent to carry any considerable portion of morbid matter in their blood before it gave way, stood some chance of life under the bleeding treatment of that day, but those of strong constitutions stood but little. These, when attacked, generally kept about until their blood became so thick and sluggish that it coursed with difficulty through the thousands of little ducts and vessels that carry life to the surface and extremities of the body, and were unconscious of their danger until the morbid matter in the blood— precipitated perhaps by the scratch of a briar or pin, or a draft of cold air or other trifling exposure—began to *clot* or congest in the intricate recesses of the brain, the liver, the pleura, or some other weak or delicate point, accompanied, of course, with pain or distress. Dr. Sangrado was then called, who proceeded at once to draw a heavy portion of the best blood from the system in order to relieve the suffering; and, having thus paralyzed the vital forces, they were next stimulated by a dose of mercury and expected to perform double duty, with their instrument (the blood) just crippled by the lancet. In other words, the horse that was striving, with all his might, to extricate a heavy load from the mire was first knocked on the head to prevent his injuring the wagon by his efforts, and then a shoulder was placed to the wheel in the vain expectation that the additional stimulus would enable the dying steed to drag it through the mud. The loss of the best blood the system could afford neutralized the otherwise good effect of the mercury, gave momentary relief to the patient just so far as life had been obstructed, relaxed the efforts that Nature was making to dispel the poisonous miasma from the blood which, in its weakened flow, went on congesting or clotting with accelerated speed. The pain or distress soon returned, and again the lancet was resorted to, alternately with doses of calomel, until the patient's whole body, deprived of its life-principle, became a mass of inert and putrid matter; and "Died of typhus fever" was generally the verdict of Death's coroner.

764. The practice of blood-letting has been, finally, pretty much abandoned, and one less revolting, but little less fatal in its operation, has been substituted by many physicians in its place, viz.: that of relieving effects at the expense of aggravating the cause by the use of opium. Instead of knocking the horse on the head under the circumstances before narrated, his efforts are paralyzed before the shoulder is put to the wheel by dosing him with poison.

765. To illustrate by another homely comparison: If a piece of cloth be run through water saturated with fustic, logwood, or other dye-wood, it will come out stained or colored. Rinse this in a brook, and the coloring-matter will quickly disappear; but drop a small lump of alum, vitriol, or other mordant in the dye-vat before the cloth is passed through it, and all the water of the lakes will not suffice to wash it white again. So, when the blood, by neglect, exposure, or abuse, has become surcharged with unhealthy matter, sufficient to interrupt its healthy flow, and begins to clot or congest, a little stimulus applied in the same direction *that the law of our nature is already striving to impel the vital forces*, will enable them to dislodge the congestion and expel the morbid matter from the blood. But introduce an opium pill or the smallest portion of morphine into the blood, and all the mercury or other cleansing stimulants on earth will scarcely purge it clean.

766. A bullock's hide once accidentally lodged on a shoal (weak point) in the River Tiber—the great artery of Rome. Against this the impurities and drifts of the river gradually *congested*, until it became a ast-anchored island. When first deposited it is probable a housewife

might, with a mere swash of her broom in the direction of the current, have so far stimulated its force as to have removed the hide (congestion) and prevented the formation of the island.

767. Before applying such a *mercurial* remedy, to be consistent with his practice as applied to the cleansing the channels of the blood, Dr. Sangrado would have first withdrawn from the Tiber sufficient water to have left the bullock's hide high and dry in the sand, and then set the woman to work with her broom; whilst Dr. *Morphina* should have advised that the swashing process should be deferred until the waters of the river were congealed by frost, or thickened by some ingenious process to the like consistency imparted to the blood by opium or other narcotics.

768. What I have said so far is mostly *theory*, which readers will, of course, estimate at what it is worth. What I am now about to say is *fact*, derived from more than thirty years' observation and experience applied to multitudes of cases with, as far as I am advised, uniform success, including bilious colic, bilious fevers, and all that class of maladies that, under the ordinary medical treatment, end in slow fevers called in the books Typhus or Typhoid, Pleurisy, common colds and sore-throat, Indigestion, and its first-born child Headache, Croup (if applied in an early stage), Dysentery, Diarrhœa, Fever Sores, and running sores generally (the fountain of which is ever the blood), cuts and bruises of the flesh (if applied immediately after the accident occurs), and, in fact, almost every acute ailment common to our climate, that commences with pain in the head, body, or limbs, or at the commencement of which the patient remarks, in a languid tone, " *I don't feel well*," with the exception, perhaps, of scarlet and lung fevers, which the remedy I shall describe greatly benefits, and lays the foundation for a certain cure, as far as my limited experience in these complaints extends, by applying additional simple treatment, viz., *packing* in the former, and certain vegetable cordials or decoctions in the latter complaint.

769. At a period when the reputation of the *blood-letting physician* I have referred to was at its height (and it was great in proportion to the scores of his victims that died, those that recovered being held in popular estimation that his skill had miraculously rescued from an otherwise mortal distemper), a hired girl living in my father's family was smitten with the usual symptoms of the prevailing malady, and Doctor Sangrado was sent for. He told my father that the girl's case was exceedingly dubious, that her organization was unfavorable, and that he had but little hopes of her recovery; still he would do all that medical skill could do to save her life. My father was opposed to blood-letting, and the doctor deferred the use of the lancet until the next day. In the meantime my father gave the girl a dose of what was then known as *Aldrich's Pills*, accompanied with a sweat. The next afternoon the doctor called again, and, after sitting a little while, inquired after the girl's health. My father told him what had been done, and that she was then apparently well and at work in the kitchen. Upon this announcement the doctor mused a few moments, and after remarking in a soliloquizing tone that " those pills are devilish things," he took up his

saddle-bags, lancet, blue pills (sure to be followed by rheumatism), opium, mercury, blisters and all, and departed, *"never to return."*

770. About this period manufacturers in the town alluded to, of which I was one, were seriously incommoded by the annual prevalence of the complaint, dubbed by Sangrado as typhus, but popularly known as *fall fever*. Business was sometimes brought nearly to a stand-still from the number of hands that were taken out of employ in consequence of long, and, in very many cases, fatal sickness. A young man or woman would leave the mill, complaining, perhaps, of a pain in the head, neck, shoulders, back, or side, or difficulty in breathing, send for Doctor Sangrado, experience momentary relief from the free use of the lancet, and, in consequence, be prostrated on a bed of languishing for· weeks or months, and probably die. I was fully satisfied, in my own mind, that both the sicknesses and deaths were, in a great majority of cases, the result of improper treatment, rather than the normal character of the malady, and greatly to the disgust of Dr. Sangrado, gave free and wide utterance to my convictions. I finally resolved to practice medicine myself, so far as I could obtain patients, from among those in my immediate neighborhood and employ, gratis ; and from that day to this, a period of more than thirty years, out of many hundreds of cases of almost every type of disease, I have never known a death to occur among those who have relied solely on the simple remedies I have furnished, nor have I known of a serious case among them all of *Dysentery*, *Pleurisy*, *Typhus* or *Typhoid*, *Brain*, *Congestive*, *Bilious*, or any other fever, except scarlet or lung fevers, of which last, as before said, my experience has been slight, and confined to my own family, in which there has been five cases of scarlet fever ; one of which was treated by two of the most renowned physicians in New York, and died in great apparent agony on the seventh day. Two of the other cases were equally severe, but all recovered without the interference or aid of the faculty.

771. For some time I relied on the "devilish pills" only in light attacks, and gave from 12 to 15 grains of calomel, with a good sweat in severe cases. I generally attended to the sweating process (which I shall hereafter describe) myself; and never, to my recollection, failed to obtain the desired sweat. The mercury stimulated the interior powers of the system, whereby the morbid matter is (as I suppose) forced from the blood into the bowels, and thus passes off; whilst the sweat, operating on the external pores of the body, in like manner as the stimulating mercury acts on the internal pores or ducts, the two forces sympathize and assist each other ; and the congestion and other causes of disease (unless it has become chronic) are wholly expelled at one operation, leaving the system as free from poisonous or unhealthy matter as is that of a new-born babe.

772. It is now nearly thirty years since I *entirely* abandoned the use of calomel, for which I substituted "*Brandreth's Pills*," which I have found, after long and varied experience, produce all the good effects of mercury, with none of its bad. Too much care cannot, however, be observed in obtaining them, as a large proportion of the *pills* sold in New

England are spurious, notwithstanding their close resemblance to the genuine and the *oaths* of the unprincipled men who vend them. To make sure of the genuine, I always obtain them from Dr. Benjamin Brandreth's own office, which is at the " corner of Broadway and Canal Street, New York," and who sends them to order, free of charge for express, for two dollars per dozen boxes. One or two boxes (or not over twenty-five cents' worth) sufficing generally to keep a family of ordinary size in Health for a year.

773. Thus any man, by an expenditure of two dollars, may keep his own family, and those of some five or six of his neighbors, in health for a year, and that with very little if any loss of time, and not a farthing's expense for medical aid. This, as a general rule, I pledge my word I know to be true by actual practice and observation—although I suppose it will not be so regarded by most readers. These pills are as efficacious in cases of hurts, bruises, cuts, sores, &c., as in other maladies. By immediately cleansing the blood they remove all danger of lock-jaw, festering sores, or congestion of the blood, at the wounded or ailing points— and nature speedily restores the injured parts. Not unfrequently, from the use of opium in some of its varied forms, or other malpractice, the morbid matter in the blood seeks to escape through vents called fever-sores. I have known instances of this kind wherein, after the patient has been in acute pains for weeks, a few doses of Brandreth's Pills have turned this current of morbid matter from the sores to the bowels, through which it has been passed off, and the patient healed almost at once. But I do not mean to be understood to say that this is the rule; as when the system has been surcharged and weakened by poisonous and stupefying drugs, nature's vital forces cannot always be rallied by any treatment that I am acquainted with.

774. I will close this long (and, as doctors will doubtlessly say, absurd and foolish) article, with a simple recipe, which, if adhered to in all its *requirements*, I know will heal at one operation a great majority of the ills we are liable to in this country, and I believe in all other countries.

775. I know that it has been used with entire effect in cases of yellow fevers; and I now have in my possession a certificate, signed by every member of a company who were nine months in the Army of the Potomac, at a time when thousands were dying around them with small-pox, and swamp fevers, and dysentery—the health of every one of whom (without an exception) was preserved, without the aid of a physician, simply by relying solely on " Brandreth's Pills," a quantity of which had been presented to the Company, with directions for using them, by their fellow-townsman, Dr. Benjamin Brandreth.

RECIPE.

776. In cases of slight hurts, cuts, bruises, punctures, &c., or slight indisposition, take from one to six BRANDRETH's PILLS, according to age and constitution; say one pill for a child one year old, two for a child of three years old, and four or more for adults.

777. Where any malady has made such progress as to cause difficulty of breathing, oppression, or severe pain in any part of the body, head or limbs, place the feet of the patient in water as hot as it can by *any pos-sibility* be borne, and throw a blanket over the knees to keep in the steam. Do not let the feet remain in the bath *to exceed* four minutes. Wipe the feet dry as quickly as possible, and rub them hard with a dry towel. Then get at once to bed, and take from one to six pills as above. (In cases of intense bilious colic or pleurisy, give six, eight, or even more, until relief is obtained, but by no means attempt to remove the pain at the expense of the life by blood-letting or narcotics.) After swallowing the pills, drink a glass of weak lemonade (or molasses and water, if lemonade is not to be had) made almost boiling, and so hot that it can *only be taken in sips;* then cover warm and a sweat will shortly ensue. This treatment will set all the vital forces of life to work, both internal and external, and not only remove the effects but the cause of the distemper, as the most ignorant cannot fail to perceive, not only by the relief that will be experienced, but from the offensive character of the matter that passes from the bowels, a large portion of which proceeds from the blood, liver, or other vital intestines. Water-gruel alone should be taken for eighteen hours after taking the pills, after which, as far as my experience has extended, patients, as a general rule, will be restored to complete health, and in a situation to eat and exercise as usual, with-out danger of relapse, for the simple reason that the blood, the seat and organ of life, is freed from all impurities, and consequently there is nothing in the system to cause a relapse; nor can sickness again ensue until the blood again becomes surcharged with extraneous and morbid matter.

778. Some readers may possibly suppose that, in accordance with *general usage*, I may have some interest other than that of a desire for the good of others in recommending "Brandreth's Pills" (which, by the by, are *always* inclosed in a certificate and directions folded around each separate box, with a *government stamp on the envelope*). For the benefit of such readers I will just say, that I have never received from Dr. Brandreth or any other person a farthing for anything done by me in relation to his pills; that I have always paid full price for every box I have had; that I have never received a farthing for any disposition I have made of them, although I have probably administered and given away hundreds of boxes—that I esteem a judicious distribution of them in a charitable point of view as of more value than an hundred-fold of the same value bestowed in money; that in case of leaving my family for any considerable season, I should do it with an easier mind if satis-fied that they would on any and all occasions—of accident or disease—resort to the foregoing prescription for cure, than I should were they left in a position to command the best medical advice (apart therefrom) in the world; and this assurance has been derived from a long and varied experience, that has fully satisfied me that there is no necessity that one life should be lost in New England, where there is now ten by what is called Typhus or Typhoid Fever—which, in fact, as a general rule, is but the ebbing away with a slow fever of the life from the blood in conse-quence of the impurities it is forced to consort with, first engendered by breathing foul air, gluttonous and hasty feeding, and other causes and

exposures, and subsequently aggravated by the malpractices of physicians—among the most prominent of which was the former practice of bleeding and parching to death with thirst, which practices were only abandoned by the faculty in consequence of an outside popular pressure, since which morphines and other narcotics have been substituted for the lancet with almost equal fatal effect, and which will be doubtlessly persevered in so long as ignorant patients measure the doctor's skill by his ability to relieve effects at the expense of aggravating the disease, instead of working them off by removing their cause.

APPENDIX.

CURES BY PURGATION.

Cure of Abram Van Wart, of Sing Sing, of Bright's Disease of the Kidneys.

SING SING, Oct. 14th, 1863.

DR. BRANDRETH,

My Dear Sir: I was taken sick two years ago with a most severe pain in my right arm and elbow. Dr. A. K. Hoffman, of this place, pronounced it neuralgia. He treated me for some time, but getting no better, advised electricity; I consented, but the shock nearly killed me, and I received no benefit whatever. After this my legs became numb and paralyzed, and my back and kidneys were tormented with most intense and continued pain. Dr. A. K. Hoffman and other physicians told me I had Bright's Disease of the Kidneys. They treated me for a long time, but finally pronounced my case hopeless. Other eminent physicians then treated me but did me no good, and gave my friends to understand that my case was incurable. So, at length, I gave up all hope, the lower half of my body being totally paralyzed and much swollen; and I suffered terrible pain in the upper part of my body. My bowels were completely constipated from the paralysis, and no medicine produced a passage, and my urine was full of albumen. This was my condition five months ago, when my wife's sister, Sally Ann Storms, begged me to take BRANDRETH'S PILLS, as she had used them herself and in her family for many years with the best effect. Induced by her and my wife, I swallowed nine Brandreth's Pills. They operated twelve hours afterward, slightly. I continued taking nine every day for several weeks, their operation constantly improving. Finding myself a great deal better, I diminished the dose one pill a day, until I got to five. One afternoon, at 3 o'clock, about three months ago, I took five pills; at 9 they commenced operating vigorously; suddenly I felt as if something gave way inside, and the stools were like egg and water mixed, several quarts of which came away, of a most disagreeable odor. The next day I felt very faint, and my neighbors came to see me die; but as soon as the faintness passed I was much better, and, for the first time in nearly two years, I was able to move and stand upon my legs. I continued taking the pills, and, in a very few days, was able to walk across my room, and now am able to walk quite a distance. I have taken altogether nineteen boxes of BRANDRETH'S PILLS, and now one pill a day is all I require. My health is nearly restored, my appetite is good, and I suffer hardly any pain anywhere, and every day I grow stronger. My neighbors look upon me as one risen almost from the dead, and I desire you to publish my case, that those suffering from paralysis and kidney diseases may know how easily they may be cured by Brandreth's Pills.

ABRAM VAN WART.

We, neighbors and relatives, certify that the foregoing statement of ADRAM VAN WART is true.

A. B. REYNOLDS, *Supervisor of the Town of Ossining.*
DAVID McCORD, *Ex-Loan Commissioner.*
J. MALCOLM SMITH, *Justice and Clerk Board of Supervisors.*
ABRAM HYATT, *United States Assessor, Tenth District.*
JAMES McCORD, *Loan Commissioner.*
RACHEL CYPHER,   RACHEL ANN SLATER,
WILBUR F. FOSHAY,   LETITIA VAN WART,
SARAH A. CYPHER,   WM. SNIFFIN.

The Methodist Society have heard the above facts stated in meeting from the mouth of Mr. Van Wart.

Mr. JOHN ARCHER, Ticket Agent at the Hudson River Railroad Station at Sing Sing, permits reference, he being fully acquainted with Mr. Van Wart and all particulars.

In Epilepsy Brandreth's Pills Seldom Fail

to cure, because they purify the blood. If we are sick from any cause we owe it to ourselves to use this remedy which Providence places within the reach of all.

NEW YORK, July 8, 1861.

DR. BRANDRETH,

Sir : A boy of mine was subject to fits from his infancy—his case was considered hopeless by the doctors, who thought he would be subject to them for life. After they had given him up, I was recommended to try your Pills, and without much faith did try them, using them according to your printed directions. Four years ago I commenced giving them to him, and to my great joy and relief he has had but ONE RETURN ONLY of his affliction since. I consider him now perfectly cured.

The extraordinary benefit they did him makes me always recommend them to my friends, and I would be glad if everybody knew their value. The cause was the worst possible; he would have been helpless and almost uselessly unfit for any kind of business from the length and severity of each attack—often lasting a whole night, and leaving him, for two or three days afterwards, entirely prostrate from weakness. Every kind of treatment was also externally applied that was professionally advised. You may, therefore, judge what good reason I have for letting you have this statement in acknowledgment for the benefit received, and for the purpose of letting those who may be hesitating under similar circumstances have my testimony in confirmation of the reliability of the other certificates, and perfect confidence like myself in the value of the Pills.

Yours respectfully,
JOHN WEBB,
18 *Beekman Street.*

Letter from General Paez, the Washington of Venezuela,

in favor of Brandreth's Pills.

NEW YORK, May 30, 1865.

Hon. B. BRANDRETH,

My Dear Sir : I have received the supply of your invaluable Pills which you have so kindly sent me. I have not only used them myself in South America, as well as in this country, for the last thirty years, never allowing myself to be without them, but have purchased them by the gross to distribute to persons upon my estates and· elsewhere, having found them efficacious in almost every variety of disease, especially those peculiar to the Southern continent. I esteem, therefore, very highly the supply you now send me, and thank you very cordially for the kind words in which you convey your generous and friendly sentiments.

I am, very respectfully, your obedient servant,

JOSE A. PAEZ.

Debility and· Costiveness Cured.

This certifies that I have used Benjamin Brandreth's Vegetable Universal Pills more than three years, and I do affirm that having used a great deal of medicine of various kinds I have found none so beneficial to my health as the above-mentioned pills.

I have been unhealthy from a child, and have had the advice and attention of the most eminent physicians, who did for awhile alleviate my sufferings, but at last their skill proved unsuccessful, and I was sinking into rapid decay, given up by my physicians, and bending over the tomb without a jot of a prospect for recovering. While in that condition a friend recommended Brandreth's Pills to me. I sent immediately and got a box, and the first dose gave me so much relief that I repeated it, and after several doses, finding my health improving, I continued to take them two or three times a week for twelve months. At the expiration of six months I thought that my health was perfectly restored, but still my bowels were irregular and dormant, so I' continued to take them as before, until the expiration of six months more, when I found, by gradually quitting, I did not need them more than once a month ; and since I betook myself to the use of Dr. Brandreth's Pills, I have had no need of a physician, except in two cases, both of which needed skill more than medicine.

During the first year after I commenced using these Pills I was very cautious both in the quality and quantity of my diet, but since that time I have generally eaten what was set before me. The Pills are the mildest in their operation of any medicine that I have ever taken ; they also produce the most powerful and free discharges of any medicine that I have ever used. And I speak from experience, that continued use will not render them ineffectual in their operation. If I take a dose and they do not operate, I continue to take them, increasing the number of Pills in each dose, until powerful discharges ensue without any pain, and in a few hours I feel perfectly well and able to attend to business.

Having derived so much benefit from the use of Brandreth's Pills, I would recommend them to all who are sick, whatever may be their diseases or complaint ; for it is manifest that nothing is more important in any case of illness than to keep the bowels regular, and it is also evident, in my own opinion, that no better medicine than Brandreth's Pills can be obtained to keep the system in a healthy condition.

R. DUNN,

No. 22 Third Street, Cincinnati.

JUNE 1, 1860.

Remittent Fever, of the Island of St. Thomas, Cured by Brandreth's Pills.

NEW YORK, May 31, 1856.

Dr. BENJAMIN BRANDRETH,

Dear Sir: It seems to me to be a duty to say that, when I was United States Consul at St. Thomas, in 1849, I used your Pills with very great advantage. I was taken with the fever peculiar to that island; the doctor bled me, and I was in very great danger of dying from that fever and the depleting. The inward fever was so great that no quantity of drinks seemed to relieve it. I was considered in very great danger, and I felt that my hold of life was really very feeble. In this condition I was recommended to use your pills. I at once took eight. Their effect was surprising. They seemed to be actuated by intelligence. I could feel them searching all round my stomach, even up to my throat; every recess of the body was aroused to action. I continued to use them daily until I had taken two boxes, containing twenty-five pills each, when I was quite recovered to my usual health.

Governor Oxholm expressed to me the opinion that the Brandreth Pills were the best medicine he had ever known; that he entirely relied upon them when he or his family were sick. He would not be without them for any money; that he believed you had been the means, by introducing them, of saving many valuable lives—a sentiment in which I concur most cordially. I desire, my dear Doctor, if you deem the above of any service, you will not be afraid to publish it.

I am, very truly, your friend,

· CHARLES H. DELAVAN,

Late United States Consul for the Island of St. Thomas, West Indies.

Cure of Dyspepsia of Ten Years' Standing   by Brandreth's Pills.

BUSHWICK, Kings Co., L. I., March 1, 1843.

This is to certify that I was taken ill during the season of the cholera, in the year 1832, and continued ailing until the spring of 1842, during which time I was severely troubled with dyspepsia, and all its various train of suffering. I became extremely emaciated, melancholy, and worn out with suffering, so that life itself seemed burdensome. I, in the meantime, applied to a number of the best physicians, who prescribed for me; and many were the bitter doses of medicine that I took, but without avail. At last I yielded to despair. The idea of taking the prescriptions of physicians any longer was useless, and I was bitterly opposed to taking pills. My friends became alarmed; often solicited me to try Brandreth's Pills, asserting that they had derived great benefits from their use. At last I was tempted to give them a trial, and it is but just to say that, after using them a short time, I began to recover, and soon was entirely restored to health: and I think it a duty I owe to the world, and to Doctor Brandreth, to make this public acknowledgment.

N. BLISS.

Mr. Bliss will be pleased to testify as to the merits of Brandreth's Pills, after an acquaintance with them of twenty-three years.

July, 1866.   B. B.

Cure of Consumption and Dyspepsia.

"HAMMONTON, New Jersey, May 7th, 1866.

" DR. BRANDRETH,

" *Dear Sir :* I have long wanted to write to you and express my gratitude for the beneficial effects that have been experienced in my own family, and in hundreds, aye, thousands of others, by the use of Brandreth's Pills. The first year my lamented friend Brockway sold your pills in Boston (1838) I called at his office. I was then in a declining state of health, and my friends, as well as myself, supposed my earthly voyage would soon terminate. Mr. Brockway urged me to take the Brandreth Pills, but having used so much medicine, with no good effect, I was more inclined to let nature take its course, and calmly submit to my fate. Mr. B. offered to give me one dozen boxes if I would try them as prescribed. By this I saw he had great faith in them, and I finally consented to take them, but not as a gift. I went home and went at it, almost hopelessly. After taking one box I began to feel better. Well, sir, when I had used up my twelve boxes, I was apparently a well, healthy man, my weight having gone from 131 pounds up to 152 pounds. I then ordered a supply, and between that time and the present I have retailed three thousand dollars worth of these invaluable pills, and am quite sure that I have thereby been instrumental in saving, not hundreds, but thousands of lives. I have given them to my oxen, horses, pigs, fowls, cats, dogs, and always with the desired effect. I have a wife and nine children, most of them born since I have used the pills. A more healthy family cannot be found. We are frequently asked how it is our children look so healthy. My wife replies that ' We raise them on Brandreth's Pills.' Now, my children overload their stomachs, get cold and out of order, like others, but they have been taught the remedy, and go and take the pills of their own accord. This I consider an important branch of their education, and feel assured, as they shove off upon the voyage of life, that they know how to take care of themselves. I was in trade at my last residence, North Lincoln, Me., for 29 years. I have been here about seven years ; I am, therefore, well known, and my statements can be verified by hundreds.

" Yours.

" C. J. FAY, P. M."

Certificate of Twenty-eight Years' Use.

NEWCASTLE, Westchester Co., N. Y., Aug. 11, 1861.

DR. B. BRANDRETH,

My Dear Sir : I am now seventy-nine years old, and for the last twenty-eight years have been a constant user of your Vegetable Universal Pills when sick, fully realizing the advantage of enforcing purgation with a medicine, which, while harmless in its nature, removes all impurities. I can safely say that the vigorous old age I now enjoy has been caused mainly by the timely use of Brandreth's Pills. I have had, in these last twenty-eight years, several fits of sickness, and occasionally some infirmity of age would press upon me. At these times I have always found your Pills a sure remedy, giving me not only health but strength. I consider them, therefore, invaluable as a tonic, with qualities possessed by no other medicine known to me. I have never, during these last twenty-eight years, used any other medicine whatever, being convinced, by experience, that none was as good. Brandreth's Pills have also been freely used by my neighbors in every kind of sickness, and have never been known to fail when promptly administered.

Yours truly,

NATHANIEL HYATT,

Justice of the Peace for Forty Years in Westchester County, N. Y.

A Man Saves His Leg.

SING SING, Westchester Co., N. Y., Aug. 24, 1860.
DR. B. BRANDRETH,

Dear Sir : Some years since a bad swelling appeared on my knee, and several physicians attended me. I kept growing worse and worse, until I was confined to my bed, a helpless cripple. Large quantities of matter kept coming from my leg, from six deep holes, together with pieces of bone. I lay in bed over one year, when the doctor came to me and said I had a very bad white swelling, and that the leg must be cut off or I would die. They wanted to cut it off then, and had brought all their instruments. I said, "No; I would die first." So they left me. Despairing of cure, I took your pills. I began with four a day, and took them every day for a month, when my knee appeared a little better. This encouraged me, and though still in bed, I continued taking your pills for four months more. I was now able to get up and go about a little with a crutch. I used the pills for three months more, when the sores all healed, and pain ceased, and I was well. I threw away my crutch, and now for the last four years I have been a well and healthy man, my leg being strong and my body sound. Words fail to express my gratitude to you.

Yours truly,
RICHARD T. BAKER.

Westchester County, ss. :
Richard T. Baker, being duly sworn, says, that the foregoing statement of his cure by Brandreth's Pills is true in every particular.
RICHARD T. BAKER.

Sworn before me, this 24th }
day of August, 1860.   }
A. JACKSON HYATT,
Justice of the Peace.

Dyspepsia Cured.

"BENNINGTON, Vt., Dec. 5th, 1843.
" *Dear Sir :* I wish you to add my testimony to the host of others that you have in favor of your valuable pills. In the year 1838, I was attacked with that disagreeable complaint, the DYSPEPSIA, which so affected me that I could not take the least particle of food without the most unpleasant and uncomfortable sensations in my chest, head, and bowels. My chest was so sore that I could not bear the slightest pressure without giving me pain. My health was most miserable ; many physicians told me they thought I was in the consumption, and that if I did not give up my business, and change climate, I could live but a short time.

" I tried everything in the shape of medicine, and consulted the most skillful physicians, but found no permanent relief. I became discouraged, gloomy, sad, and sick of life ; and probably, ere this, should have been in my grave, had I not fell in with your precious medicine. A friend of mine, who had been sick of the same complaint, advised me to try your pills : but, having tried most other medicines without obtaining any relief, I had but little faith that your pills would be of benefit to me ; but at his earnest solicitation, I procured a box and commenced taking them.

" The first box produced little or no effect, and I began to despond, for fear that your medicine would prove like others that I had taken; but my friends urged that one was not a fair trial, and I purchased a second, and before I had taken the whole box I began to experience a change; the pain in my chest began to be less painful, and my food did not distress me as much as formerly. I went on taking them until I had taken six boxes, and my DYSPEPSIA WAS GONE, and my expectation of an early DEATH VANISHED, and I felt like a 'NEW CREATURE.' I was then, and am now, a healthy man; I have never since been troubled with Dyspepsia. I have administered your pills to the members of my family, and to my friends, and in all cases with good success. You can publish this if it will be of any use to you.

"I am, dear sir, truly yours,

"J. L. COOK,
"Publisher of the State Banner."

Remarkable Case in which Fifty-two Pills were Used before the Bowels were Opened.

John Pickett, living at 553 First Avenue, New York, aged 27, of robust constitution, from a severe wrench was laid up. His back pained him as if the muscles were torn. His bowels, kidneys, and bladder seemed paralyzed. For seven days nothing passed his bowels, spite of all the remedies administered by his three doctors, who told his wife they could do no more, and he would die. She was advised, as a last effort to save him, to give him Brandreth's Pills. So she procured a box, and gave him four pills every four hours. She rubbed the pills down to powder under a knife on a plate, and then mixed with molasses. She continued this treatment until she had administered *fifty-two* pills, when they operated, and the man's life was saved.

Observation Particular in respect to above Case.

It is right here to call attention to the fact that while, in the first instance, this great quantity of Brandreth's Pills were required to produce a thorough cleansing of this man's

PARALYZED BOWELS,

two pills every day thereafter were all-sufficient to keep them open until his health was established.

Thus we see how important a medicine Brandreth's Pills are; suitable for the most trying emergencies of bodily affliction, as for the most simple disorder. Always safe yet always sure.

They are indeed a century in advance of all other purgatives.

Fever and Ague Cured.

Mr. John Y. Haight, Supervisor of New Castle, Westchester County, New York, desires the attention of those interested. He says: "I was, about two years ago, attacked with fever and ague, which, notwithstanding the best medical advice, continued to sorely afflict me for six tedious months; I became yellow as saffron, and reduced to skin and bone. Medicine and physicians were abandoned in despair. As an experiment, I concluded to try a single dose of six of Brandreth's Universal Vegetable Pills on an empty stomach, early in the morning. The first dose seemed to arouse all the latent energies of my exhausted frame. Their purgative effect was different from anything I had ever used or heard of. At length this effect ceased, and I seemed lighter and breathed freer. That evening I was indeed sensibly better and slept soundly all night. The next day I followed the same course and took the same number of pills. I continued to take the pills in this way about three weeks, when I found myself entirely cured. It was two years ago, and I have had no return. My health has been surprisingly good, and I have used no medicine since.

Mr. Carpenter, of Gouverneur, New York, sixty-four years of age, says he has used Brandreth's pills for thirty-four years; administered them first to his coachman, who had Fever and Ague; gave eight the day after the chill; chill and fever less severe; gave eight more the next day, and so every other day, until the chill and fever did not return, which was in about eight days from the first attack. He then gave four every other day another week, when the man was entirely restored to his usual good health.

He was himself attacked, took them in the same way, and was cured in less time; has used no other medicine for thirty-four years; found them always every way reliable for himself and for his family when sick; has recommended them to thousands with the best results; feels confident that every family would have a larger average of health if these pills were used in the place of calomel and other hurtful remedies.

The following is an extract of a letter from Hon. CALEB LYON, of Lyonsdale, now Governor Lyon of Idaho, to Dr. Brandreth:

"My sincere thanks are due you for the boxes of Brandreth's Pills that you were so kind as to send me previous to my departure for the East; and a more efficient medicine as a preventive of disease upon the miasmatic shores of the Danube, or the plague-stricken cities of Egypt and Asia Minor, I do not believe was ever used. My whole party took them freely, and while others were ill and delayed, we kept well. Enclosed you will find the translation of a letter from Achmet Hallilla, an Arab Sheik, to whom I presented several boxes.

" 'Peace be unto you and length of days; thy medicine (Brandreth's Pills) was a fierce foe to Azrael, both in pestilence and caravan sickness; the little orbs were rich with the wine of health; let the maker wear this golden circle, that he may know I was wounded with the arrows of disease, but am now healed.

" ' May he grow in the sunshine, and dispensing blessings be the most blest.
(Signed) " 'ACHMET HALLILLA.' "
Brandreth's Pills are both sugar-coated and plain.

Paralysis of the Legs, of Seventeen Years' Duration, Cured by Brandreth's Pills Alone.

Extract of Consul Graham's Letter to Dr. Brandreth, on file at 294 Canal Street.

General T. has a brother over forty years of age, whose legs have been paralyzed for seventeen years, so that he could not walk a step. He has tried all sorts of remedies, and been under the care of various physicians, all of whom have pronounced his case incurable. I gave my friend a box of Brandreth's Vegetable Universal Pills, with the printed instructions ; his brother took them, and was so pleased with the effect that he prevailed upon Messrs. Zimmerman & Frazer to let him have a few dozen boxes. He has now taken some thirty or forty boxes, and is so far recovered that he CAN WALK WITH A CANE, and has full faith that he will recover entirely. He is so enthusiastic in favor of the pills, that he has cut your likeness from some of the package-labels and has posted it over his table, and frequently burns a candle before it (he is a Catholic); and when his friends come in he points to it, saying that this is the true " saint," " *my saint;* all the rest I value nothing in comparison." This gentleman entirely recovered the use of his limbs, and is now one of the healthiest and soundest men in Buenos Ayres.

Captain Berry, formerly of the New York Custom House, had also lost the use of his legs, and was obliged to use crutches. He resorted to Brandreth's Pills; three months' vigorous use cured him of his rheumatism entirely.

Cancer Cured.

Mary H., wife of L. D. Grosvenor, of the United Society, Harvard, Mass., was cured of a cancer of many years' standing. "The prospect of terminating my life by the ravages of that insufferable scourge of humanity, the cancerous tumor, was certainly prevented by the timely and persevering use of Dr. Brandreth's Medicine, and a wonderful cure effected."

Isaac W. Briggs, of 145 Suffolk Street, New York, says he has used BRANDRETH'S PILLS for thirty years, having commenced to use them in February, 1836, for dyspepsia and affection of the kidneys. He took Brandreth's Pills every day for thirteen months, and in March, 1837, became a perfectly sound, healthy man. Mr. Briggs will be pleased to answer any questions on this subject.
July, 1866.

UNITED STATES SANITARY COMMISSION,
WETHERSFIELD, WYOMING COUNTY, N. Y., June 27, 1865.
DOCTOR BRANDRETH :—This certifies that I have used your celebrated Pills for over twenty years, personally and in my family. When we are sick, instead of sending for a doctor, we use Brandreth's Pills. I believe if every one would adopt the same course, the doctors would have but little to do. I have traveled in fifteen States, and been in the army sixteen months, and necessarily exposed to much disease, yet by the use of your Pills occasionally, have secured my health through the biting winter's frost and the scorching summer's heat.

In fact, Doctor, I feel, with your Pills in my pocket, safe from the attacks of disease. They seem to cleanse the blood and regulate the system, whether it be troubled with dizziness, diarrhœa, or costiveness. When out of sorts, I use them, and they always cure me. I would not be without them for four times their cost.

I send this to you that others who know me may profit by it, wishing to do good to my fellow-beings.

N. HIGLEY.

Dyspepsia and Costiveness Cured.

D. J. TENNY'S CASE.—*New York Mentor,* January 14, 1860.— Whether the Brandreth's Pill is ever convertible into blood we will not now discuss. But our chief object at this time is to give a statement of a gentleman who says he has taken one of the Brandreth Pills for at least sixteen months, daily, or about 480 days in succession, and who says that at the end of that time he considered himself cured of Dyspepsia, attended by a constant costive state of the bowels, which had troubled him for a long time.

This gentleman, Mr. Daniel Tenny, resides at the Astor House, in this city, and has been in the enjoyment of excellent health ever since he was cured by this treatment. He is an intelligent man, and there is no doubt of the truth of his statement. This proves, at least, that as many as one of the Pills prepared by Dr. Brandreth can be taken for nearly 500 days in succession without harm, and at the end of that time a dyspeptic and costive habit of body may be perfectly cured. This could not be said of any of the cathartics in use by those who style themselves the *Regular Faculty.*

Asthma Cured by Dr. Brandreth's Pills.

The following cure of Asthma by the use of Dr. Benjamin Brandreth's Pills is authenticated by seventeen well-known respectable citizens of Greenwich, Conn. :

This will certify that Thomas S. Brown, who had been for some time previous much affected with asthmatical symptoms, was taken suddenly worse on the 12th of June last : he began to cough and raise phlegm, and in the course of twenty-four hours expectorated nearly two quarts of thick white jelly-looking matter. Three physicians pronounced it a nervous humid spasmodic Asthma, and after prescribing for some time, to no effect, the three consulted together, and finally declared that they could do him no good ; it would and must result in consumption, and death would ensue, and that in a very short time. The pain was excessive in all parts of his body ; and the difficulty of breathing was such as almost to cause strangulation. He was reduced to a mere skeleton, and finally gave himself up to death. After being in this miserable state nearly two months, he saw an advertisement of Dr. Brandreth's Vegetable Universal Pills, and immediately sent by Captain J. Waring, of Greenwich, for a 25-cent box, and found relief in the course of a few days. It is proper to say that he commenced with two pills at night, and two in the morning ; he found relief the second day, and encouraged thus to persevere with larger doses, he was soon able to sleep comfortable, and now, having taken them for about four months, according to the directions, is entirely recovered, and so far as we can judge, entirely in consequence of taking the above Pills, which we have also used in our families, and have found them invaluable.

JAMES R. MEAN,	JAMES MOORE,
DANIEL S. BETTS,	HANNAH HITCHCOCK,
JOHN II. REYNOLDS,	JAMES MEAD,
ABEL PALMER,	THOMAS BERTRAM,
REV. R. PALMER,	ISAAC OLMSTED,
JOHN R. PALMER,	P. V. T. JESSUP,
HENRY BEWSLEY,	STEPHEN WARING,
SAMUEL JESSUP,	AUGUSTUS LYON,
	JOHN LIMPRY.

Mrs. Mary Blanchard, 206 Clermont Avenue, Brooklyn, was cured of Asthma of long standing by
BRANDRETH'S PILLS.
She is acquainted with other cases of persons cured of Asthma by the same remedy, and kindly permits reference.

Painters' Colic Cured.

DR. BRANDRETH,

Sir:—I am a painter by trade, and have frequently been troubled with slight attacks of colic, arising from contact with lead in the forms it is used in my business. My eyes have also been made somewhat weak from the same cause. Your pills have been my only medicine, and they have never failed to restore my health. For all the diseases incident to a painter, I think Brandreth's Pills a certain remedy. My journeymen, by my advice, always take them whenever their arms become paralyzed, or their bowels constipated, and they have been cured by a few doses. Painters will find your pills invaluable.

Yours, &c., DENNIS NORTON.

SING SING, March 23, 1865.

Saint Vitus' Dance Cured, of Twenty-five Years' Standing, with Brandreth's Vegetable Universal Pills.

SIR: With the most grateful feelings and the highest consideration for you, I sit down to state one of the most remarkable cures perhaps you have ever received, and effected, sir, entirely with your never-to-be sufficiently praised Vegetable Universal, and, I might add, life-restoring Pills.

The gratitude I feel makes me scarcely able to state the case, which would not, I am sure, be believed, were it not universally known in the town of Wareham, where we reside, and the miserable condition my dear wife, Lucy Hooker, has been in for the last twenty-five years, now restored to health and to her family, when for so many years she was considered to be beyond all human aid.

For the last twenty-five years my wife has suffered from Saint Vitus' Dance, and a complication of diseases which the doctors only seemed to continue to make worse instead of better. Calomel and bleeding, tonics and blisters, then calomel and bleeding, tonics and blisters again. Every doctor round the country at all famed was tried, until finally, she receiving no benefit, I thought I would try the mineral doctors no more, and therefore took her to Boston to Dr. Thomson. She went through several courses of his treatment, and appeared to gain some thereby. But alas! she soon became as sick as ever. I

13

then was obliged, she becoming suddenly worse, to send for two of the Wareham doctors again. They told me candidly she was beyond the powers of medicine, and that she must soon sink under her diseases. What was I to do? I had often been recommended your pills, but always held them in contempt. ONE MEDICINE and ONE DISEASE I could not understand. I told your agent, Abishia Barrows, of Wareham, what the doctors said. Again he strongly recommended the pills. I talked to my wife about them; she said she would try, if there was any hope—hoped they might be blessed to her, but that she was resigned. I went for a box, and when I returned one of her doctors was in the room. He made a deal to do about it, said she could not bear them, they were too strong for her, she could not bear any kind of physic, that she would die in all probability from the effects of the first dose. The more he said in opposition the more Lucy was determined to try them, and actually took a dose of four pills in his presence, and while he was holding forth against them. Away went the doctor and reported through the town that I was killing my wife by giving her those BRANDRETH'S PILLS—those Prince of Quack's Pills—those Impostor's Pills—and created quite an excitement. In the meantime she was receiving the benefit.

The first dose of four had a most wonderful effect—no wonder at the state she was in. The corruption was indeed dreadful. She took six the next night, and the same results. Instead of their causing weakness, she became stronger, and able to sit up a little. She persevered, sometimes taking as many as twelve at night and seven in the morning. When her pains were severe she took larger doses, and she did the same if the appearance of the evacuations was bad—in fact we followed your printed directions most carefully.

Sometimes she became worse—all the worst symptoms of the disorder presented themselves. Often at such times have I trembled lest she should die; but by persevering with the pills she soon recovered; and after every attack of this kind she seemed to be more firmly established in the recovery of her health, or rather her health seemed stronger after each of these attacks. At first, not only the doctors opposed her using the pills, but all her friends and relations; they all considered that the pills would surely accelerate her death. But long since the tide of opinion has changed, and those who most opposed now most strongly recommend them.

It is about sixteen months since she took the first dose. She has used in all one hundred and fifty-two boxes, all purchased of your agent in this place, Abishia Barrows. I consider that she is like one raised from the grave, to bless myself and family, and give your pills and a kind Providence all the praise. She has not enjoyed so good a state of health since she was a child, certainly not since we were married.

The doctor who saw her take the first dose, I understand is entirely converted to your principles of curing diseases by continued purgation, and is trying to find out what your pills are made of. But I believe he uses your pills in his practice—in fact I feel sure of it.

The cures which have been made in our region since my wife's recovery are truly surprising. Every one that feels sick thinks of no other medicine than Dr. Brandreth's Pills. I hope, sir, you will come and favor our town by a visit; you will find many grateful hearts to welcome you.

In the hope that you will live long to benefit mankind, I and my wife join in our mutual kind wishes and grateful feelings, and remain,

Very respectfully,

WILLIAM HOOKER,
LUCY HOOKER.

WAREHAM, Barnstable Co., Mass., May 23, 1838.

Yellow Fever Cured.

A gentleman, with whom I am well acquainted, writes as follows: "In 1838, at New Orleans, at the St. Charles Hotel, while at table taking dinner, before the soup was removed, I was taken with dizziness, dimness of sight, and confusion of ideas; in short, all the symptoms of yellow fever, though well five minutes before. I asked a waiter to lead me up to my room, for the confusion of mind and dizziness was so great, that I could never have found the way alone. When there, I took eight Brandreth's Vegetable Universal Pills, and laid down. I was watched carefully, and for three or four hours was partly delirious; but in four hours the pills began to work, and my mind was clear enough to know my danger. Bleeding was recommended. 'Do you think,' said I to the doctor, 'I want depleting?' 'Your life is not safe without it,' was the reply. 'Then I will take eight more Brandreth's Pills,' said I. Those on the top of the first eight, with plenty of Indian meal gruel, carried me out of all danger, and half a dozen medium doses cured me entirely in less than a week. Those who want to be safe, should take a few doses of pills as a preventive."

Tenea, or Tapeworms, Entirely Eradicated with Brandreth's Pills.

READING, FAIRFIELD COUNTY, CONN.

DR. BENJAMIN BRANDRETH:

Dear Sir—I have been troubled with the tape worms for twelve years; many have come from me, from twenty to thirty feet long—more or less every day of shorter ones—every two or three weeks I had a sick time from them—pressure at stomach—heavy load—many have crawled from me while at work—injured my health so much that I was not able to work one half the time—spent a great deal of time and money in consulting physicians and taking their prescriptions—have been reduced very low by taking medicine, without effect—last fall heard of Brandreth's Pills as a Cure All—had but little faith in them, but was determined to try any, everything, I could find at all probable to cure, thinking that without some remedy I must be destroyed by them. I procured one box, took one dose, and *one worm came from me ten feet long;* took the second and third, which cleaned them all out, and I have not had one since. I have, however, taken several boxes of pills since, but have seen no appearance of worms. It is now ten months since, and I have gradually recovered my health, and am now able to attend to my business as usual, and have no doubt that they are all extinct. When I was afflicted with worms, I wanted to consume three times as much food as I would if in good health. Now I take my regular meals, and am hearty and enjoying good health, and able to do a good day's work. The last worm that came from me was twelve feet long. I have not the least doubt that it was Brandreth's Pills (your valuable Vegetable Medicine) that effected the cure, as everything else that I could hear of was tried without effect.

Yours very respectfully, and grateful servant,

AARON T. DIMON.

JUNE 20, 1838.

The above person is well known in Fairfield County. John B. Sanford, of Bridgeport, Conn., has assured me of his respectability.

Cure of Pimples on the Face of Three Years' Continuance.

Dr. Brandreth :

Dear Sir : For some considerable period I have been troubled with an impurity or acridity of the blood, which seemed to be past cure. My face, in consequence, presented an unseemly collection of pimples. I was abstemious, and seldom tasted any beverage stronger than water, and yet, with all my care as to diet, my blood got no better, and my appearance continued the same. My face all the time seemed as if it was held near a fire ; it seemed as if something was on it that might be brushed off. It was very annoying, and caused me much anxiety, not because it interfered with my personal appearance, which it did, but because it more or less affected my health, which was beginning to break down. I took very little medicine ; but when the above state of things had remained about the same for three years, I was induced to use your pills. I took them, in all, about one month—every day, or nearly so—taking no higher dose than five pills, and sometimes only one. I think, altogether, I did not use over four boxes. They cured me completely. My face is free from all pimples and inflammation, and my complexion perfectly clear. Gratitude has induced me to render this account, which you may publish.

I am, with respect, yours, &c.,

N. H. BAKER.

Sing Sing, *March* 30, 1855.

The following modest note from Mr. Bemis, of Dudley, Mass., for a supply, tells its own story :

Dudley, December 7, 1853.

B. Brandreth :

Dear Sir—I have sold all the Pills I had of yours, and the money is ready when you will send my receipt. Please to send more Pills as soon as you can —send to Webster Station. I have sold $117 worth of your Pills, and they give universal satisfaction.

Yours, with respect,

PHINEAS BEMIS.

Brandreth's Pills Never Failing in Diarrhœa and Dysentery. Read.

Battery Anderson, Sept. 9, 1864.

Dr. Brandreth, New York : Please find one dollar enclosed, for which send me that worth of your Pills, as I have used and given all I had. These Pills have cured all who took them for the diarrhœa in a few days. Some had the disease two or three months. The army doctors had failed to cure in all of these cases.

I have found your Pills to be never-failing in diarrhœa, bilious affections, headache, and costiveness. How is it the Sanitary people do not give out your Pills ?

Yours, with great respect,

PAUL P. DUFOUR,

Co. A, Thirteenth Heavy Artillery, Bermuda Hundred, Va.

Captain Isaac Smith, of Sing Sing, says, thirty of Brandreth's Pills, taken according to directions, cured him of a very severe bronchial affection, after other means had failed, and he wishes his numerous friends to know the fact.

Extract from a letter dated Dawson, Iowa, April 24, 1866, to Dr. Brandreth, from Andrew Logan, Esq.:

"My wife became an invalid. Our physician represented her case as incurable. I then called two other physicians, and the three held a consultation and pronounced her case consumption. I then discharged all the physicians and determined to trust to your Pills. I got five boxes, which she took according to the printed directions. By the time these were used up, there appeared a change in her condition for the better. I then bought fifteen boxes, and she continued to take them for three months, when her health was entirely restored."

Original letter at 294 Canal Street.

Persevere in the Good Work.

The Rev. Ezra Wilmarth, East Wilson, N. H., says: "He has seen the salutary effects of Brandreth's Pills in many cases, and is fully convinced of their great value;" that he "thinks it his duty to recommend them wherever he knows there is sickness, and is confident that they are calculated to promote the general health of mankind."

Nervous Debility and Bilious Headache.

Mr. Webber, whose case is mentioned below, is still living, a fine healthy man of over 67 years:

William Wood Webber, of Grigg Street, Southsea, in the Borough of Portsmouth, England, bell-hanger, voluntarily cometh before me and maketh oath and saith, that he was for five years and upward dreadfully afflicted with a nervous debility of his whole system, attended with a bilious headache which prevented him (deponent) from attending to his business the greater part of that time. He (deponent) has sometimes been so violently affected as to fall down senseless, which had nigh once put an end to his existence. In this melancholy state he was recommended to take Brandreth's Vegetable Universal Pills, and after taking them for four or five weeks, according to the directions, he was perfectly cured. It is necessary and essential to observe that after taking them six or eight times he was much worse; but Dr. Brandreth informed him that such would be the symptoms, and prevailed upon him (deponent) to persevere, which he did; he therefore went on, as above stated, and the most beneficial results followed. It is now six months since deponent was quite cured, and he has had no return of the said disorder, but keeps in the enjoyment of perfect health, which he entirely attributes to Brandreth's Pills, the Vegetable Universal Medicine.

WILLIAM WOOD WEBBER.

Sworn at Portsea, in the said borough, this 15th day of December, 1831, before me,

D. SPICER, *Mayor.*

Indigestion and Disordered Liver.

Brandreth's Pills are warranted free from all mercury or other mineral. A gentleman writes:

"I have for years been afflicted with disordered liver and indigestion, and have been restored after years of suffering, merely by the use of some fifteen boxes of the Brandreth Pills. For several years I have been more dead than alive; I have crawled about, for my locomotion could not be dignified by saying I walked. I had the best advice, but was blistered, bled, took blue pill and calomel until my mouth was sore, dieted, and drank mineral waters. At last I saw hope wiped out of my doctor's and relatives' looks—it was clear I was doomed. In fact this was to be expected; for when I did get up in the morning, I was more dead than alive; I was unable to attend to any business, and exertion of any kind seemed too much for me to endure. In this sad state I read J. W. Webber's case, and also Mr. Cooke's, of Bennington; these letters, with the advice of a friend, induced me to give the Brandreth Pills a trial. I began with only two pills, which purged gently; in a few days I took two more, they also operated mildly; then I took four, feeling some apprehension about my bowels; they operated finely, bringing away very slimy stools. I rested for a day or two, and then took two more; then I took six, and at last I became fully convinced of the efficacy of purgation, as a cure for disease. I have taken as high as eight pills in twelve hours—but the dose must be in proportion to the sickness—inflammatory cases require strong doses, and all serious sickness where pain is present, the same. But with weak persons the plan is to begin easily, and sort of feel your way, taking larger doses as you proceed. This method in the use of Brandreth's Pills has cured me, and restored to health one who had prepared himself for the grave."

Letter from Arnold Buffum,

THE PHILANTHROPIST.

CINCINNATI, OHIO, April 15, 1843.

Dr. Brandreth:

In the course of my life I have suffered often and much from sickness; I think I have been under the care of physicians more than twenty different times, for weeks at a time. But for the last five years I have employed a physician but once, and then only for a single day; not, however, because I have been exempt from frequent illness, but because I have found a far more speedy and effectual remedy in thy Pills, than I ever found in the medicines administered to me by my physicians. Wherever I go, I constantly carry a box of them with me, or at least a few of them wrapped in a paper in my vest pocket; and whatever illness comes upon me, I invariably find relief from the use of them.

Having been much occupied in travelling and public speaking, I have frequently taken severe cold, which before I used these pills, invariably resulted in soreness of the throat and chest, and a severe cough; but latterly, though more exposed than ever, when I have taken a cold, by taking one or two pills at a time for two or three nights, I have *invariably* succeeded in removing all soreness of the throat and chest, and in effectually preventing the cold from settling on my lungs so as to produce a cough.

Once during last winter, while travelling on horseback, and subject to much exposure, I was suddenly seized with a very sore throat, high fever, and entire prostration of strength and spirits,—by the use of two doses of the pills, and drinking freely of cold water, a copious perspiration was kept up, and in forty-two hours one of the most severe attacks which I ever experienced gave way ; and in two days more I was able to pursue my journey. At another time, continual exposure and daily exercise in public speaking brought on a severe lameness in the small of the back and kidneys, which became so exceedingly painful that I was forced to speak sitting ; not being able to stand on my feet; at length the soreness extended quite through me, and the pain became so severe that I never closed my eyes during a whole night, and several times during that night I had serious doubts whether I would live till morning. I took seven pills, which went to the seat of the disease, and as by magic, seemed to lay hold of it, and carried it all off, so that I attended a meeting on the same evening, and spoke without pain for more than two hours, and the pain has not returned since. I regard this as one of the most extraordinary cures that I have ever known, and I can truly say that, in a similar case, I would not exchange Brandreth's Pills for all the medicine of the drug store. I have used the Pills, and administered them to others on various other occasions, and, as far as I know, in no case without complete success. Especially have I found them altogether superior to any other medicine I have ever tried for colds, coughs, and soreness of the lungs. I consider that the maker of them especially serves the great cause of humanity, and I shall recommend them wherever I go.

Thine respectfully,
A. BUFFUM.

In October 1843, Aaron Hamilton of Sing Sing, Westchester county, was taken suddenly sick in the night with great pain in his bowels and stomach. He took six Brandreth Pills, and in two hours took four more. In a little time he threw up two worms, and passed several downwards. He has enjoyed good health since.

St. Vitus' Dance and Scrofula Cured.

SING SING, 3d January, 1843.

· DEAR SIR :

It is with gratitude and esteem that I address you for the purpose of informing you of the beneficial effects which your Pills and External Remedy have had in restoring one of my sons to health, who had been sorely afflicted winter before last with St. Vitus' Dance, and for a period of ten months he was entirely helpless from the terrible disorder. He was also subject to the Scrofula in his neck. By the use of your Pills freely, and also applying the the External Remedy to the enlargements upon his neck, he has become entirely cured. He has been now well over a year ; and I trust, by the blessing of Divine Providence, he will continue so.

You are at perfect liberty to make what use you please with this communication. I consider it a duty I owe to you to make it, and hope it may be the means of extending the usefulness of your most excellent medicines.

I remain yours, respectfully,
II. M. REQUA.

To DR. BENJAMIN BRANDRETH,
Spring Hill, Sing Sing.

Indigestion and Bilious Affection Cured.

SING SING, January 14, 1843.

DEAR SIR :

This will certify that I have used your Vegetable Universal Pills for indigestion and bilious complaint which had almost proved fatal to me. I had been under what was supposed good medical treatment, and used various advertised remedies, but without any good effect. I then made trial of your celebrated pills, which gave me immediate relief, and soon effected a perfect cure. I have since used them in my family with the best effect. They are the best and easiest purgative we ever used.

I am, respectfully, yours,
NICHOLAS FOWLER.

DR. B. BRANDRETH,
Spring Hill, Sing Sing.

———

SING SING STATE PRISON, Feb. 4, 1843.

DR. BRANDRETH,

Dear Sir : About four years since, I had a very severe attack of the piles. I tried almost every remedy, but without any good effect upon my painful disease. I thought I would try one box of your Vegetable Universal Pills. I done so ; and before I had taken all the pills it contained, I began to feel the good effects of them ; and by the time I had taken four boxes of pills, I was entirely cured, and have never since been troubled with the painful and truly unpleasant disease. I entirely attribute my cure to your valuable and inestimable pills.

Very truly yours,
R. LENT,
Architect, Sing Sing State Prison.

———

SING SING, Jan. 24th, 1843.

DR. B. BRANDRETH,

Dear Sir : If you alone were concerned in the present statement, the greater inducement for making it would be removed, for of course no testimony can strengthen you in your convictions in relation to the value and efficiency of your Pills, which have already proved such a blessing to the thousands who have used them ; but I have looked out upon this vast expanse of creation, encircling in its arms, as it does, thousands bowed down with sufferings similar to my own, who would gladly hasten to the same source that restored my health, if they were persuaded that they would meet with the same happy result. Therefore, Sir, it is that those thousands may be convinced, and profit by their conviction, as I have done, that induces me to state before the world a period of suffering, such as few have, and I hope few ever will know, and the permanent relief I received from your Pills; but how to begin, I hardly know, to describe those extreme tortures that seized upon my arms, shoulders, side and face, having about ten years since contracted a very severe cold, causing a very severe fit of sickness, attended with an affection of the Liver, as was supposed, which was the consequence of my taking a great quantity of medicine—and I must say, I have not seen a well day since, until I commenced taking Brandreth's Pills. For the last ten years I have been afflicted with what is commonly called Salt Rheum and Erysipelas, at times covering and seeming determined to devour my whole body, and by making use of various means was enabled to check the disease from time to time, until early in June, 1841, my disease assumed a very different appearance; and unpleasant as the task now is to me, I will, for the sake of spreading light and knowledge in the world, give a few of the particulars of my case : swelling and painful affections of the joints, tumors formed under the skin with burning lacerating pains, and finally coming out in horrible sores, covering nearly the whole of the right arm, and penetrating almost to the bone, and spreading to my face, covering nearly half including the nose, making for the time an entire wreck of that organ ; from thence to my shoulder and side, and my whole body and limbs swollen in the most frightful manner. Residing at this time in one of the western cities of New York State, I had recourse to most of the eminent Physicians of that part of the country ; and the most that they could do was to pronounce the disease a scrofulous affection, which it seems they were not prepared to combat. A change of air and climate was recommended, and in traveling I became acquainted with a lady from Sing Sing. She advised the use of Brandreth's Pills—but supposing that they could be of no use to me, as I had tried so many things, I thought little more of them at that time ; but after having endured the most excruciating tortures, and incurring great expense, I was, thank God, about six months since, by reading one of Dr. B.'s advertisements, and what I had heard about them, induced to purchase a box of Brandreth's Pills. Jealous of the article, I resolved not to have my imagination at all busy, but nevertheless to give them a fair trial, which I did, by taking according to the directions accompanying each box, as far as my feeble state would admit, two or three boxes. Overjoyed at the discovery of an article which I well knew improved my health, used them secretly for a few weeks, but becoming convinced that Brandreth's Pills would cure me, I made bold to declare it.

Sir, are you alone concerned to know it? I think not, for I know that the medicine that possesses the power to cure me is capable of conferring the same blessings upon thousands of others suffering, perhaps dying ; therefore, these are all concerned to know that they can be cured. In fact, all are concerned in the discovery of anything that tends to promote the happiness of the human race, for we are social beings and cannot suffer alone. Persons may doubt this statement as I have doubted similar ones, but be assured it is but too true ; and in giving it, I have unsolicited, to you, sir, and the world, if you choose to publish it, discharged a duty which I felt incumbent upon me in making it known for the benefit of those who choose to believe it, as I believe that I have been cured of a scrofulous affection of the worst possible character and of long standing, by the use of less than twenty boxes of Brandreth's Universal Vegetable Pills, at an expense of less than Five Dollars, instead of chasing phantoms at a greater advance in fees, without any good results ; and when I look into the past, upon these solitary days and sleepless nights, I thank a kind Providence that it is as well with me as it is, and I thank you, sir, that you are enabled by your scientific researches to minister to our infirmities.

RACHEL TURRELL.

Fits Cured.

This may certify that my son, of five years old, was attacked with epileptic fits, in 1837, and continued to be troubled with them for more than one year. After every other remedy had failed I tried the Brandreth's Pills, which effected a cure in about six months, and he has not been troubled with them since.

DAVID CHAFFEE.

GRAFTON STREET, August 2, 1843.

Mr. Wilson, of 135 Christie Street, for twelve years was afflicted with Chronic Rheumatism, and for the last three years was not able to walk; has taken twelve boxes, the pain has entirely left his feet and knees, so that he is able to walk with comfort.

Miss W*****, a young lady residing in Hubert Street, had a severe pain in her knee, from which she suffered excruciating pains for upwards of three years, which confined her to bed almost all the time. Dr. Mott and several others of the faculty had bled, leeched, and blistered to no effect; by taking Brandreth's Pills she has perfectly recovered the use of her knee. Observations on the above would be superfluous.

Mr. G. Miller, of Harlaem, in September last, was dreadfully afflicted with Fever and Ague; the attack generally came on him every day about 12 o'clock; the disease had debilitated him in such a manner that his recovery was doubtful. A gentleman who has tested the goodness of Brandreth's Pills, in his own family, persuaded him to try the medicine. After the first box the Fever was perfectly cured, and by continuing taking the medicine for about six weeks, perfect health was restored.

Benj. Weeks, of Westchester, was violently afflicted with Dyspepsia; he could not take any food without the most unpleasant sensations in his chest, head, and bowels. His chest was so sore that the slightest pressure gave him pain; his life was most miserable; numerous were the medicines used; and the skill of the first physicians tried in vain; as a last recourse he took Brandreth's Universals, and in two months they effected a perfect cure.

Worms.

A young woman a short time since took these Pills for a violent pain in her side. After three doses she parted with a worm fourteen inches in length and one inch round; she has since been perfectly well, and has kindly allowed Dr. B. to refer any one to her.

It is a fact that there are good remedies, but it is very doubtful whether there are many good physicians. Extraordinary cures in which Brandreth's Pills have effected a perfect cure after the most eminent medical men had altogether failed:

Mrs. Luther, of North Third Street, near Second Street, Williamsburg, for seventeen years was seriously afflicted with a violent pain in her left side, which often became very bad. The side was wearing to all appearance away, and just over the seat of the pain was a place you might have laid an egg in. Extreme debility and general bad feelings were the consequence; she could do nothing for herself and family with pleasure; no relief was experienced from anything used until July last, when Brandreth's Universals were recommended, and immediate relief was experienced, and on the 31st of December she assured Dr. B. the Pills had perfectly restored her health, and that her side was become like unto the other. Mrs. L. stated many other particulars, which, were there space, would be mentioned.

Cure of Terrible Ulceration.

SECOND HOUSE FROM TENTH AVENUE, TWENTY-EIGHTH STREET, }
New York, Nov. 2, 1842. }

Dear Sir: Last January I was taken suddenly with pain in my left side in the night, and my wife had to get up and steam it, but the pain got no better; I then sent for Dr. Adams. He ordered a poultice of bread and yeast, and then a lump began to form about six inches from my arm-pit. Dr. Adams gave me pills which did me no good, and the pain still became more severe. At this period Dr. Adams brought another doctor with him, but I still continued to get worse, and although several other physicians came to see me, yet I continued to grow worse and worse. Dr. Adams opened at one time the abscess which first commenced under my arm, and which had extended to my hip-bone and thence to the small of my back, and from thence to my shoulder-blades. Being poor, I sent for the dispensary doctors, and they attended me, but I continued to get worse, and the ulcers were some of them, such as I could see, more than half an inch deep. The doctors, both dispensary and the others who visited me, only a few days before you called upon me, told me it was ten thousand to one whether I recovered or not—that I might not live through the night. This was in the early part of February. I had not been out of bed since the beginning of January. At this time, the latter part of February, my wife went to see you, and beg you to come and see me. You dressed my ulcers for me that night—it took a yard of linen to dress them once. You left me two boxes of pills, which I used as you directed me, and my wife dressed me with your Universal Salve, and rubbed the callous places with the Liniment. In two months I walked to your office in Broadway, from Twenty-eighth Street, corner of Tenth Avenue. I came after that, seven or eight times for you, to see how my back got on, and to receive your further advice. I went on getting better every day, and my ulcers one after another got well, until the latter part of July, when I went to work, being a sound man, with the exception of having nearly lost the sight of my right eye, during my sickness, which, however, gradually gets better and better from the use of your pills. I send you this letter that you may publish it; and should any one wish to inquire any particulars of my extraordinary cure, they can see me where I live, which is the second house from the corner of Tenth Avenue, in Twenty-eighth Street.

I remain, dear sir,

Yours very respectfully,

PATRICK BRALLEY.

To Dr. BENJ. BRANDRETH, 241 Broadway, New York.

EDMESTON, OTSEGO Co., Jan. 4, 1839.

DR. BRANDRETH:

Dear Sir: I feel it a duty I owe to the public, as well as yourself, to inform you of the astonishing efficacy of your truly valuable pills. I was attacked about the 1st of November last with the prevailing bilious or typhus fever, violently. The pain in my head and back was most excruciating. I took first six of your pills, then eight, ten and twelve at a dose twice a day, yet found no relief. My wife then read your directions to me, after which I took seventeen, then twenty and twenty-two. I continued to take twenty morning and evening for four days, when I found the disease yielding and the fever literally broken up; I then gradually diminished the quantities according to your directions. In two weeks I was out again.* I used no medicine but the pills.

---

* Others who pursued the ordinary course were confined from six to twelve and fourteen weeks.

There has since been a number of cases of the same fever in my neighborhood, where the patients have followed the same course. J. E. used no medicine except your pills, according to your directions in "violent diseases," with the same happy effect. I took fifteen boxes; another twelve, and others ten and down to four. Some used drafts upon the feet.

Yours truly,
WATERMAN BURLINGHAM.

MELBOURNE, VICTORIA, 1st June, 1858.

MR. BLANDFORD, *Agent for Brandreth's Pills, Melbourne:*

DEAR SIR : Having had a severe attack of inflammatory rheumatism, by which I was confined to my bed for several days, during which time I suffered the most agonizing pains in my side, back and limbs, and was fearful that I should be confined to my bed for a long time, my husband brought me one of Dr. Brandreth's pamphlets ; after reading it carefully, I concluded that I would try the pills, which I used as directed. I have been using them three weeks, and I am happy to say that to Dr. Brandreth's Pills I owe my recovery to health and strength. I feel stronger and better than I have done for a long time, and I am convinced that the disease is eradicated from my system.

If you deem this letter of any use, please publish it.

I am, dear sir,
Very respectfully yours,
MANDY WAYMAN.

LITTLE BAY STREET, SANDIDGE.

MELBOURNE, 1st Aug., 1858.

MR. J. T. BLANDFORD :

Dear Sir : I am a mason by trade, and for some time past have felt almost unable to attend to my business. Three weeks ago, on my way home in the evening, I stepped into a water hole and got quite wet, from the effect of which I took a severe cold, my whole body became much swollen, my breathing became very difficult. I had sharp pains in my chest, and in fact when I called on you at your office I considered myself in very great danger. I bought two boxes of Dr. Brandreth's Pills, and took six pills in the office and six more on my return home. In about five or six hours I discharged several quarts of water, and felt greatly relieved. I have continued to take the pills, and am happy to say am quite well. I consider the Brandreth Pills the means of saving my life. I have heard them called the Poor Man's Medicine of America, where they are so celebrated. I trust they will be known as such here. I will never be without Brandreth's Pills as long as I can obtain them.

Please publish this letter. I am anxious that the people here snould know where to get a medicine that they can rely on.

I remain, dear sir,
Yours respectfully,
JOHN FLANNIGAN.

HOWARD STREET, NORTH MELBOURNE.

PARK STREET, SOUTH YARRA, Aug. 20th, 1858.

SIR : This morning, having mislaid my spectacles when the morning's *Age* arrived, I took it up merely to endeavor to read the large type of the leading article, but judge my astonishment when I could, with facility, peruse the smallest type. This extraordinary fact I attribute to the use of Dr. Brandreth's Vegetable Universal Pills. Make any use you please of this communication.

Yours very truly,
JOHN HARRISON.

Letter of the Rev. Ezra Wilmarth, in favor of the Brandreth Pills.

EAST WILTON, N. II., July 27, 1836.

DR. BRANDRETH:

My Dear Sir: Having recently become acquainted with your valuable pills, and seen their salutary effects in a great variety of cases, I take the liberty of addressing you, stating my conviction of their value. Although I have heretofore been unfavorable to nostrums, I am fully convinced of the value of yours.

I am a minister of the Gospel, of the Baptist denomination, in this town, and pastor of a church, and am well known; therefore, I hope my recommendation of your Pills will be of some use in causing those who know me to make trial of them, as I feel confident they are calculated to promote the general health of mankind.

Wishing you abundant success in your attempts to benefit the world,

I am, with high respect,

Your obedient servant,

EZRA WILMARTH.

Bilious Remitting Fever and Dysentery Cured.

PATERSON (New Jersey), Aug. 18th, 1836.

Sir: I write this out of respect to you for your excellent Pills, for both I and my family think it a great blessing that we have met with them again in this country, because we knew them to be excellent and good; when at Leeds, in England, there it was always said if any person was sick, get a box of Brandreth's Pills and they will cure you.

Sir, I have been sick of a bilious and remitting fever, for which I got three boxes, and they have done me more good than all the physic ever I took in my life; for before I took them I was almost gone with a liver complaint; and now I am as well as ever I was in my life. In my family we have had three attacked with the dysentery; they (the Pills) cured them in two days, so that we have all of us great occasion to praise Dr. Brandreth's Pills.

I am, sir, yours very truly,

And greatly obliged,

RICHARD HAMPSHIRE.

Asthma Cured.

Mr. John Benist, of No. 69 Chapel Street, New York, was afflicted with a dreadful asthma for nine years, during which time he was unable to lie down in bed, and frequently was gasping for breath, expecting every coming hour would be his last. He applied to several of the first physicians in New York, none of whom gave him the least relief. At last, Brandreth's Universals were strongly recommended, and in the course of a short time he found great benefit, and by continuing the Pills, he is now quite well, and able to attend to his business; indeed he is perfectly restored to health.

Dyspepsia Cured.

Newburgh, N. Y., Feb. 14, 1836. Dr. Brandreth—*Sir :* The many flatter-ing notices you have received from respectable individuals, of the success of your Vegetable Universal Pills, render it unnecessary for me individually to eulogize, or those who are ignorant of the specific to censure. Having had ocular demonstration as well as bodily, I cannot refrain from expressing and publicly acknowledging the signal result and final cure of that dreadful disease known as Dyspepsia; hoping such persons as may be afflicted with the above disease, this notice may influence some to make the experiment. You are at liberty to refer them to me voluntarily on my part.

I remain your friend,

JOHN A. STEVENS.

Rheumatism.

A gentleman who had lost the use of his limbs with Inflammatory Rheu-matism, and was so miserably afflicted that he could not turn in bed without assistance—the pains were violent in all parts of his body, but especially in his breast, back, arms and feet. This person took no other medicine than Brandreth's Pills—for two weeks he took 12 pills per day, and often as many as 20, and in three weeks he was able to get out; and now, having persevered with them so as to produce copious evacuations every day, is at this time per-fectly cured; it is not two months since he was first taken ill. Now, Dr. Brandreth would ask, would this have been the case with your bled man? with the man to whom mercury has been administered? No! he would have been in bed months, and his convalescence would have been tedious. The above gentleman is highly respectable, and can be referred to.

A Running Ulcer of Three Years entirely removed with Eight Boxes of Brandreth's Pills.

Edward Brown, son of Mr. James Brown, St. James Street, Kingston, Ulster County, for three years had a running ulcer in his hip, which obliged him to be carried about; the doctors were in daily attendance, and the best advice was had from New York. All did not relieve the poor child, who was not expected to recover. Brandreth's Pills were commenced with four months ago, and a decided change was effected before the third box was finished, and now, having taken eight boxes, is quite well.

A little boy, aged four years, swallowed a pin, and, as a matter of course, his parents were much alarmed. His father called on Dr. Brandreth, who recommended him to give the child five or six pills per day, and no bad con-sequence would arise. This advice was taken, and on the fourth day powerful evacuations having been kept up, the pin was discharged, and not in the least corroded. Reference can be given to the parents, who are highly respectable.

Mrs. S., in East Broadway, has been afflicted for nearly eight years with a bad leg, which prevented her going about. The sore was larger than the palm of the hand—she had had recourse to various doctors, who frequently healed it up, but in a few weeks was as bad as ever. Brandreth's Pills were recom-mended, and in a short time her leg was perfectly healed, and she is again able to walk with pleasure and comfort, and the leg has every appearance of being perfectly sound. Reference as to the above can be made to Mr. Aaron Swartz, grocer, corner of Pike Street and East Broadway.

Difficulty of Breathing Cured.

Danbury, Conn., March 8, 1836.—Dr. Brandreth—*Sir :* Will you be good enough to send us some more of your Vegetable Universal Pills ? there are many persons here taking them for every complaint, and all find relief. I can say they are the best medicine I ever took, and I have tried almost everything, but found no relief until I took your Pills. My difficulty of breathing is greatly relieved, and I am getting well. Many are taking them here for the same complaint, and find them very good.

Yours, respectfully,   ELIZA MORRIS.

Piles Cured.

Messrs. Coggershall & Walters, of New Bedford, have forwarded me the following facts of that most painful and unpleasant disease, the Piles. The original letter can be seen at 187 Hudson Street. Mr. McFarlane, of New Bedford, has been laboring under that most dreadful disease, the Piles ; he has had them upwards of two years—has tried various things from different doctors, to no effect. Brandreth's Vegetable Universal Pills were had recourse to, and a complete cure is effected. He is now quite well.

(*From the Louisville Enquirer.*)

Liver Complaint Cured.

NEWARK, Dec. 25, 1836.

DR. B. BRANDRETH.

Dear Sir : Having been afflicted for ten years with a most dreadful liver complaint and dropsy, and tried every remedy that could be thought of, I gave up all hope, went into the country, left my business, to die in peace ; but hearing of your invaluable medicine, I was induced to try it, not expecting to be any better. To my surprise, I had scarcely taken one box before I felt relief. I have since taken three boxes, and now I am well, by the blessing of God and the use of your medicine. If you think this will be any service to let suffering people know this fact, you are at liberty to publish the above.

Yours, with kind respect,
(Signed,)   LEWIS TOMPKINSON.

Dysentery and Deafness Cured.

AUGUST 20th, 1835.

Sir : Allow me to express my grateful feelings for the benefit I have experienced in your Vegetable Universal Pills in the cure of Deafness, which I have been subject to nearly thirty years. I have frequently been under eminent aurists in London, who have invariably syringed me, and who have all said no other mode of treatment would be of service. The latter part of May I again lost my hearing, with continual unpleasant noises in my head. It was with difficulty I could hear any one speak ; knowing you were an English surgeon, I applied to you to be syringed, thinking that was the only remedy; you refused to operate, but told me a box of your pills would have the desired effect, and I was induced to try them, especially when I found that many persons had been cured of the same complaint. I have taken two boxes, which cost me fifty cents, and am happy to say, am completely cured. The dose I took was two or three at night, and twice during the time I took five. They never inconvenienced me in the least, and were remarkably easy in their operation—I certainly can recommend them to any one laboring under the same unpleasant disease.

Permit me likewise to say my eldest daughter, two weeks since, had a dreadful Diarrhœa or Dysentery on her, which in two or three days reduced her frame, and I thought would have sent her to the grave. I immediately applied to you to know if the Vegetable Universal Pills would have the same beneficial effect on her as they had on myself; you told me to persevere and they would make a cure—I had confidence in them, and am happy to say, by her taking from four to eight pills every night, the dreadful disease left in about a week. She is now well, and getting up her strength very fast. She took no other medicine whatever; she continues occasionally one or two pills at night. My family had used the Hygeian Medicine for upwards of twelve months, and found they could not leave them off, as Costiveness and Piles were sure to follow. Thank God, your Pills leave no such enemies behind them. I have no hesitation in saying, that your Vegetable Universal Pills are the safest and best medicine myself or family ever took. Make what use you think proper of this communication, and you are at liberty to refer any one to me, and I think I am only doing my duty in thanking you, through divine mercy, for the benefit received.

I am, sir, yours very truly,
JAMES LANCE,
250 Eighteenth Street, near Broadway.

Certificate of JOSEPH GOULDEN, who has known the above Pills forty years:

I hereby certify, that I have known Brandreth's Vegetable Universal Pills for upwards of forty years; they were used in my family connections, in the County of Dorset, England, since the year 1796, many of whom they cured of old standing complaints.

JOSEPH GOULDEN.
BRIDGEPORT, Feb. 18, 1836.

Disease of the Prostate Gland Cured.

Henry Lathrop, of Edmonston, Otsego County, New York State, a respectable farmer, was afflicted for more than a year with this most painful, and generally incurable disease. Some of our highest medical men pronounced his case incurable, and advised him to settle his affairs, and patiently await the result, as it was not in the power of medicine to save him. Mr. Lathrop, before he went home, called upon me, and having stated his symptoms, I told him what his disease was, and in this I agreed with the doctors who had said he was incurable. But I also told him I felt confident that if he would persevere with my Pills they would cure him. Mr. Lathrop proved his confidence by purchasing six dozen boxes, which he took home with him, and in about *three months* he returned to me in New York City a cured man, having used the Pills as I directed. In fact, he said he never was better in his life. This was in 1835. Since that period Mr. Lathrop has administered the pills to upward of a thousand persons, all of whom, he assures me, have derived the most astonishing benefit from their use.

___

NEW BEDFORD, Nov. 7, 1835.

DR. BRANDRETH—

Sir : About eight weeks past I saw some of your Pills, and read one of your wrapping-papers, but thought it was, as thousands of such things are now-a-days, a mere speculative, money-catching thing—still I was advised to try them by persons who said they were most RIGHTEOUS PILLS. I was, however, faithless of their value; but my complaint grew so violent that I purchased two boxes, took them according to the directions, and found that they helped me much. My neighbors, knowing how long I had been afflicted, were anxious to know the result, and I informed them that I had received great benefit from the two boxes, which would induce me to purchase more. My wife for a long time had been in a poor state of health. She also took some, and found great benefit. And now, sir, excuse me while I detail some of my complaints, the main body of which seem as though the main springs of life were all fettered. DYSPEPSIA or INDIGESTION, Weakness of the Lungs, Nervousness, Rheumatism, SICK-HEADACHE, ASTHMA, GREAT LOSS OF APPETITE, LANGUOR, TREMOR, COSTIVENESS, etc., etc. Such have been my varied symptoms, but I must and will say, that I never took such medicine as your Pills, which seem to touch all parts of my complaints. I intend to persevere with them, and you may send me 500 boxes, which you must charge at the wholesale price.

I am, sir, yours respectfully,
SAMUEL S. ALBRO.

___

Piles Cured.

Messrs. Coggershall & Walters, of New Bedford, have forwarded me the following facts of that most painful and unpleasant disease, the Piles—the original letter can be seen at 187 Hudson Street. Mr. McFarlane, of New Bedford, has been laboring under that most dreadful disease, the Piles. He has had them upward of two years—has tried various things from different doctors to no effect. Brandreth's Vegetable Universal Pills were had recourse to, and a complete cure is effected—he is now quite well.

___

NEWBURGH, N. Y., Nov. 4, 1835.

Dr. BRANDRETH—

Sir : I was induced some time since, by the persuasion of a friend, to try a box of your Pills. From the immediate relief and happy result I have received from the same, I cannot but recommend them to my friends, and particularly to all invalids who may be afflicted with costiveness, not to DESPAIR until they have given your Vegetable Medicine a trial.

Hoping you may be the means of making us poor creatures happy, and add to your popularity and wealth,   I remain your friend,
J. W. SWIFT.

You may refer, or make what use you please of this letter.—J. W. S.

14

Extraordinary Cure of Rheumatism, Diarrhœa, and Affection of the Lungs.

John Shaw, of Pembroket, Washington County, Maine, being duly sworn, says that he was taken violently sick about six months since. The pains in his head, breast, back, left side, and instep being so bad that he was unable to help himself, and was taken into the Chelsea Hospital in the City of Boston. That after being in said hospital five weeks, Dr. Otis said he did not know what was the matter with him, and that he could do nothing for him, nor could he prescribe any medicine. That he, therefore, was conveyed from the Chelsea Hospital to the Sailor's Retreat on Staten Island. That he was there physicked with all sorts of medicine for a period of four months, suffering all the time the most heart-rending misery. That, besides the affection of his bones, he was troubled much with a disease of the lungs. Sometimes he would spit a quart of phlegm in the day. Besides this affection he had a bad diarrhœa, which had more or less attended him from the commencement of his sickness. That at times he dreaded a stool worse than he would have dreaded death. That he can compare the feeling to nothing save that of knives passing through his bowels. After suffering worse than death at the Sailor's Retreat on Staten Island, the doctor told him that medicine was of no use to him—that he must try to stir about. At this time he was suffering the greatest misery. That his bones were so tender he could not bear the least pressure upon the elbow or upon the knee; that his instep was most painful; that, as the doctor said he would give him no more medicine, he determined to procure some of Dr. Brandreth's Pills, which he did from 241 Broadway, New York. That he commenced with five pills, and sometimes increased the dose to eight. The first week's use so much benefited him that the doctor, not knowing what he was using, said, " Now, Shaw, you are looking like a man again. If you improve in this way you will soon be well." That he found every dose of the Brandreth Pills relieved him; first, they cured him of the pain when at stool; that they next cured the diarrhœa, and finally the pain in his bones. That the medicine seemed to add strength to him every day. He told the doctor yesterday, the 11th inst., that he felt himself well, and also that he owed his recovery to Brandreth's Pills, under Providence—that he had taken the medicine every day for nineteen days. That the doctor told him if he had known he had been taking that medicine, he should not have stayed another day in the house. He considers it his duty to make this public statement for the benefit of all similarly afflicted, that they may know where to find a medicine that will cure them.

JOHN SHAW.

John Shaw, being by me duly sworn this 12th day of April, 1842, did depose and say, that the foregoing statement is true.

JOHN D. WHEELER,
Commissioner of Deeds.

Cure of Insanity.

NEWARK, March 8, 1838.

RESPECTED SIR : I have long felt it resting on my mind as a duty, to communicate by way of letter to you, sir, the great benefit I have received from using your invaluable Pills; they have proved a great blessing to my health. For the last two years I have had my health renewed by taking them after other physicians had failed in their efforts to relieve me of a disease that was fast tending to dropsy, and bordering on to madness of mind—insomuch I was pronounced insane by most all who saw me. As I was incapable of having any charge of my family for nearly one year, a number of times I made an effort to take my life, but was prevented from so doing by that ever-watchful Eye that never slumbers nor sleeps. I am a living monument of the free mercy of the Lord to all who were witnesses of the disordered state that I was in when your medicine was thrown within my reach, and faith was given me to believe that it would relieve. I commenced taking it every night, and the first change I perceived about me was on the night after taking three doses. I felt a singular sensation in my ear, and on rubbing it, something gave way, that proved to be hard congealed wax. I felt such a relief of distress from my head, that I knew not what it could mean for some time, for the sound of my own voice appeared like another, and all sounds seemed different to my hearing from what they had for years past; and for two weeks following the quantity of wax that came from out my ears would to many be pronounced too incredible to be relied on, unless they had seen for themselves, and my blood began to circulate more freely through my system, by gradually taking the pills which before had nearly ceased to move through my veins, and it appeared to me that my life was at times departing from the body. I could find nothing that animated or cheered my mind; any way life had become a burden to me, but as my confidence strengthened in persevering with the pills, I found my life daily returning, and invigorating both body and mind, to the unspeakable joy of my family and friends; and since they have proved such a blessing to me, I have felt it my duty to recommend them to all with whom I have intercourse. Standing myself as a witness of their virtue in producing health of body, which, beyond a shadow of doubt, will give clearness of mind and ideas, which cannot be clear if those organs where knowledge lies are obstructed by disease, which thousands of our fellow-creatures are suffering under, and are still made worse by the treatment of our most popular physicians of the present day, by taking blood, and giving many things that are daily undermining and ruining the constitution forever, from having that strength that is natural for us, if we pursue the right course to obtain it by simple remedies instead of those of another kind, which is so unnatural as bleeding. The argument you lay before the public, and the experience I have had for myself on this important subject wherein life is at stake, has thoroughly convinced me that bleeding is injurious, and can and ought to be dispensed with, as it has been ascertained to a certainty that other means have been discovered that have the desired effect in producing health without proving so pernicious to the constitution as those mentioned.

I have been instrumental of convincing many to take them, but the most are bound by that strong cord of prejudice which will not so much as admit plain facts to be true, but endeavor to paint them in a different color from the original ones given; but I am encouraged that the time is nigh at hand, that people are awaking from their slumbers, and seeking after truth in all things respecting this life, as well as the life to come. It is true that error abounds on all sides, but we know that truth is of divine origin, and will prevail in spite of all opposition that is thrown in its way by all who love not our Lord Jesus in sincerity of heart, and are making every effort to amass wealth by imposing on the public in various ways to deceive the unwary; but let them beware and take heed to themselves, that the curse of the Lord is upon their riches if their eye is not single to His glory and the good of their fellow-men. It is love that has urged me to speak in so plain a manner to one who is an entire stranger to me, and I hope it may be received by you, sir, as coming from one whose mind has been freed from prejudice, knowing that the motive I have in view is the good of my fellow-beings, whose welfare I feel deeply concerned in. Although moving in a very humble and obscure sphere of life, to which many are placed, may the Lord greatly bless and strengthen your efforts in the cause that you are engaged in, is the prayer of my heart.

You are at liberty to make use of these lines as you think best.

MARGARET E. A. SHATLAND.

DR. BRANDRETH, New York.

St. Louis, November 28th, 1837.

GENTLEMEN : I deem it a duty which I justly owe, not only to you, but to the whole community, to acknowledge the beneficial effects which have resulted to myself from the use of that highly serviceable medicine, Dr. Brandreth's Vegetable Universal Pills.

About eight months since I was suddenly taken with the *Dropsy* in my feet, the surface of which was likewise covered with the *Tetter*.

I had repeatedly taken the advice, and followed the prescriptions of several eminent physicians of St. Louis, but derived no benefit therefrom.

I had also tried many experiments, and used every medicine that could be suggested, but without any visible abatement of the swelling, and they remained in this unnatural situation until my sufferings were alleviated by the aid of Dr. Brandreth's Pills. Shortly after I had commenced taking your medicine I discovered a visible alteration for the better; the swelling gradually subsided, the Tetter entirely left, my bodily health daily improved, and my feet once more returned to their natural size.

Two months have elapsed since my cure, and my feelings now warrant me in saying that through your instrumentality I have exchanged a painful disorder for a good sound state of health.

That suffering humanity may read, and benefit from this disclosure,
I beg to subscribe myself, yours gratefully,
MARGARET BROWN,
St. Charles Street, St. Louis.
To Messrs. TOUSEY & MICHAEL, *St. Louis, Mo.*

———

CARROLTON, Greene County, Ill., Oct. 5, 1837.

GENTLEMEN : I beg leave to inform you that my sister was taken about three weeks since with a violent intermittent fever ; at my request she took two of Dr. Brandreth's Pills, which did not affect her otherwise than by creating a faint sickness at the stomach. The next day she increased the dose, which operated powerfully. She took the third and fourth doses, after which she had no return of the fever, her strength increased rapidly, and her health has been good since.

A sister of my wife had been in a decline for several months with strong symptoms of a confirmed consumption. She commenced taking Dr. Brandreth's Pills, and before she had taken two small boxes in doses of three and four per day, a decided change for the better appeared. She still continues their use, and the glow of health is fast taking the place of her late consumptive expression of countenance. She will persevere in their use from a positive conviction that her health will be perfectly re-established thereby. Other individual cases I could mention. Suffice it to say, that *all who have used* the Pills to my knowledge praise them.

Very respectfully yours,
LUCIUS S. NORTON.
Messrs. TOUSEY & Co., *St. Louis.*

———

NEW ORLEANS, 14th Jan., 1838.

"He that is wise is wise for himself, and he that scoffeth (at Dr. Brandreth's Pills) alone must bear it."—Listen, oh, ye incredulous! hearken unto the voice of your friend, and neglect not the counsels of those who have learned wisdom from experience. Know, you that are slow of heart to believe, that I am a man who has suffered many afflictions from a hereditary diseased system.

From my youth up I have never known what it was to enjoy a MOMENT OF HEALTH, till lately. My disease has been a chronic headache and a severe debilitating weakness and faintness at the pit of the stomach, which diseases have been in a great measure removed by taking only TWO BOXES of Dr. Brandreth's Pills. I can now say, and with truth too, that I know what health is by experience; and I would that I could raise my voice so high that all the earth might hear. Then would I proclaim the virtues of this invaluable medicine. But what is my aim in all this? Is it that I am *interested* in the sale of Dr. B.'s Pills? Most assuredly, no; I am in no way connected with their rise or downfall; but I recommend them for the benefit of mankind, and especially to those who are to receive the most benefit from their use, my fellow-citizens of the South.

S. FRIEND.

———

GRAND GULF, March 6, 1838.

Mr. JOSEPH B. BROCKWAY,
    Dear Sir: We wish you to send us some more of Dr. Brandreth's Pills, for we are entirely out. Since the people have found out we keep them they are called for every day. Send them by the first opportunity, and
Oblige yours, &c.,
WHITEMAN & McFARREN.

———

WARRENTON, Miss., March 1, 1838.

Mr. J. B. BROCKWAY,
    Agent for the sale of Brandreth's Pills.
    Dear Sir: Enclosed we hand you ten dollars, the amount of the bill with which you furnished us some time since. The pills we find very saleable, and the demand for them is very great; in fact, so great is their reputed efficacy and virtue here, that we should feel ourselves in some degree guilty of crime, if we were to deprive them of so valuable a medicine. We wish you to send to us by some safe conveyance—by the captain or clerk of some boat in the trade—fifty dozen boxes Brandreth's Pills, and forward your bill to us on the usual terms.
Very respectfully, your obedient servants,
JOS. TEMPLETON & CO.

———

PORT GIBSON, Feb. 27, 1838.

Mr. JOSEPH B. BROCKWAY,
    Dear Sir: Enclosed you have ten dollars in payment for fifty boxes of Brandreth's Pills, left with me some time since by your agent.
    For some length of time after receiving the agency, there was but little demand for the article, as people were afraid of some deception; but since it has become known, the demand for it is rapidly increasing. I am now nearly destitute of the article, and as I have daily calls for it, wish you would send me a supply by Mr. O'Neilly—20 doz. boxes would not be too large a quantity.
Respectfully yours,
D. Y. THOMAS.

———

Mrs. Elwell's Case.

MRS. ELWELL, then of MIDDLEFIELD, OTSEGO Co., N. Y., was seriously attacked with inflammation of the stomach and bowels. She was given over by her physician, and a consultation of doctors was called. The decision was that she must die. She, however, partially recovered, but her stomach was in a very deranged state. Very little action could be produced on the bowels by the most skillful of the profession. She continued for many months under the treatment of one doctor after another, gradually growing worse, and so truly deplorable was her situation for four months before she tried the Brandreth Pills, that nothing passed her bowels except by the aid of the most powerful cathartics. Sometimes eighteen of one kind of pills were given to her, then say a dozen of another, and a portion of some other medicine, before action could be produced, and then so great was her distress that, for the whole of the four months above alluded to, she invariably fainted when anything passed her bowels. In January, 1837, she thought she would try Brandreth's Pills, and sent to my office in Cooperstown for a box. She took four pills. On going to bed, her husband enquired as to the effect of her new medicine. She replied, " that she did not feel any effect at all." He then said, that in the morning, if she took a dozen more, he guessed they would operate like all the rest of her medicine. She answered, she did not know but it would, for she did not expect anything would cure her. However, early in the morning her bowels were moved, and without pain or distress, and consequently without fainting, to the utter astonishment of Mr. Elwell, and the great joy of his wife. In the course of a few hours, they operated four times equally easy, and the consequence was she did not lie down through the day more than one hour. She had not for months been able to sit up one hour in a day. The next evening she took another dose of four pills with the same happy effects. On the third evening Mr. Elwell called on me and purchased a large supply of the pills, related the above facts, and said he never would be without the pills in his house if they could be obtained. It is now two years since the above facts occurred, and Mr. Elwell informs me that his wife soon recovered her health, that he has never had occasion to call in a doctor for her since, and that her health is now very good.

                                                       ELISHA FOOTE.

COOPERSTOWN, Feb. 22, 1839.

Annual Report of Mr. Sinclair Tousey, General Brandrethian Agent.

                                    LOUISVILLE, October 18, 1837.

Dr. BRANDRETH :

    Dear Sir : It is now one year since I opened an office in this city for the exclusive sale of your Vegetable Universal Pills, the sale of which since that period has increased beyond my most sanguine expectations; I have been compelled to establish an additional office in the city of St. Louis, Missouri, for the more convenient supplying of that section of country. I was induced to become your agent here in consequence of being convinced of the unrivalled health-producing qualities of your pills. My aunt they effectually cured of what is commonly called a Sick Headache, of about thirteen days' standing, which had often confined her to her bed for several weeks at a time. My mother they entirely cured of a violent pain in her side, with which she had been afflicted for several years; myself they completely cured of habitual costiveness. These, together with numerous other cases that came under my observation while at New York, convinced me of their efficacy in every form and symptom of the only one disease, for I am a firm believer now in Brandrethianism. The pleasure I feel in making them known to my fellow-beings is more than I can well describe. I presume, sir, that you are aware that your Pills were not known to any extent anywhere to the West of the Alleghany Mountains previous to my introducing them in Louisville; taking this into consideration, together with the fact that I am located in a fortress of M. D.'s (there is a medical college here) it makes my success and their unprecedented sale appear truly surprising.

It affords me great pleasure to state that in every town where I have introduced these valuable pills that they have generally been received favorably, and their sale and popularity have invariably increased beyond all precedence, until scarcely any other medicine is used or thought of.

The thousands of cures that have been effected by their use, together with thousands of testimonials received in their favor, have not only gone beyond my expectations, but they have perfectly astonished the bigoted enemies of the Brandrethian theory, and has, I am very happy to inform you, caused many, very many, who were formerly its bitterest enemies, to become its most zealous advocates. More than thirty-seven hundred of the most respectable of our citizens have voluntarily come forward and testified to the virtues of your medicine from their own experience.

It now becomes my duty (which I think a pleasure), as your general agent for this section of country, to transmit you testimonials of a few of the very numerous cures effected by the use of your pills which have come under my own observation, and had I the liberty to use the name of every individual who has testified to their extraordinary virtues, it would not only astonish the Regulars, but it would cause the foundations of Esculapian practice to quake with fear, besides filling at least one large volume. This, however, is not at all necessary, as the fame of the medicine is now spreading with such unparalleled rapidity that ere long its happy influence will be universally appreciated throughout the civilized world, and the only question invalids will ask will be, " Where can I get Dr. Brandreth's Genuine Pills?"

Case I.—BILIOUS FEVER.

Louisville, November 16, 1837.

Mr. S. Tousey—*Sir:* I feel it a duty which I owe, not only to you but to the public generally, to acknowledge the great benefit which I have derived from the use of the Pills for which you are agent. I was attacked about six weeks since with chills and fever, from which I recovered in about three weeks, when I was almost immediately attacked with a bilious fever, from which I had great doubts of ever recovering. Fortunately, I was induced by some of my friends to give Brandreth's Pills a trial; and I now find myself, after the free use of these Pills for a few days, perfectly restored in health and able to attend to my business as usual. After finding the happy effects of these Pills upon myself, I was induced to give them to one of my children—a girl eight years old—who had been ill for some time, apparently in a deciine. It gives me pleasure to inform you that she is gradually getting better since we first used the Pills, and I hope in another week to apprise you of her complete recovery.

I am, sir, very respectfully yours,

FELIX WOOD.

Case II.—DISEASE OF THE LUNGS.

Mr. Summers, City Pump Maker, has been afflicted with the above complaint for seven years; he tried a great many medicines before commencing with Brandreth's Vegetable Universal Pills, but never derived any benefit compared to what he received from them. He strongly recommended them to all as the best family medicine he ever used. Mr. Summers is well known in Louisville.

Case III.—FEVER AND AGUE.

Mr. H. Humphrey was violently attacked with the Fever and Ague, and after using but four boxes of the Pills he found himself perfectly cured and able to attend to his business right off. Such is the extraordinary efficacy of your health-restoring medicine, which makes friends of, and creates health in, all who use it. Long life to its maker. N. B.—Mr. H. resides in Third Street.

Case IV.—ERUPTION OF THE SKIN.

Mr. James Conklin was afflicted with an eruption of the skin, together with severe pains in all parts of his body. He used several highly recommended medicines previous to trying our Pills, but all to no purpose; he has used only a few boxes of them, and is now entirely free from all eruptions, his skin being now perfectly cured, and his body is quite healthy in every respect—no pains, appetite good, sleeps well. As many as fifty or sixty cases of eruptions of the skin have occurred where your Pills have been used and cures effected in this city.

Case V.—GENERAL DEBILITY.

Mr. John Downing's wife has been troubled with a general debility for a length of time; she has tried a few boxes of Brandreth's Vegetable Universal Pills, and finds them of great benefit. She is encouraged to persevere with them, being convinced that they are the best medicine she ever tried—the opinion of all.

Case VI.—DYSPEPSIA.

Mr. James Allen, residing in Clark Co., Indiana, has been afflicted with Dyspepsia for several years; he has tried but three 25-cent boxes and is much better, his appetite being restored, and his chest is free from pain with which he was troubled so much. His digestive organs are become healthy—that is all, but that is everything.

Mr. Stockton, the writer of the following letter, 's well known in this quarter of the country.

Case VII.—CHILLS AND FEVER

Mr. S. Tousey : I am compelled by an impulse of gratitude to acknowledge, not only to you, but to the public generally, the beneficial effects produced upon my son by the free use of Dr. Brandreth's Vegetable Universal Pills, for which you are agent. About six months since, my son, 15 years of age, was very suddenly attacked by that vile disease called Chills and Fever. He was occasionally so violently stricken with it, that I had given him up, and thought all medical aid was useless. I was prevailed upon by my friends and acquaintances to give Brandreth's Pills a trial, but it was a long time ere I was convinced of their efficacy ; I almost detested the idea, but my friends perseveringly persuaded until I was compelled to yield, and I am happy to inform you that after the free use of these pills only thirteen days, he was thoroughly cured and restored to sound health, and I am now perfectly convinced that they are the best medicine extant. Very respectfully yours,

E. F. STOCKTON.

Louisville, 20th September, 1837.

Case VIII.—SWELLED LIMBS.

Mr. H——h has been afflicted for about 5 years with swelled limbs, accompanied by very violent pains in every part of his body; he was unable to attend to any business or obtain any rest by night. These symptoms were produced by an excessive use of calomel. He used several bottles of Swain's Panacea and other remedies, but to little or no effect. He commenced with your Pills a short time since, and a few days ago he informed me the swellings had subsided, and the pain entirely left him. The Pills, to use his own words, "made him feel like a new man."

In addition to the above, I would state, I have known a great many other cases similar to the above, where Brandreth's Pills have been used with the same happy results, all of which go to prove the extraordinary power of your medicine in removing the most inveterate diseases from the system. ·

Case IX.—LIVER COMPLAINT.

MORGAN COUNTY, KENTUCKY, Aug. 19, 1837.

MR. L. TOUSEY,

Sir: It becomes my duty to acknowledge to you, and through you to the public, the great benefit my wife has derived from the use of Brandreth's Vegetable Universal Pills. About three years since my wife was brought very low with an attack of the Liver Complaint. A physician was employed, and after prescribing some time to no effect, he gave us this consoling information, that he could do her no good, and he thought nothing else would. After continuing in this miserable state some months, I was induced, from an advertisement which I read in the *Louisville Journal*, to give her some of Brandreth's Pills, thinking they could do her no harm if they done her no good ; and it gives me pleasure to inform you that, contrary to our expectations (for we considered her beyond the reach of medicine), she began to recover, and is now quite well. Should you consider this of any service to you, you are at liberty to publish it.

Respectfully yours, &c.,

T. SMITH.

Case X.—INFLAMMATORY RHEUMATISM, LOSS OF APPETITE, &c.

Mr. James Johnson, residing in Grant County, Indiana, suffered for about three years with Inflammatory Rheumatism ; at times his feet were so much swollen that he could not get on his shoes ; besides this he was troubled with costiveness, being sometimes three or four days without a passage. In addition to this he had scarcely any appetite ; he had advice and medicine from several physicians, but without any benefit, except for a short time. He expected he never would again be blessed with good health. After reading numerous testimonials in favor of Brandreth's Pills, and hearing them very highly recommended by some of his neighbors who had used them, he was persuaded to give them a trial, and now, after having used them about five weeks, he finds himself able to put his shoes on and walk about as he used to do. Besides this his appetite is perfectly restored, his bowels also being regular and healthy. He says that he has an excellent appetite, and thinks Dr. B. should have a monument erected to his memory for discovering so good a medicine.

The following letter, from the Rev. M. W. Sellers, will no doubt be read with interest. Mr. Sellers is well known to numbers of our citizens here:

CASE XI.

MR. S. TOUSEY,

Dear Sir: I send you the following account of my case, and hope it may be of service to you in prevailing upon other persons to give Dr. Brandreth's Pills a trial. In the fall of 1833 I was attacked with a severe pain in my breast, which continued to increase until a pain in my stomach and side took place, which brought me very low. I took different medicines to remove it, but to no effect. I then applied to Drs. Luster and Constant, of Louisville. They pronounced it a severe case of Dyspepsia and Liver Complaint. I commenced using their medicines, and found great relief in my side and stomach. I was in hopes a cure was effected, but the pain in my breast still remained. They then tried external applications to great length, with no success; and last winter the pain had become more violent. Mr. R. Barnett, of your city, informed me of Brandreth's Pills. I told him I had tried the Hygeian Pills without deriving any benefit; he told me BRANDRETH'S PILLS WERE THE BEST. I then applied to you, as you may recollect, for some of these pills. It appeared to me at the time that my strength was so fast declining that I could not live long without some relief. I commenced using the Pills, and shortly afterwards I was attacked with the pleurisy; and as bleeding had become such a habit I was persuaded to be bled, but mended slowly, and at length I was more violently attacked with the same complaint again. It seemed to me that I could not live long. However, I took eight of Brandreth's Pills, and in the course of a few hours I felt better. I then took twelve more, and have had no pain in my side since. This encouraged me to continue their use for the pain in my breast, and I mended very fast. In one month I gained ten pounds in weight. I enjoy good health at present, and feel myself perfectly restored. I can say that Brandreth's Pills were the first medicine that appeared to relieve the pain in my breast, and in any case of sickness I would rather use these valuable pills than any other medicine that I know of. By experience of said pills in my family, particularly in my own case, I know them to be good. My mother who lives with me, nearly seventy years of age, has been afflicted with a urinary complaint for about ten years, and by using these Pills during the last summer is now entirely well. I have known several cases of fever and ague, two or three cases of scarlet fever, and other diseases that the human family is daily subject to, cured by the use of these pills; several of my neighbors are using them for the breast complaint, and all find relief. I have no doubt but a great many other cures would have been effected by perseverance with the pills, but there is one great difficulty they labor under—timid purchasers commence using them and take one or two small doses, just about enough to make them feel a little queer, and get frightened and then away to the doctor, who takes great care to cry down the pills, knowing it stands them in hand to do so.

I reside in Lettersburgh, Clark County, Indiana; I have been a resident of said county more than twenty years, eleven years of that time I have been a minister of the Gospel, of the Baptist denomination. I am aware of the great opposition these pills labor under; but let me ask one question, viz.: What food is best suited to our nature and health? I think the answer is, the vegetable. Then do not let us be opposed to the vegetable kingdom for our medicine.

M. W. SELLERS.

OCTOBER 22, 1837.

Annexed I send you extracts from letters received from my agents, which make the proof in favor of your Vegetable Universal Pills almost overwhelming.

The following extract is from the Postmaster at Henderson, Kentucky, dated

HENDERSON, October 14, 1837.

The fame of Brandreth's Pills is on the increase here, and I am daily receiving assurances of their efficacy in every complaint—fever and ague of a most aggravated nature has been in almost every case speedily and effectually cured.   Yours, &c., &c.,
                                                (Signed,)   P. H. H.

The following is from the Postmaster at Hutsonville, a small village in Illinois, dated August 16th, 1837 :

As regards Brandreth's Pills, I believe they give universal satisfaction; at all events, I cannot keep them on hand long—almost every person who has bought of them' recommend them to their friends and continue themselves to use them—the last lot you sent me of fifteen dozen boxes did not last sales of two weeks. I have sold upwards of ten dollars' worth in one day, at retail.

The above speaks volumes in their praise. Another agent writes : They are deservedly becoming so popular that I shall be able to vend a great quantity of them. I could furnish you a valuable receipt of their efficacy from experience in my own family. Not only this, but the whole neighborhood bear testimony of their beneficial effects.

In conclusion, I send you the annexed letter from H. Foster, Esq., my agent at New Albany, five miles below Louisville :

NEW ALBANY, November 23d, 1839.

CASE XII.

Mr. S. TOUSEY : Your favor of 20th ult. was duly received as to the success of Dr. Brandreth's Pills; I can state, in general terms, that I have sold about 160 dozen boxes of these pills, and have made a great deal of inquiry of those that have used them, and find they have been very beneficial to this community. I can recommend them with the utmost confidence. I can here state that last fall, when I became an agent, my wife was in a very low state of health, and had a very distressing cough; she was apparently on the eve of going into a consumption—the use of ten boxes of the pills entirely restored her, and she has never failed since that time, when indisposed, to receive benefit from a single dose.   I am yours, &c.,

HUGH FOSTER.

You will perceive by the above testimonials that your medicine is justly in high repute in this part of the country, as it must be everywhere where it is introduced. I could, as I stated above, had I time and space, extend the list of testimonials of its efficacy to several hundred pages.

I would state that I have sold, during the year past, nearly eighty-five thousand boxes of your Vegetable Universal Pills, and have not the least doubt but I shall be able to dispose of more than double this quantity during the coming year, as those that have been sold have established a reputation for them that will last as long as the body of man is subject to indisposition.

My office in Louisville is 99 Fourth Street, near Jefferson ; and in St. Louis at 56½ Market Street, near Third.

Wishing you every success, I remain, sir,
                                        Respectfully yours,
                                                        S. TOUSEY.

To DR. BENJAMIN BRANDRETH, New York.

PLEASANTVILLE, Mt. Pleasant, Westchester Co., June 10, 1859.
Dr. B. BRANDRETH,

My Dear S r: I have long been a friend of yours, because I verily believe your valuable pills saved my life. I have recommended them for nearly twenty years, and don't want any others in my store. In 1849 I took a heavy cold, and being much exposed for some days afterwards, it settled on my lungs. For three months I was terribly troubled with a hacking cough and profuse night sweats, and reduced almost to a skeleton. I took various syrups and cordials, but found no relief. At last a friend, Jesse Baker, of Miles' Square, Westchester Co., said, " Hammond, why don't you try Brandreth's Pills, they may help you." I bought a box, and took some. They purged me freely—my last dejection being a thick,-viscid, yellow matter. I found myself greatly relieved at once, and within a week got entirely well. I recommend your pills to everybody, and they always do good. I shall always sell them, and I think they are the best medicine in the world for coughs, colds, consumption, and all kinds of sickness, for I know them by experience, having administered them to over one hundred cases of disease, and always cured.

Yours truly,

W. H. HAMMOND.

Jaundice Cured.

Mr. Benj. J. Stebbins, a highly respectable and well-known farmer of Pawlina, Dutchess County, N. Y., writes July 9th, 1859, that he was prostrated with jaundice every spring and fall for years, in spite of all the efforts of physicians; that he was cured by a few doses of Brandreth's Pills, and "has never suffered from the disease since."

See page 21 for testimonial from Supervisor Bissell, of Newcomb, as to cures of small pox; also, page 46, from sixty soldiers; and page 151 as to cures of rheumatism.

These testimonials are selected running through a period of nearly forty years, and to those who would learn have significance.

B. BRANDRETH.

ASIATIC CHOLERA:

Purgatives the only Treatment with Hopes of Cure.

OPINION OF

SIR THOMAS WATSON, M. D., F. R. S.,

Professor of Theory and Practice of Medicine in KING'S COLLEGE, London.

It is well known by the reading public that for forty years, Dr. Brandreth has recommended Brandreth's Pills for the cure of Asiatic cholera and all lax affections of the bowels, because they remove poisonous and offending matters safely from those important organs; he being opposed to the use of opium and astringents on the principle that they dam up the disease in the body and lessen the chances of recovery.

Dr. Brandreth, as early as 1834, says the Asiatic cholera is, in all cases, without exception, connected with a poisonously contaminated state of the blood or condition of the system, that will not maintain a healthy action of the heart and organs generally, causing a feeble circulation, shown by the pulse, which hardly beats over forty in a minute, which occasions stagnation in the blood vessels, and an accumulation in the vessels of the stomach, bowels, and liver, from which the evacuations are simply exudations.

These symptoms arrest the secretions generally, but of the liver and kidneys in particu'ar, and constitute, in fact, the essence or essential attributes of the disease. He asks: What are the indications to be fulfilled, or the requirements of a rational treatment?

Restore excitement to the heart and secretive organs, by divesting the blood of its poisonous qualities through the organs of the stomach and bowels, thus cleansing the liver and the kidneys, and restoring the heart to its proper action.

With this view he recommends

Brandreth's Pills as the Remedy,

as universal experience has testified they excite the liver and all the secretions; in fact, their stimulating operation is general upon the whole system—upon the heart as well as upon the most remote membrane. These pills, therefore, in his opinion, fulfill the purpose of a sure, because rational treatment.

After forty years of effort against the established practice, it is indeed a great gratification to know that his principles of cure have received the indorsement of the greatest light in the medical world. Sir Thomas Watson, M.D., F.R.S., recommends EVACUATION AS THE CURE FOR CHOLERA, and condemns the use of opium and astringents.

So early as 1831, Dr. Brandreth advocated the same method of cure which was successfully carried out in London. The same practice was very successfully enforced in New York with Brandreth's Pills in 1834 and 1835, and again in 1848 and 1849. In June of this latter year the most undoubted evidence of their great curative qualities in Asiatic cholera was published editorially in the *New York Sun,* say June of that year. In 1853 and 1854, in 1865 and 1866, they were

(221)

the reliance of hundreds of thousands of families, and have seldom failed to cure Asiatic cholera, perhaps never when used in season. In fact, all recovered who took them early, while those living where the disease was raging never had it, who used them occasionally, though constantly exposed.

Yet Brandreth's Pills are not pretended to be an absolute preventive of the disease; nevertheless, common sense will tell every one that if a drain be opened and left free from filth, when a sudden addition of impure matters run that way, it would not overflow and poison the whole town, like one in a less free condition. So those using Brandreth's Pills, during the presence of cholera, will be safer than those who carry in their systems a load of impure humors, on which the disease may settle, and which Brandreth's Pills would have removed without causing any weakness, but actually appearing rather to increase the customary vigor. This same principle of evacuation, of purging, of cleansing, is equally applicable to rheumatism, bilious, and all painful diseases whatsoever. It has been tested by "time," and has not been found wanting. In fact he has strong reason to believe that the same high authority above quoted will ere long give in his adherence to the curative method of treatment by means of purgatives.

Asiatic Cholera.
Sir Thomas Watson on its Diffusion, Pathology, and Treatment.

A valuable addition to our scant knowledge of the origin, nature, and disseminating media of Asiatic cholera has been issued from the press. Sir Thomas Watson, Bart., M.D., F.R.S., setting a commendable example to the medical profession, has published a revised edition of his "Lectures on Medicine." How necessary for the guidance of the pathological students who sat at the feet of Sir Thomas Watson a revised edition of his lectures had become, may be gathered from the fact that when the former edition was published—prior, be it observed, to the great visitation of cholera in 1865-6—the learned doctor told his pupils, "whenever a suspicion arose that cholera was present in the community, not to try, in cases of diarrhœa, to carry off the presumed offending matter, but to quiet the irritation, and to stop the flux as soon as possible by astringents, aromatics, and opiates." Whereas now, while still entertaining no doubt that the true indication of treatment is to "stop the flux as soon as possible," he believes this may be best effected "by carrying off the offending matter."

Sir Thomas prepares the minds of his readers for the changes some of his opinions have undergone by observing that the last great visitation of cholera was "more fertile of instruction on many interesting points relative to the disease than any of the three preceding epidemics." In one very important particular Sir Thomas's views remain unchanged. He always held, and imagines that few of the original doubters remain unconverted to the doctrine that epidemic cholera is catching. He contends that it results from a material poison which is portable, capable of being conveyed from place to place, and communicated from person to person, or from inanimate substances to which it clings, such as articles of furniture or clothing. That the morbific matter floats also in the air, and may be wafted about by its currents, is a general and well-founded belief. Dr. Bailey says that when it travels over great distances, it uses the vehicle of human intercourse; but that it may be diffused over smaller space, as from one part of a town to another, or from a tainted port to a ship anchored to leeward, by the movements of the atmosphere. With this opinion Sir Thomas concurs, and he adduces in support of it the following facts:

The long migrations of the disease are not made rapidly. Its rate of progress never exceeds, and is often slower than that of modern traveling. Its primary appearance in an island or a kingdom is always at its outer boundary. In our own country, for example, it first planted its foot in a seaport town on the east coast, over against the mainland where cholera was raging, and whence ships had very recently arrived. The same is true of its subsequent visitations. On the other hand, the crews of vessels sailing from healthy places remained free from the disease until they have entered an infected port, or held intercourse with an infected shore.

Confirmation of these statements is given by Dr. Bryson, in his statistical report of the Royal Navy, published in 1868. He says:

The medical records of the service have been searched in vain to discover an instance in which either cholera-morbus or yellow fever made its appearance amongst the ship's company unless one or more of the men or officers had previously—within at most twenty-one days—been exposed in some house, ship, or locality where the infectious virus which emanates from persons ill of the one or the other of these diseases existed. The spontaneous origin of either malady far away from an infected locality is unknown in the naval service.

This may be taken as conclusive, as it seems to be equally clear from the examples cited by Sir Thomas, that the atmosphere forms one of the vehicles of infection. For instance, the towns of San Roque and Gibraltar, five miles apart, were abruptly smitten by the plague, not only on the same day, but almost at the same moment. At a small town near Toulon the plague fell upon the place in the night, and thirty cases occurred simultaneously on the following day. A curious circumstance in connection with this impregnation of the atmosphere with choleraic poison was recorded in the *Dublin Morning Register* respecting the first epidemic—that of 1832:

In the demesne of the Marquis of Sligo, near Westport House, there is one of the largest rookeries in the west of Ireland. On the first or second day of the appearance of cholera in this place, I was astonished to observe that all the rooks had disappeared; and for three weeks, during which the disease raged violently, these noisy tenants of the trees completely deserted their lofty habitations. In the meantime the revenue police found immense numbers of them lying dead upon the shore near Erris, about ten miles distant. Upon the decline of the malady within the last few days, several of the old birds have again appeared in the neighbourhood of the rookery; but some of them seemed unable, from exhaustion, to reach their nests. The number of birds now in the rookery is not a sixth of what it was three months ago.

During the outbreak at Constantinople, in 1865, a similar migration of birds took place. It was observed that all the sea-gulls which used to flit over the waters of the Bosphorus deserted the place, nor did they reappear till the disease had departed, and the atmosphere had become pure once more. A striking proof that the air may be a vehicle of infection—that the poison may enter the lungs with the breath—is furnished by the fact that two pilots took the disease in consequence of having their open boat towed by a ten-fathom rope at a considerable distance astern of the steamship England, on board of which cholera was raging. They were never on board the vessel. Both of them had cholera, and one of them died of it. Both took the disease home and transmitted it to their familes, near Halifax, where the disease had been unknown for many years.*

Notwithstanding these proofs that infection may enter the lungs of healthy bodies, it is still doubtful whether the disorder can become epidemic, except in certain conditions of the atmosphere. Mr. Glaisher has observed that each epidemic in London has been attended with a particular state of atmosphere, "characterized by a prevalent mist, thin in high places, dense in low." He goes on to enumerate other atmospheric characteristics observable during the prevalence of cholera:

---

* A thin piece of muslin or a silk handkerchief tied over the mouth, would have prevented these pilots from taking the disease.

A dense torpid mist, and air charged with the many impurities arising from the exhalations of the river and adjoining marshes ; a deficiency of electricity ; and (as shown in 1854) a total absence of ozone, most probably destroyed by the decomposition of the organic matter with which the air in these situations is strongly charged.

More horrible than the knowledge that cholera may come to us in the air we breathe is the conjecture, now reduced almost to a certainty, that we may eat and drink the poison and so obtain the disorder—THAT THE DISCHARGES FROM THE ALIMENTARY CANAL ARE AT ONCE THE MAIN OUTLET FOR THE POISON, AND THE CHIEF SOURCE OF INFECTION. Dr. Snow has shown how easily portions of the rice-water excretions may come to adhere to our food during its preparation or consumption ; and the disgusting fact has been made too certain by the unchallengeable disclosures of the microscope that the water supplied for domestic purposes by the London water companies habitually contained visible particles of human ordure. In all the visitations of cholera the disease was least virulent where pure water was obtainable. Mr. Simon reported that " the population drinking dirty water appeared to have suffered three and a half times as much mortality as the population drinking other water ;" and the sudden, rapid outbreak of the disorder in the east of London, in 1866, was distinctly traceable to the unfiltered and infected water supplied by the East London Water Company.

With respect to the propagation of the disease, Mr. Simon uses this strong language :

It cannot be too distinctly understood that the person who contracts cholera in this country is *ipso facto* demonstrated, with almost absolute certainty, to have been exposed to excremental pollution. Excrement-sodden earth, excrement-reeking air, excrement-tainted water—these are for us the causes of cholera.

Mr. Simon hopes that " for a population to be poisoned by its own excrement will some day be deemed ignominious and intolerable ;" and he says that the local conditions of safety are, above all, these two :

First, that by appropriate structural works all the excremental produce of the population shall be so promptly and so thoroughly removed, that the inhabited place, in its air and soil, shall be absolutely without fæcal impurities; and, second, that the water supply of the population shall be derived from such sources, and conveyed in such channels, that its contamination by excrement is impossible.

It is shocking to think it should be otherwise now. (But no man can receive the disease unless there be those matters in the system capable of receiving it. All do not have it. How many ? May the number not be increased ? Certainly by using Brandreth's Pills.) See page 589, Vol. 2, of Sir Thomas Watson's Lectures, 1870, London, Longmans, Green & Co.

" Half a tumbler of fresh cholera dejecta found its way into a vessel of drinking water, the mixture being exposed to the heat of the sun during the day. Early the following morning nineteen persons drank from this pitcher. (The water attracted no attention either by its taste or smell.) They all remained perfectly well during the day, ate, drank, went to bed, and slept as usual. One next morning was seized with cholera. Two were attacked the second morning. On the third day two more were attacked. The remaining fourteen remained in their usual health, and were altogether untouched by the disease." These fourteen had nothing in their bowels or blood on which the disease could fix and germinate. And this is how Brandreth's Pills save you from the cholera, for these fourteen persons used Brandreth's Pills as their regular medicine when sick.

THE POISON OF THE DISEASE THE CAUSE OF THE THICKENING OF THE BLOOD, NOT THE PURGING. READ THIS PART WITH GREAT ATTENTION. Our knowledge of the morbid anatomy of cholera has become more complete and more exact in consequence of the post-mortem inspections, in cases of death during collapse, made by Dr. Parkes, Dr. Johnson, Dr. Sutton, and others. It is acknowledged on all hands that the primary and special danger in cholera lies in its ██iod of collapse. Now it was a very natural and plausible theory which attr██u'd this state of collapse to a drain upon the blood by the profuse and repeated fluxes from the stomach and bowels, whereby the blood, being robbed of its more liquid ingredients, and made thick like tar or treacle, became incapable of flowing freely, if at all, through its natural channels ; and thus the circulation coming ultimately to a stop, life stopped also. And the practice suggested, and put in force, as a direct corollary to this theory, was that of endeavoring to arrest the destructive flux by astringent drugs, and by opium, to sustain or urge on the lingering circulation, and to restore the spent strength and the lost animal warmth by alcoholic and other stimulants. Upon similar grounds was advocated the dilution of the thickened blood by water injected into the veins. IT IS AFFIRMED, ON THE OTHER HAND, THAT THE CONDITION CALLED COLLAPSE IS NOT DUE TO THE EXCESSIVE DISCHARGES FROM THE BODY ; THAT THOSE DISCHARGES ARE REALLY ELIMINATIVE OF THE POISON OR OF THE PRODUCTS OF THE POISON WHICH CAUSED THE DISEASE, AND ARE TO BE PERMITTED OR EVEN ENCOURAGED RATHER THAN CHECKED ; AND, THEREFORE, THAT ASTRINGENTS AND OPIATES CAN DO NO GOOD, BUT ARE, ON THE CONTRARY, POSITIVELY HURTFUL.

Sir Thomas combats the first-mentioned theory, and quotes Dr. Parkes to prove that the most hopeless cases are those of collapse after very scanty discharges or with no discharges at all. Says Dr. Parkes :

It may confidently be asserted that there is no one who has seen much of cholera who does not know that, exclusive of the mildest forms of the disease, a case with little vomiting or purging is more malignant and more rapidly fatal than one in which these are prominent symptoms.

Castor Oil and Purgatives Recommended.

Now as to treatment. Dr. Johnson, of Liverpool, also holds that "the phenomena of cholera result from the entrance of a peculiar poison into the blood, where it probably undergoes a rapid process of self-multiplication, and spoils certain of the blood constituents, which are then ejected through the mucous membrane of the alimentary canal ; that the feelings of general oppression and *malaise* sometimes experienced before the onset of the bowel symptoms are indicative of blood poisoning ; that the copious discharges are expressive of the efforts of nature to throw off a noxious material, and really form, therefore, a necessary part of the process of recovery ; and that if the pouring forth of the vascular excretion be checked (as it can perhaps be by opium), the risk of fatal collapse is thereby increased. He declares that the results of his own practice, founded on these views, have amply justified them ; and a considerable body of other evidence has now been furnished in support of the same plan. Sir T. Watson thinks it is plain that, if " elimination " be a condition of recovery, the method of elimination is nature's method, which art may help or hinder—help by the cleansing method, hinder by the astringent. It should be remembered that one dreadful symptom of cholera consists in very painful cramps of the larger muscles of the body, produced, it may be assumed, by the choleraic poison. Dr. Johnson supposes that the stoppage of the blood is caused by the same poison acting upon the muscular fibres of the minute pulmonary arteries. The thickening of the blood is a consequence, and not a cause, of the arrested circulation and the collapse. The true explanation of the fact that mere diarrhœa, however profuse, does not thicken the blood, is probably, as Dr. Johnson suggests, that water is rapidly absorbed from the soft tissues, to take the place of that which escapes from the alimentary canal. Such is the theory which Sir Thomas Watson thinks a reasonable one. He says: " It is founded on a true analogy; it is consistent with the symptoms noticed during life, and with the conditions discovered after death. We may therefore legitimately regard it, until fairly refuted, as a sound as well a most ingenious and important theory. In truth, it derives strong confirmation from the fact that it unlocks, like the right key, the whole of the pathological intricacies of the disease. Thus, the emptiness of the systemic arteries accounts for the extinction of the pulse at the wrist, for the cadaverous sinking of the eye-balls and falling of the features, for the blueness and coldness of the skin, and for the absence of syncope. The circulation stops, not from debility of the heart, as in exhaustion, but in consequence of a direct mechanical impediment to the onward course of the blood. We can understand the importance of brandy against this condition; and how, on the other hand, bleeding may help, both by relaxing the spasm and by unloading the distended right heart, to restore the circulation.* In this explanation Dr. Johnson presses, plausibly enough, the singular effect of the injection of fluids into the veins of these patients. It appears that, to be most influential, the fluids must be hot; and he concludes that they act not only by diluting the morbid blood, but chiefly relaxing, through their warmth, the spasm of the smaller arteries. The blood then flows on again, and the symptoms of collapse are for a time removed. Again, the husky whispering voice is owing not to muscular weakness, but to the small volume of the tidal air in the respiratory currents. As but little venous blood reaches the lung-tissue proper, there is but little demand for air to meet and decarbonize it. The respiration accordingly becomes shallow, and the vocal pipe, feebly blown through, refuses to speak. Under the temporary impulse of the warm injections, the voice regains its usual tone and note."

It is evidently wrong to dam the choleraic poison and its products within the body. Even when those products have, in one sense, been separated from the system, they may produce highly noxious effects if they remain shut up in the stomach or bowels, there to ferment and decompose. Admitting, as we must, that a minute quantity of the morbid excretions swallowed with water may suffice to produce the disease, a large quantity retained, through weakness of the expulsive powers or otherwise, can scarcely be harmless. Rather may we expect that its expulsion will tend to liberate the patient from danger and discomfort; just as the opening of large abscesses, and the discharge of foul pus and imprisoned gases, are often seen to rescue, as if by magic, a sick man from apparently impending dissolution.

Having arrived at these conclusions, Sir Thomas has not far to seek for confirmation of the theory. Dr. McCloy and Dr. Robertson testify that—

Of 375 cases of cholera admitted into the Liverpool Parish Infirmary in the last epidemic, 161 proved fatal—a gross mortality, under all the modes of treatment adopted, of 42.93 per cent. Of these cases, 91 were treated with astringents and stimulants, camphor and iced water, applications of ice, and hypodermic (opiate) injections; and the mortality per cent. of these cases was 71.42. Eighty-seven cases were treated with purgatives, and with a liberal use of food and alcohol; and the mortality was 41.37 per cent. One hundred and ninety-

* This advice as to brandy and bleeding is bad, and will do hurt if followed; but worse than all will be the effect of the injection of fluids into the veins. When the disease is treated by purgatives, vegetable purgatives, by

Brandreth's Pills,

the collapse never occurs, everything arranges itself by nature's own efforts, she having been assisted by means of Brandreth's Pills, which never weaken.

seven cases were treated with castor oil only, and the mortality was 30.45 per cent. Dr. Brandreth affirms that over 90 per cent. recover when treated with his pills.

Now, if this theory and practice in respect of cholera be true and right, the practice ought to be right in respect of the associated diarrhœa also ; and so, indeed, it is. Those who have largely tried it, strongly affirm that it is right, inasmuch as it is eminently successful. Dr. Johnson avers that he has found it so. And the concurring testimony of Drs. McCloy and Robertson confirms the soundness of the theory and practice. Their experience of diarrhœa was very extensive. Several thousand cases came under their observation in various dispensaries in and near Liverpool. Many were of a most severe choleraic type. The treatment they adopted was generally evacuant in its nature."

Had Brandreth's Pills been used in the place of castor oil, the mortality would not have been over ten, and probably less than five per cent. ; in fact, on persons of sound constitutions, not one per cent.

Remarks upon Cholera, Fevers, Small Pox, &c., &c.

I now take pleasure in placing before the public a word further in reference to this disease, and other maladies arising from poison in the blood, among which I place cholera, small-pox, scarlet fever, yellow fever, typhoid fever, fever and ague, and all fevers without exception, including rheumatical and diptherit- ical. The maladies arise in the human body from the absorption of a specific poison, which seems capable of multiplying itself according to the condition of health of the patient when stricken down. Common sense tells us how little water it needs at the commencement of a fire to put it out, and the same prin- ciple is applicable to the getting out poison from the human body. A little energetic medicine in the beginning will do wonders in ridding the body of the poison, which much may be unable to achieve when it has got under a full head- way. So when a thing hurts, remove it, and in a choleraic attack, without the loss of a moment's time. We know that thousands of persons are living whom Brandreth's Pills have cured of this terrible disease, and we have the highest medical authority for their use. Such authority, indeed, tells us that the state of collapse is not due to the excessive discharges in cholera, but to the poison, which prevents the formation of carbonic acid by the union with the oxygen of the blood; heat is not generated, but the blood remains charged with carbon, paralyzing the action of the heart, causing the slow pulse so observable in this disease, the dark skin and ghastly expression of countenance so awful in collapse. Then apply yourselves to the removal of the poison—and Brandreth's Pills are the remedy, safe, energetic, and sure; safe, because they only act upon what is contrary to health ; energetic, because they act according to urgency of symp- toms; sure, because they never fail to produce purgation if given while sufficient vitality remains. Wait not for advice, but swallow six or eight at once, and continue with more or less according to urgency of disease, being guided also by bill of directions which are around each box. When you have produced bilious stools, or the disease moderates, the patient is safe. But Brandreth's Pills will do better for you than many doctors, and as much as any can. The diet should be good chicken broth, or from fresh mutton or beef. My opinion is, that broth made from sheep's head is the most appropriate of all in affections of the bowels. It should be simmering a long time; until the meat leaves the bone. When the pills have operated very thoroughly, ten drops of spirits of camphor in a half a wine glass of water seems to soothe, and can do no harm. But no spirits or astringent medicines should be used, because they dam up the poison if any remains, which may occasion a relapse.

This seems to be a very easy method of treatment, and though the cholera is a frightful malady, yet, treated with purgatives, is a simple affair, and usually curable. But are purgatives indeed a proper remedy? Let us see. *The greater the amount of the intestinal discharges, the greater is the sum of poison removed, and the greater the chance of recovery;* while the most hopeless and fatal cases are those patients who have very scanty discharges, or no discharges at all. If the terrible collapse were owing to the drain upon the blood effected through the intestinal discharges, it would be prolonged, deepened, and rendered more perilous by the continuance of those discharges. But patients recover from a state of collapse, Brandreth's Pills operating at the time; even in cases where they have not been used, and when the evacuations were allowed to go on without trying to stop them by opiates or astringents, the patients have recovered from collapse. This fact and our experience proves that in using Brandreth's Pills we are really aiding and following

Nature's own Plan of Cure.

Poison *in the body,* the aim should be to *get it out;* that done, the patient is safe. When Brandreth's Pills cannot be obtained, castor oil may be used; but it must be fresh, for rancid oil will make matters worse; and remember, castor oil is very prostrating, while Brandreth's Pills have a tonic and strengthening effect immediately the operation is through, and even measurably while it is going on. Sometimes there is severe sickness of the stomach; for this, very hot boneset tea, or HOT water is good, and Allcock's Porous Plasters to the chest and all around the diaphragm. The great object is to get the pills down. If the patient cannot swallow pills, rub them to a powder and mix with molasses, and give four every two hours until they evidently operate. This effected, you will have warmth on the surface, which was before chilled by the approach of death.

Diet, abstinence, and water, wisely employed, will do a great deal, and sometimes restore health. But this is obtained under the direction of able and learned physicians, whom the poor cannot have because they cannot pay the price. Now, Brandreth's Pills will do as much, often more, when used according to the printed directions which are around each box, than the greatest doctors can do for you. I humbly believe them to be

The Medicine of Providence.

And all can have them for Twenty-five Cents a box, and which could not be prepared for a dollar by any druggist, if prepared in a small way. Never be without those pills in the house; it is having them ready when you are first seized with cholera, or dangerous sickness, and taking them at once, that saves trouble, and nips the disease in the bud.

In conclusion, I beg the patient to submit to no injection of warm water in the veins, which takes away every chance of recovery; to no subcutaneous injection of morphia; to no bleedings, leeches, or blisters; to take no calomel, opiates, or astringents. A bandage of flannel may be placed around the body; two or three Allcock's Plasters are better yet. And I tell you if these directions are followed which I have given above, ninety-five per cent. of those who are attacked with cholera will recover, and I believe a larger proportion. The great thing to be remembered is to always have

Brandreth's Pills

about you, so they may be used at once, before sickness of stomach or cramps come on. The poison absorbed into your body being the cause of cholera, the beginning to take it out is the beginning of the cure, so lose no time in having to send for the pills.

The public servant,
B. BRANDRETH.

JANUARY, 1872.

PRINCIPLES OF CURE.

Thoughts on the Structure, Wear and Renewal of the Human Frame.

LIFE, existence, the power to feel, feeling : who but God the Father created it, who " Breathed into man the Breath of Life, and man became a living soul ?" The life is in the blood ; the blood is life.

Experience and reason tell us the importance of pure blood ; no impure blood can carry the " life " our great Creator intended us to possess. We will try and compile some words upon the principle of gaining health, and some words on the structure, wear and renewal of the human body.

The mighty oak proceeds from a small acorn. Whence does it derive the nutrition which makes it grow ? From appropriate fluids contained in its mother earth. Whence do the ostrich and fowls of the air and of the water come ? Verily from an egg. All fluid but the shell. Here we see a few weeks of the needed warmth converts the yolk and white of the egg into an organized being hardly less wonderful in structure than that of man.

The oak obtains direct growth from the earth, while man derives his growth from the blood of his mother, which, though all fluid, provides the babe with bones, flesh, hair and the horny nail. Physiology teaches that all parts of the body were originally from blood ; or that at least they were brought to the growing organs by means of that life-giving fluid.

The most ordinary experience tells the thoughtful mind, that at each moment of life, in the animal body, a continued change of matter, more or less accelerated, is going on ; that a part of the body is transformed into unorganized matter, loses its condition of life, and must be again renewed. There is sufficiently decisive ground for the opinion, that every motion, every mental affection, is followed by changes in the chemical nature of the secreted fluids ; that every thought, every sensation, is accompanied by a change in the composition of the substance of some part of the body. Wonders surround us on every side. The mighty power of steam, and the continuous speed of the electric current are now understood, but the formation of a crystal, of an octahedron, is not less incomprehensible than the production of a leaf or a muscular fibre ; and the production of vermilion from mercury and sulphur is as much an enigma as the formation of an eye, or the hair or nail, or the reparation of a bone from the substance of the blood. We know exactly the mechanism of the eye, but neither anatomy or chemistry will ever explain how the rays of light act on consciousness, so as to produce the power of seeing. •

We must believe that God works through the laws of Nature by immediate intelligence producing results, marked by evidences of design. No laws with which man is in the least acquainted, can tell how atoms group themselves into the form of eyes, ears, and limbs ; becoming instruments of optics, of acoustics, and of locomotion, or organs of thought and emotion. And we also believe the light that has been given us on the subject of purgation, as tending to the cure of disease, has been derived from a source which we will now call Providence. We know the principle is true, and that its enforcement in a human body causes to be thrown out what is hurtful, often preserving and restoring to health, what

otherwise would have become disorganized and dead. Thousands of men and
women are to-day alive and well, who, but for this practice, would have been in
their graves, or in an abject condition of disease.

We know the milk of the mother gives nutrition and growth to the child.
Physiology teaches that the milk is derived from the mother's blood. Wonderful adaptation! the food of the mother becomes changed into blood, which
provides milk for the child's sustenance, growth, and for the hardening of its
bones.

The chemical components or equivalents of an egg, of milk and blood, are
nearly the same. Every part of an organized being may therefore be said to
be derived from blood or its equivalents.

Waste and Repair.

The body wears. Movement causes waste. The hardest steel wears away
when used. So also the body wears away, but unlike the steel, it is renewed
faster then it wears away in a child, which is the occasion of its growth. It is
a great truth, we die daily; but the food consumed also supplies us with new
life daily. These are marvellous facts; this decay and renewal are among the
wonderful mysteries of the Almighty.

We know the hair and our nails grow. Mark your finger nail near the root.
Day by day it advances towards the end; at length we pare the mark away.
The whole nail has been renewed, the growth was supplied, the waste was
repaired. The same waste, the same renewal occurs in the nose, and all other
parts, though we cannot mark the change as in the finger nail.

Where the Reparations Are.

The substance which is to form the nail is in the blood; as perfectly mixed
as a grain of salt is dissolved in a glass of water. As the blood circulates in
the small vessels at the root of the nail, this nail substance deposits and organizes
itself, and replaces what is worn away. The hair is also renewed by materials
from the blood deposited in the roots of the hair; so the bones; and so the
fl sh; and so with all other tissues and parts of man's body. Each part receives
its needed supply of new material. Thus the eye retains its fire, thus the tongue
its power of utterance, the brain the power of thought.

Analogy tells us even the brain, the organ of thought, wears, and is renewed
by the blood, which circulates and renews all the parts of the body alike,
whether it be brain, spinal cord, the eye, the bones, the flesh, the hair or the
nail.

The blood carries new material to repair the waste, and it reloads itself with
worn-out parts which it discharges through the appropriate vents. When the
new materials are greater than the waste, the child grows; or the man spreads.
When the waste is exactly equal to the new material, the body remains of the
same size and weight. These facts indicate that the substance of all the
organs and parts of a living body are present in the blood. It is therefore important to our well-being that this life fluid should be free from imperfections.

For if the blood does not contain all the needed ingredients, or if it should
contain more, it cannot renew the different parts according to their requirements. Deformed and ill-made people owe their infirmities to the blood of
their parents; pure blood can do no otherwise than make perfectly organized
beings, thus we may estimate the value of certain means to make the blood
perfect.

FOOD PROVIDES FOR THE SUPPORT OF EXISTENCE, and supplies all the parts of
which blood is made.

SUBSTANCES WHICH CONTAIN AND SUPPLY NUTRITION ARE FOOD.

Healthy food possesses substance, because the stomach cannot grind it well without it possesses this quality. Too fine food makes the stomach weak; it cannot use its muscular power, and debility of the stomach follows. If we do not walk, our legs soon become weak. To be strong, organs need exercise. When food is digested, part makes blood; the refuse passes off by the bowels, the kidneys, and the skin. Our stomach, if properly supplied, continually prepares new blood, which renews all the organs, carrying vitality to the hair and nail as well as to the head, with its master-organ, the brain. Every part is each moment of our lives changing, the worn-out parts carried away, and new parts supplied, whether good or bad. Here we see the necessity of eating and drinking several times a day. We constantly wear and constantly repair. Such is the law of our being.

WORN-OUT PARTS MUST BE EXPELLED.

The worn-out parts must be expelled from the body daily, or the blood will become impure. We may comprehend this by an inquiry respecting new-born children. They have taken no food by the mouth, and yet when born their bowels and bladders are full. Whence did these secretions come? They came evidently from the blood of the mother, which made their bodies. We also know that sick persons, who eat no food for days, have evacuations by the kidneys and bowels. These parts are also the worn-out parts of the blood and body.

The blood is in fact a messenger, capable of taking, when there is a supply, to every part of the body what it needs for renewal, and also carries back to the bowels, kidneys and skin, worn-out substance to be expelled from the body.

We therefore must admit that every part of a human body is made from blood; and that it wastes and is repaired; that food makes blood which is distributed with singular intelligence to all the various organs.

HOW IMPURE BLOOD GETS INTO THE CIRCULATION.

The bowels may be costive; in this case there is an absorption into the circulation of gases and gummy substances, which are a great cause of poison to the blood. Should the kidneys fail to do their work, another source of poison to the blood is developed. Again, should the perspiration be checked, matters flow back upon the blood which soon load it with impurities. Suppose only the feet, by cold, cannot perspire, and their fetid exhalations flow back upon the blood. If all these outlets—the skin, the kidneys, and the bowels—do their work even imperfectly only, for a short time, it is evident that the blood will be burdened with noxious matters, which must interfere seriously with the circulation, and soon clog up the smaller vessels, so that only a small amount of blood can pass. Soon the lungs, the intestines, the stomach and the brain, will sound an alarm. You will have pleurisy, inflammation of the bowels or severe cholic, violent headache or sick stomach, because the worn-out parts of the body, instead of being carried out by those avenues nature designed, are shut up, poisoning the blood, thus causing it to become impure.

Other causes besides these produce impurity of the blood. The food may not be healthy; digestion may be imperfect; troubles, grief, anxiety miasmas from swamps or other exhalations; breathing close air in crowded rooms; staying in too hot rooms; all these causes tend more or less to vitiate the blood. Grief, fear and anxiety, *hurt by making the blood to circulate slower*, and soon produce a very serious injury to the composition of the blood, occasioning stubborn fevers, and various derangements of the body and mind. Some are born with a larger portion of corruptibility than others, who are consequently more exposed to be attacked by disease. These unfortunates seldom live to an advanced age, unless their constitution improves, which is often the case by applying the proper remedy at the proper time.

Synopsis of Proceeding.

All the parts of the body proceed from, or are made from the blood.

All the parts of the body waste or wear, and are renewed by blood made from the food.

That the blood is a messenger that carries a load both ways: *i. e.*, It carries new blood to supply new material, and brings back to the bowels, the kidneys and the skin, worn-out material, to be discharged out of the body.

The retention of these worn-out materials are the source of impure blood, and therefore the source of disease.

Worn-out parts must be removed by Nature or Art.

If there be a daily addition of what is wanting, and a removal of the worn-out parts, present health may be preserved, and even lost restored.

The most important avenue of the cleansing process of the blood is the skin. Vastly greater in weight of worn-out parts go off by this channel than by the bowels and kidneys combined. So, when the perspiration is checked—known by the coming on of some sudden pain, accompanied usually by a cold feeling which finally takes the form of a violent chill—now no time must be lost in restoring it, by placing the feet in hot water, and taking from six to eight of

Brandreth's Pills, or two or three Sarsaparilla.

* This simple plan will prevent the sad consequences which may otherwise occur, and which often terminate in affections of the lungs or bronchi, that no art or medicine perhaps may cure.

Excessive labor or excitement or mental application sometimes is the occasion of sudden attacks of sickness. This is produced from too great a quantity of the worn-out parts of the body remaining in the circulation, the returning blood being unable to carry them to the proper outlets for their removal from the body.

Bad air breathed, infallibly corrupts the blood; contagion, touching bodies infected by disease; and excesses of all kinds, whether of drinking, eating, labor, &c., are a source of impurity of the blood, and more or less injurious, according to the greater or less strength of the constitution.

Pure and Impure Humors.

The humors are the various individual fluids of a living body. In man they comprise four-fifths of the whole weight, or thereabouts. They may be divided into two kinds, the good and bad. The ground may be considered the pure blood; the bad the impure blood. From these are made the bile, the lymph, mucous, slimy, and synovial fluids, which give smoothness and limberness to the joints, and suppleness to various organs. Pure blood makes all the fluids healthy and good; impure blood makes, in time, all the fluids unhealthy and bad. That is, pure blood makes us well, bad makes us sick.

The humors are soon corrupted from any cause which interferes with the regular habits of the body, for in them the germ of corruptibility resides.

---

* See Dr. T. R. Hazard's letter of advice.

But pain is the certain sign that the humors are getting depraved. You must not wait too long before the remedy is taken. We should never forget that when the principle of corruption obtains the control, life ceases; for corruption is the extinguisher of life.

Mucous, Slimy, Synovial Secretions.

Healthy mucus keeps and preserves the suppleness of the membrane or covering which lines the mouth, the stomach, the intestines, the interior of the bronchi, the ear, bladder, the uterus, and the lining of the veins and arteries. The synovial fluid lines the joints and acts as oil does to machinery. Slime, I think, has its offices, but they are more vague. These secretions are all derived from the blood, which are healthy when the blood is good, and depraved when it is impure. Thus in colds, coughs, bronchitis, whooping coughs, mucus becomes phlegm, and is very troublesome. The mucous discharge flows from the nose, ears, bladder. It is seen in catarrhs and in other diseases. Its source is abated when the blood is purified, and gives no further trouble.

Bile.

Bile is a secretion from the blood, and is a very important humor. It unites with and separates the dreggy excrementitious parts from the food (chyme) before it becomes chyle, which feeds the blood with new materials, *new blood in fact.* It acts much the same as white of eggs does in clearing syrup. Bile is secreted more in hot weather than in cold, and is usually more needed, because more fruits and vegetables are consumed, and it separates the refuse from the healthy parts.

How Decline (otherwise a Consumption of the Lungs) is produced.

We have seen how good blood is the source of health. Now, when this element of life is imperfect, it cannot supply health; the hair may fall off, the joints will be stiff; the skin will become sallow or of a dirty tint; the breath will be of bad flavor; the eye will be dull; the change in the solid parts of the body will be seen—the flesh will be flabby, and the bones painful. Because bad vapors or undigested elements in the blood, are condensed upon the various organs, and serve to make them grow or repair their waste, it is plain that organs made with a greater or lesser proportion of such materials cannot be sound. If the bad condition of the blood continues but for a few days or weeks, the body will be out of sorts and debilitated. Should this state remain for a considerable time, the whole of the body will be renewed with imperfect blood, and the individual's health will have become prostrated. He will be said to be in a decline. No organ seems more affected than another, except the lungs—there is always a cough and mucus raised—the person is said to have bad health,—is in a decline.

Sound health needs no other name: bad health has every degree, from a headache and costive bowels to a complete breaking up of the entire system. Bad health in some appears to be a decaying condition of the whole body, one organ or part being affected very much in the same sort of a way as another.

Pure and Impure Blood.

Pure blood may be compared to clear water; impure blood to muddy water. If you pass muddy water through muslin, you soil it; continuing this process, you cover it with thick mud.

The blood passes through all the tissues and organs of the body, even the bones, and something of a very similar nature takes place in regard to them that takes place in regard to the muslin. If the blood is impure, more or less dirt is left behind it.

Should an organ, or part of the body, be weaker than the rest, there a greater quantity of impure matter will settle, and go on rapidly increasing. Here is the source of our humors, swellings, enlargement of glands, boils, running sores, catarrhs, lung affections, fevers, intermittent and otherwise.

We know this must be so, for these diseases are cured by purgation with Brandreth's or the Sarsaparilla Pills or innocent purgatives, which take dirty humors out of the body, and if they were not there, they could not be removed; being there, we know they were left there by the blood. In these cases, purgatives have, in forty days, taken out of a human body 100 pounds of most impure matter; we know they could not have been in the bowels; they were part of each individual texture and fibre of the whole frame. This man was perfectly restored to health, though supposed beyond all hope of recovery.

We have seen sometimes in the blood a natural tendency to free itself from impurities by vomiting, by sweating, and by spontaneous purging. It is these hints improved upon, and a remedy made in accordance therewith, that usually results in producing a radical cure.

Collections of Impurities.

The presence of impurities is not always a source of pain. The aggregation of humors in a large tumor is often without pain. While sometimes great suffering is occasioned by an inconsiderable swelling; the fact is that the pain is the consequence of two causes; the biting acrimony of the humors, and the natural sensitiveness of the part upon which they settle.

Nature may be Assisted, but she Cures, and sometimes alone.

We have said nature sometimes frees herself from the humors which trouble her, without any aid. A sickness now and then defies all the methods of relief, and yet subsides upon some few pimples breaking out about the corners of the mouth or elsewhere. This proves the necessity occasionally of local applications. We see also that persons of strong constitution, and young, suffer for days with pains in the limbs, loss of appetite and fever, who suddenly get better after a cholic followed by slimy, bilious stools.

IMPORTANT MEDICAL FACT.

The relief produced by these natural intestinal evacuations were the original line or guide to this practice of Purgation, which enforced with our purgatives, or other appropriate medicines, is destined to be adopted by the entire civilized world, at no very distant day.

Cures Effected by Expelling Humors.

When nature cures, it is by some evacuation. There is always something to be seen. Either rash, pimples, slimy humors, or bilious discharge. There is always an appeal to the senses.

All can Comprehend.

Animals of the brutal race, whose habits we can note when they are sick, eat those herbs which open their bowels, by which means they become cured.

From these facts and reasoning we are satisfied that Purgatives are the sheet-anchor of curatives, and we have no doubt their use dates before the flood. But we know that David said, "Purge me with hyssop, and I shall be clean;" and St. Paul, "Purge out the old leaven, and ye shall be a new lump." It is true these are illustrations spiritual, but how could they have application unless confirmed by practical experience in the body of matter?

The purgative method is capable of being comprehended by both learned and by the unlearned. It needs no study; it is founded upon common sense, and is applicable to all disease. While so easily understood, it is nevertheless of great value, because it teaches us how we may cure one's self when sick. Those who know a purgative cures by its purifying effect upon the blood, are more sure of health than those who put their faith in other methods without this purifying treatment.

How a Good Purgative Acts.

A good purgative penetrates the whole mass of the blood. During the time of penetrating, whether one hour or six, no effect whatever is felt. When the impregnation is perfect, the blood begins to deposit its bad parts in the vessels which lead to the bowels. In from one to four hours the effect of from four to eight pills will be over. The body usually feels relieved of a load, even after the first purgation. How then shall we feel after twenty? We shall feel well, renewed, disenthralled; our sensations will be those of our early youth; every organ of the body will rejoice in itself, and because it has been thoroughly cleansed.

A good purgative never expels any but the dirty parts of the body or of the blood. Good purgatives cleanse all organs to the capacity of their strength, as a piece of soap cleanses according to the weight and the dirt it has to remove.

Importance of a Speedy Supply of Food after Purging.

After purging, the blood must be supplied with new material. This should be done quick. If you take out, you must replace by good warm oatmeal or Indian meal gruel, and while the purgation is progressing, if possible. Then eat your breakfast as usual after a little nap. In two or three hours, it will be well if a half a pint or pint of good plain soup or broth is taken, made from fresh meat. This helps the purgation, and fills up with sound fluids the place of the nasty ones evacuated.

By using purgation in this way every day for several days together, and then resting for a few days, doing this alternately, the whole body can be renewed much sooner than in the ordinary course of nature. Some intelligent men have said in from two to four months. This is a short space for re-making the body. In from six to twelve months I have no doubt it can be soundly re-made, provided Brandreth's Pills, or Sarsaparilla Pills be the purgative. By purgation a larger portion of humors are expelled than would be without; if these humors are replaced with wholesome, easily digested food, it will make new bone, new nerve, new skin, new lungs, and, in fact, every fibre and substance of the body will be altogether new and without blemish.

Follow the Path Indicated by Nature.

From what has been said in the preceding pages, "We know, and from what we see and feel, that our bodies are subject to get out of order, inducing pain, and tending to their destruction. In this disordered state we observe nature providing for the restoration of order, by producing some salutary evacuation of the poisonous matter. She brings on a crisis by stools, vomiting, sweat, urine, expectoration, &c., which often ends in the restoration of healthy actions. Now, experience has taught us, also, that there are certain substances, by which, applied to the living body internally or externally, we can at will produce the same evacuations, and thus do, in a short time, what nature would do but slowly, and do effectually, what perhaps she would not have strength to accomplish." When, then, we have seen a disease relieved by a certain *natural* evacuation, we may reasonably expect a cure of it by the use of such substances as have been found by experience to produce the same kind of evacuation or movement. Thus fullness of the stomach is relieved by vomits, affections of the bowels by purgatives, colds by a spontaneous sweat. So, when we are sick, if the trouble is above the diaphragm—the line which separates the chest from the bowels—we may take some boneset or bitter herb tea, or other tea without sugar or milk. Boneset is the best tea to take. If a vomit is needed, this produces vomiting. The medicine that we advocate, however, is one which experience of many years has proved seldom fails to suit the case, wherever located, whether in the chest, the head, the bowels, or the limbs; and the great advantage is, that under no circumstances can it harm. The celebrated Dr. Lull, of St. Lawrence county, N. Y., who used the medicine for over thirty years in his practice, says: "The BRANDRETH's PILLS reduce, lessen and expel the principle of disease; and in proportion as they effect this great object, they increase the principle of life. That being purely a vegetable compound, they invigorate, purify, and cleanse the blood, correct and regulate all the secretions, and, by purgation, discharge the whole mass of morbid matter from the body *without reducing the strength.* If one hundred of the most enlightened physicians were to unite their individual skill, it could scarcely do so much to cure as a dose or repeated doses of Brandreth's Pills."

In a book of " Authorities," comprising the opinions of upwards of two hundred physicians, published by B. Brandreth, M.D., in 1867, Dr. Hazard, of Newport, R. I., says: "It is now nearly thirty years since I *entirely* abandoned the use of calomel, for which I substituted Brandreth's Pills, which I have found, after long and varied experience, produce all the good effects of mercury with none of its bad. One or two boxes of those pills will generally keep a family of ordinary size in health for a year. Thus any man by a small expenditure may keep his own family in health for a year, with very little, if any, loss of time, and not a farthing's expense for medical aid. This, as a general rule, I pledge my word, I know to be true by actual practice and observation. These pills are as efficacious in cases of hurts, bruises, cuts, sores, &c., as in other maladies. By immediately cleansing the blood, they remove all danger of lockjaw, festering sores, or congestion of the blood at the wounded or ailing points. Not unfrequently, from the use of opium in some of its varied forms, or other malpractice, the morbid matter seeks to escape through vents called fever sores. I have known instances of this kind wherein, after the patient had been in acute pain for weeks, a few doses of Brandreth's Pills have turned the current of morbid matter from the sores to the bowels, through which it has been passed off, and the patient healed almost at once. But I do not mean to be understood to say that this is the rule; as when the system has been surcharged and weakened by poisonous and stupefying drugs, nature's vital forces cannot always be rallied by any treatment that I am acquainted with."

Thousands of pages of testimony can be produced like the above, showing the claims which Brandreth's Pills possess upon the confidence of the public. INDEED, LITTLE SHORT OF MIRACLES HAVE BEEN WROUGHT BY THEIR USE, IN EVERY FORM OF DISEASE. It is well known now in the United States and throughout South America that they are the safest and most reliable purgative known. We take a dose of these pills, which in a short time are absorbed by the blood, *on which it acts much the same that white of egg does on syrup, separating the impure parts from the pure.* Should there be any unpleasant sensation some hours after a dose, remember it is not the pills which occasion them, but the humors which are put in motion. So soon as the impurities have left the intestines, the unpleasant sensations stop. Therefore, we know it is the humors which occasioned the pain, and not the pills. One thing the patient may rely upon, that Brandreth's Pills never expel any but unsound humors— humors which make us sick and which must be expelled.

After a good purging, the blood must be purer than it was before; but remember you cannot continue to improve, unless you replace the matters removed by good food. *You cannot starve and be benefited by purgation.* When by a moderate meal the blood has been supplied by new material, then the improvement in the general feeling will be decided. By continuing every twenty-four or every forty-eight hours this process, the whole mass of the blood will in time become entirely renewed, provided care is taken to replace the impurities removed by healthy food. Healthy food, in fact, is as important as the medicine. All the taking out in the world will not cure, unless you replace what is taken out by nutritious food.

A Cure easy before Humors have settled.

Health is soon restored by this course when the humors are simply floating along with the circulating mass of blood, which is the case in all recent attacks of painful affections of all kinds. But when the case is chronic, occasioned by congestions, deposits, tumors, ulcers, dropsy, &c., the cure will be more tedious, or by the use of morphine or veratria, or any other anodyne or poison which fastens the depraved humors in the blood, making them more difficult for purgation to detach, as is the case after fevers, &c., &c. After purgation, the blood passes through diseased parts and gets foul again by cleansing them from a further quantity of their impurities. If it was pure before entering a diseased organ, it will not be so on leaving it. So, after some days or weeks, as the case may be, we must begin purging again, by carrying off through the intestines the corruption it has contracted in the diseased parts; on passing through them again, it will remove another portion of the evil matters. Thus, if the purging is repeated at proper intervals, the whole of the evil matters will finally be passed off by the bowels. It is merely a question of time; the tumors, the congestions, the dropsies, will as surely disappear as water from a vessel if constantly bailed out.

FISTULAS, RUNNING SORES, SCROFULAS, RHEUMATIC AND OTHER CONSTANT PAINS, ARE A CONSEQUENCE OF A SETTLING OF THE HUMORS. BY USING BRANDRETH'S PILLS, THE BLOOD BECOMES PURER. AS IT CONTAINS LESS IMPURITIES, IT DEPOSITS LESS UPON THE PARTS AFFECTED, AND THE INTENSITY OF THE DISEASE DIMINISHES. BY CONTINUING THE PILLS, A TIME WILL COME WHEN ALL THE IMPURITIES ARE TAKEN OUT OF THE BLOOD, AND NO MORE DEPOSITS ARE MADE. THEN THE DISEASE IS CURED.

The same rule is applicable to discharges of all sorts, as fluor albus, running at the ears, catarrhs, diarrhœas, dysenteries, etc. In these cases, the humors are in the blood, and it throws them out in any way it can. Brandreth's Pills, in these cases, always cure by perseverance. Of course, good, easily digested food is indispensable.

Thus, we see by purging with Brandreth's Pills, the entire fabric of the body can be entirely renewed, reconstructed, and renovated. The defective portions removed and remade from the food consumed.

In very painful diseases, such as inflammatory rheumatism, and inflammatory affections generally, the wise course is to use the pills in such doses as will produce energetic purgation. Also, in cases of stubborn costiveness the same rule must be observed.

Many persons have used these pills for supposed incurable diseases, and have continued to live on quite comfortably to what had been their lot before they used this great medicine. At length their constitutions underwent a change, and they recovered their health completely. The pills were taken once a week in some, two or three times a week in others; again, in some not oftener than twice a month with the same happy result. One thing is certain, that the body never gets used to Brandreth's Pills. After every dose the blood is freer from bad qualities than it was, and this is soon well understood and acts as a guide in their further use.

Synopsis of Proceeding.

Brandreth's Pills are digested, and their active purgative separating quality circulates with the blood, passing thus through every part of the body, which, thus stimulated, deposits its impurities in the organs communicating with the intestines. By continuing the process, the whole body becomes renovated and renewed, all its bad parts being purged away and new parts remade, which occupy the places of the old unsound ones removed.

Remarks General upon Blood-Vessels in Health and Disease :

FOOD, APPETITE ; NEED OF RESTRAINT, AND THE WISDOM OF GENERAL MODERATION WHILE USING PURGATIVES; EXCELSIOR MEDICAL COLLEGE—ITS OBJECTS; HOPES OF A SOUNDER MEDICAL KNOWLEDGE FOR THE PUBLIC.

WHEN in health our veins and arteries are full of good blood, while persons whose bodies are diseased have often less good blood than foul humors. *The more impure humors the less blood.* The abundance of impurities are indeed often so great that hardly sufficient good blood remains to continue life. Here we see the evil principle of sickness nearly extinguishing the good principle of health. In these cases of feeble vitality we have to feel our way. Two Brandreth's Pills night and morning, with an occasional dose of four or six pills, will be sufficient as a commencement as a rule, being careful to supply the patient with nutritious food. Slops, as gruel and broths, in much quantity, are apt to turn sour with patients of this class. Beef tea and mutton chops, tenderloin beef-steak, and broiled chicken agree, and should be supplied. The usual food is often all that can be obtained ; good roast or boiled mutton or beef, even if cold, should form part of the diet, is easy of digestion, and makes good blood. The more appropriate the food, and the more it is relished, the sooner a return to health may be expected.

EXCELSIOR MEDICAL COLLEGE.

Before long I hope to see a certain corporation of the State of New York endow a hospital where the poor may come and use Brandreth's Pills under the direction of experienced nurses, and where the most appropriate variety of victuals and drink will be amply supplied, and all without any expected return but the blessing of THE BOUNTIFUL.

Milk.

Milk toast may form part of the diet if it agrees with the patient, but milk is not deemed the most appropriate food while using the Brandreth Pills. And cold vegetables and cold water had better be abstained from while the *pills are in you,* as well as fruits generally, which are apt to lay heavy or turn sour. Some persons who have used Brandreth's Pills extensively say these things never hurt ; perhaps not, but they do not give the medicine a fair chance.

They certainly interfere, to some extent, with the intended action of the purgative effect, and call greatly upon the vital forces, beside *running the risk* of colics. I remember once being called to a man in the night suffering from griping pains, which his family took for inflammation of the bowels. I found he had taken four Brandreth Pills before going to bed, for costiveness, and ate a large half-ripe apple at the same time. There was no help for it. I gave him ginger tea and six more pills. *It was wind.* In half an hour he got rid of the trouble, and in future will be careful to eat apples at a proper time and ripe or cooked.

In using Brandreth's Pills or any purgative, the intention is to operate upon the bowels, to obviate costiveness, remove some fulness or settling of humors from the head, or other part. To effect this object you desire the full action of the medicine, which is a very important feature in purgation. Cold bathing and cold vegetables and fruits, or cold water, *are sure* to *retard* the effect. You take a purgative to purge; cold applications, externally or internally applied to the body, have the tendency to measurably hinder this action, and, therefore, to use them at such a time is pulling the wrong way for your health. When you use Brandreth's Pills, if possible use warm comfortable diet. Whether of meats or drinks, these help the medicine and the cure. Ordinary diet and ordinary washing may be adopted with moderation. But because you may wash in cold water, even bathe, if that is your *daily practice*, you need not be dabbling in the water for an hour. If you do bathe, bathe quickly while using the pills, and what is of equal importance, dress quickly. Because a drink of cold water will not hurt you, you need not drink a quart without taking it away from your mouth.

The proper plan is the day a purgation is taken, even one Brandreth's or one Sarsaparilla Pill, it is not well to eat any raw fruit, lettuce, cabbage, radish, even watercress is best abstained from. But if you do partake of these things, let it be in great moderation.

THIRST A GOOD SIGN.

Thirst is a good sign when Brandreth's Pills are used, and proves they are doing good. Suppose the patient can get nothing but water. In this case let him drink only a little at a time, so that the stomach shall not get chilled. But the patient must be in a poor case who cannot procure a piece of bread well toasted, and put hot into cold water. THIS IS TOAST WATER. Now toast water is always proper when you are under the operation of Brandreth's Pills, and can usually be procured. Some people say plain water sours, but toast water never. Let such use toast water; it is simple and good. Use intelligent judgment, and neither your diet nor your habits need feel restraint while you are using Brandreth's Pills, which are all vegetable and innocent.

Patients who have done the medicine most credit are those who understand its use best. In nearly all these cases it has been their own intelligence which has taught them. Both Brandreth's and the Sarsaparilla Pills *are innocent*, and warranted free from all poisonous ingredients whatever. A person of sense soon learns how to adapt the dose to his case and constitution. Also the best diet to quickly make new blood to supply the place of the bad humor removed.

Synopsis of Proceeding.

The more impoverished the blood, the weaker the patient; therefore greater necessity for nutritious food. Broths, gruel, not so good for the weak as beef tea beefsteak, mutton chops, chicken, oysters, &c. When good things can be got and relished, the road to health is straight; when they cannot be obtained, or when obtained not relished, the road to health is very crooked.

Agitations, Low Spirits, Despondency.

The approach of a radical change for the better in the condition of the blood preceded by want of appetite, despondency, flying pains, sometimes in the chest, between the shoulders, small of the back.

In these cases we recommend an Allcock's Porous Plaster, to the chest, side, or back ; it seems to act locally very slightly on the skin, producing a tonic effect, but infallibly does good and helps the restoration to health ; sometimes the want of appetite is referable to a peculiar agitation of the humors. In these cases a little hot or cold boneset tea is often serviceable, and for heartburn and sour stomach cannot be excelled. Many persons are subject to fits of heartburn, and sour stomach, and attacks of wind, whose health is otherwise good. Hot herb tea relieves these difficulties at once, and without any trouble. But always remember that a cure depends upon freeing the body of acid humors by purging.

Cancerous Affections.

The Sarsaparilla Pills were originally made to relieve the terrible burnings and prickings of the stomach which arise from supposed incipient cancer or scirrhus of the stomach. Hundreds carry the germ of cancer in them. These unfortunates have before them, by ordinary practice, usually a slow and painful death. The Pills take hold of the roots of the disease and drag them out.

Nervous and Chronic Cases.

In cases of supposed ulcers of the lungs, in carbuncles, in boils, in ulcers of the legs, in fever sores, in white-swellings, and in all cases of debility and scrofula, when Brandreth's Pills do not produce decided benefit after a few doses, we would recommend the Sarsaparilla Pills, which have a similar, but not the same effect. They are a peculiar purgative, and take hold effectively in these cases. Brandreth's Sarsaparilla and Buchu should also be used by all persons affected as above. It is true that we have wonderful cures where only the Brandreth's Pills were used ; in these cases the patient had invariably a good appetite, but when this is not present our rule is at fault. For to cure by taking out, you must put in. If you purge, you must eat. So when you cannot eat you must try these other remedies, which often restore your appetite, when the road to health becomes straight by the use of Brandreth's Pills alone.

Acute and Chronic Disease.

If we are taken suddenly sick, that is what is called acute disease. *Never take one or two pills in these cases;* valuable time is lost and the strength wasted. You want several doses of pills of from four to eight each, according to the bulk of individual. Dr. Hazard's method is excellent. See bill of directions, and also Book of Authorities, paragraphs 776 to 778.

Chronic disease is when it has been of some standing ; then you feel your way, and even other applications may accelerate a recovery as stated above. These will be more fully referred to when we speak upon each disease under its particular heading.

Fatigue, Prostration, Weakness.

Should prostration be experienced during a course of Brandreth's Pills, yet, if the same goes off after a sleep, you may be assured it was only fatigue. Yet the proper method is to moderate the dose if the purgation has been thorough. Even to suspend its use for a day or two. If you find your health is gaining, you may continue to rest.

The following texts are presented as a proof that purgation was the great reliance in ancient days. But it may be said that the purging mentioned is spiritually applied, not bodily. True, but it *was*, figuratively applied; from whence the figure? Why, from its known effect in the human body. We therefore expect that these texts will be taken as *Bible Proof* of the excellency of purgation as a purifier, as a restorer to health of a tainted diseased body, a making of it " clean"—*i. e.*, restoring health by cleansing :

Psalms 51 : 7.—Purge me with hyssop, and I shall be clean, wash me, and I shall be whiter than snow.

Psalms 65 : 3.—As for our transgressions thou shalt purge them away.

Psalms 79 : 9.—Deliver us, and purge away our sins for thy name's sake.

Mal. 3 : 3.—And he shall sit as a refiner and purifier of silver; and he shall purify the sons of Levi, and purge them as gold and silver.

Matt. 3 : 12.—He will thoroughly purge his floor, and gather his wheat into the garner.

1 Cor. 5 : 7.—Purge out therefore the old leaven, that you may be a new lump.

2 Tim. 2 : 21.—If a man therefore purge himself from thee, he shall be a vessel unto heaven, sanctified and meet for the Master's use and prepared unto every good work.

Heb. 9 : 14.—How much more shall the blood of Christ, who through the Eternal Spirit offered himself without spot to God, purge your conscience from dead works to serve the living God.

Heb. 1 : 3.—Christ, when he had by himself purged our sins.

Prov. 16 : 6.—By mercy and truth iniquity is purged, and by the fear of the Lord men depart from evil.

Isa. 6 : 7.—And he laid it upon my mouth, and said, Lo this has touched thy lips, and thine iniquity is taken away and thy sin purged.

Isa. 27 : 9.—By this therefore shall the iniquity of Jacob be purged.

Ez. 24 : 13.—In thy filthiness is lewdness; because I have purged thee and thou wast not purged, thou shalt not be purged from thy filthiness any more, till I have caused my fury to rest upon them.

5 Pet. 1 : 9.—But he that tasteth these things is blind, and cannot see afar off, and hath forgotten that he was purged from his old sins.

John 15 : 2.—Every branch in me that beareth not fruit, he taketh away ; and every branch that beareth fruit he purgeth it that it may bring forth more fruit.

Ez. 47 : 12.—And the fruit thereof shall be for meat, and the leaf thereof for medicine.

Peter 11 : 9.—Hath forgotten that he was purged from his old sins.

Purgation the Oldest Curative Means.

For five hundred years the Romans had no Doctors; they cured themselves, when sick, by purgatives, by baths, and diet. The purgative method is the oldest curative means, and dates from the earliest period of the world. Other systems and theories have died out, while this has lived on, and now, by means of the Excelsior Medical College of New York, we hope will in time absorb all other systems of medicine AND BECAUSE IT IS TRUE. Opposition and misrepresentation must be expected ; reformers do not usually have smooth roads. But let me speak for my disciples—OUR TRUST IS IN GOD, our cause, and our energies, and the intelligence of the age. Is it to be understood that Brandreth's Pills are the only purgative remedy we recommend ? Our experience of these Pills converted many of us to a full belief in the purgative doctrine. We believe in them, and know they are capable of great things, as restorers to health, by purging foulness from a diseased body, and therefore deserving of attention by all who need such aid. But we believe there are many other valuable purgatives, alteratives, as well as other excellent assistants for the cure of disease, which will be referred to in a future article, and the Sarsaparilla Pills is one other, which see next page.

Remarks by our Philosopher.

But no medicine alone cures disease. In fact perhaps it were better to only claim that the best only takes away the impediments to the recovery of health, the depraved humorers from the blood. Purgatives, whose action is innocent, are all that is really called for, in connection with PURE AIR, and all the exercise the body can bear, with plain food. Even bad cases of consumption, have been cured by this method. The late Dr. Marshall Hall facetiously observed :
"If I were seriously ill of consumption, I would live out doors day and night, except in rainy weather or mid-winter; then I would sleep in an unplastered log house. Physic has no nutriment, gasping for air cannot cure you, monkey capers in a gymnasium cannot cure you, and stimulants cannot cure. What consumptives want is air, not physic—pure air, not medicated air—plenty of meat and bread."

If to this treatment, the doctor had added Allcock's Plasters, when a local tonic or strengthener was called for; and the use of a purgative or alterative when the bowels needed assistance, the fame of his advice, would have caused thousands of consumptives to regain their health, whose forms are now in the grave. Brandreth's Pills, and the Sarsaparilla Pills should be always handy for the consumptive.

This method of cure by cleansing the blood has had great success, and each day is becoming more favorably known. All disease is due to an alteration of the humors. In other words, some one or more of the humors of the body have become vitiated; and to cure the disease and reduce pain, must be by taking out the bad and replacing with good humors from the food. The health cannot be impaired without affecting the blood, and the blood will again affect the health. Thus we go from bad to worse. We eat to repair our losses; if the digestion is good we soon recover our health, but if not, our blood gets worse and worse, and then it is only by purgation that we can recover the balance and get our bodies again on the road to health.

In fact, evacuations are the true means by which the purity of the humors can be recovered, because by the bowels must be expelled the poisons from the blood, whose presence threaten life. Some persons have an idea that purging takes out from the body elements other than those which produce disease. It may be so with some purgatives, but not with those we employ. Ours remove only evil or depraved humors, which are replaced by sound new blood from an ordinary meal. And the treatment continued usually soon restores the blood, and all the humors, to that state of pureness which constitutes health.

The medicines that are safe and sure are BRANDRETH'S PILLS or the SARSAPARILLA PILL (sole Life Addition). These medicines, separate or together, will be found worthy. They come well recommended by millions of our citizens. And have the largest sale of any pills in the world.

Prepared by B. BRANDRETH, M.D., Sing Sing, N. Y. Principal office, Brandreth House, and sold by all druggists. Price, 25c. with full directions.

INDEX OF DISEASES.

244   INDEX OF DISEASES.

INDEX OF AUTHORS QUOTED.

246   INDEX OF AUTHORS QUOTED.

PARAGRAPH.

Johnson, Jas...................482, 493
Kennedy............................652
Kingslake.....................258, 259
Kirkland...........................396
Kramer............................ 740

Laennec...........................624
Lane..............................
Lanza......................... 672-673
Lawrence..........................651
Leeson.......................711, 712
Lemazurein........................467
Liebig............................727
Lind..............................403
Lloyd.............................498
Louis, Ch. A..................641, 642
Louis, E. H 643

Mackin.......................692-697
Magendie.....................713, 714
Markham...........................
Magennis..........................231
Marx..............................622
Martin.......................424,426
McIlwain..........................646
McCullock.........................568
McKenzie..........................581
McLeod............................674
Mead..............................543
Meterius.......................... 87
E. Miller.....................219, 220
Mitchell..........................390
Moore, I..........................237
McMullen.....................320-324
M 'icus, Pathology...........435-446
Me 'icus..........................277
Miller.......................205-207
Monot and Henderson..........579, 580
Moore, G..........................644
Morgan, Chas.................344-348
Morgan, G. F.................653-656
Mosely............................396
Manneley.....................666, 667

Nickoll...........................499
Nooth.............................221

O'Berne......................260-279
Œcterlein.........................740

Parey.........................66-100
Paris........................545-552
Parisé............................645
Patterson.........................278
Pearson......................279-281
Pennington 391
Philip............................

Pickford.....................758-760
Pidduck...........................687
Pott..............................228
Potter.......................271-273
Power........................274, 275
Pring........................505-516
Pringle......................193-201
Pricards..........................238
Pritchard....................447-449

Redman 396
Reeve.............................232
Rhazes............................ 64
Richter......................675-679
Robertson....................203, 204
Rush.........................368-409

Sanctorius...................101-120
Sara.........................698, 699
Savaresi..........................239
Say...............................396
Schultz......................680, 681
Scudamore....................559-562
Selle.............................208
Shaw.........................500, 504
Sherwood..........................726
Skimshire.........................222
Stephens..........................582
Stoker.......................583, 585
Strack............................434
Sutton.......................223, 224
Sydenham.....................152-166

Taylor............................700
Tuomey.......................424-426
Tainsh............................240
Tyro..............................256

Unwins.......................323, 324

Vage.........................241, 244
Vandeswieter......................256
Velpeau 592
Vogel.............................701

Waddley...........................276
Waddy........................702, 705
Walsh 349
Watt.........................359-364
Wegg..............................733
White.............................225
Whydt............................598
Willan............................192
Williams, C. J. B............682-684
Williams, Robert.............647-650
Wilson, Andrew...............459-479
Wilson, J. A.................715-723
Woodward.....................235, 236